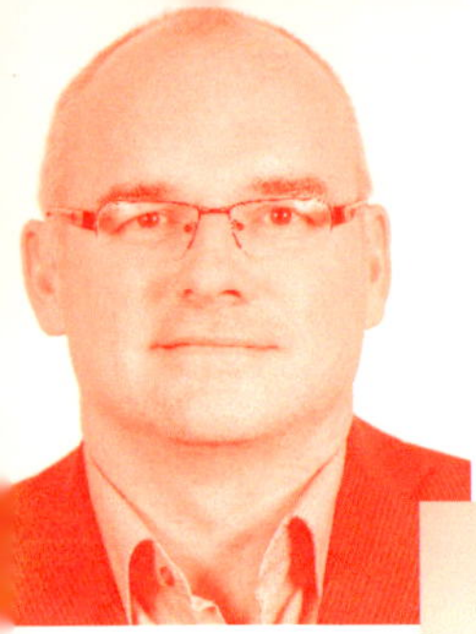

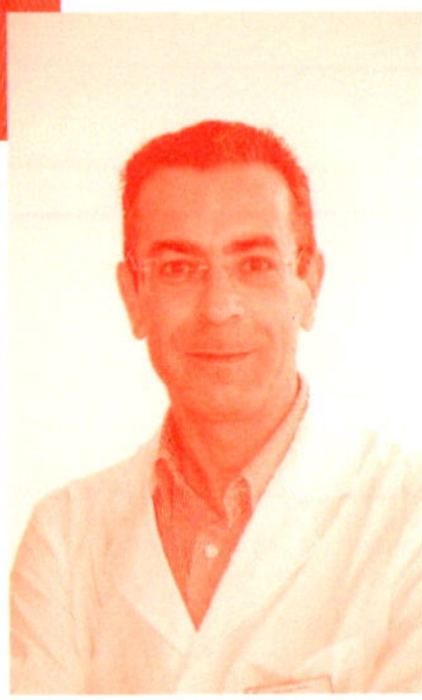

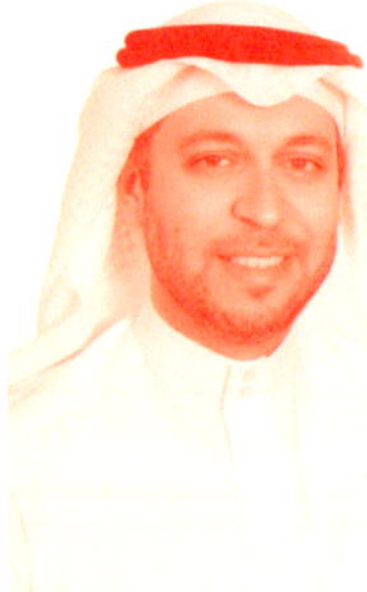

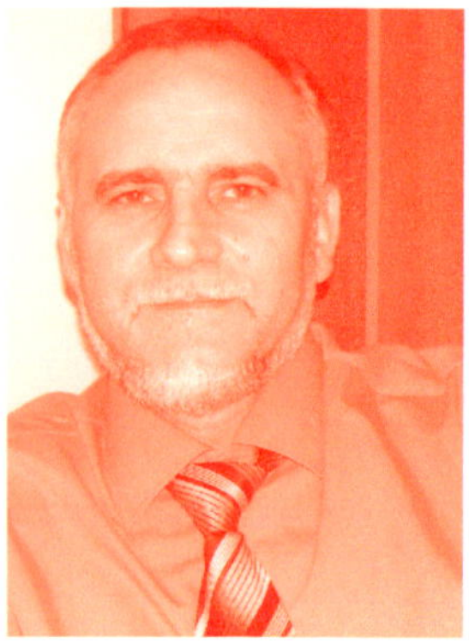

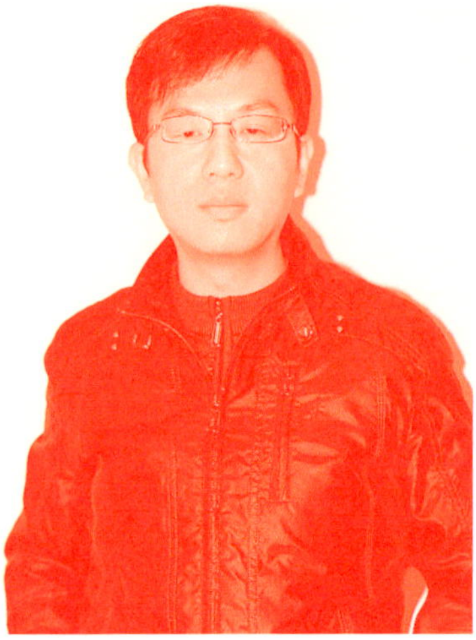

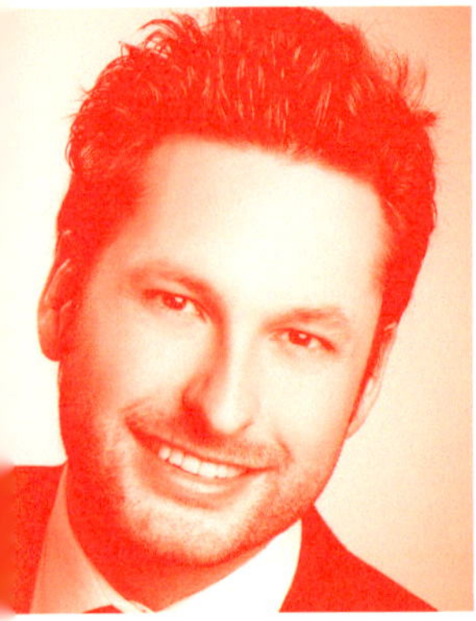

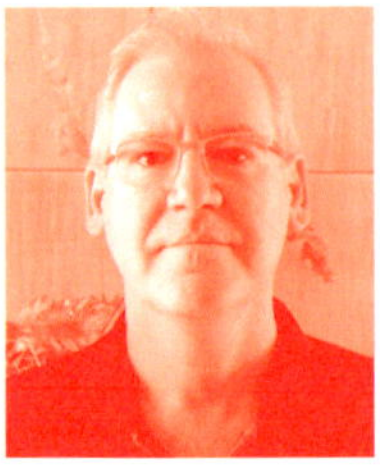

IntechOpen

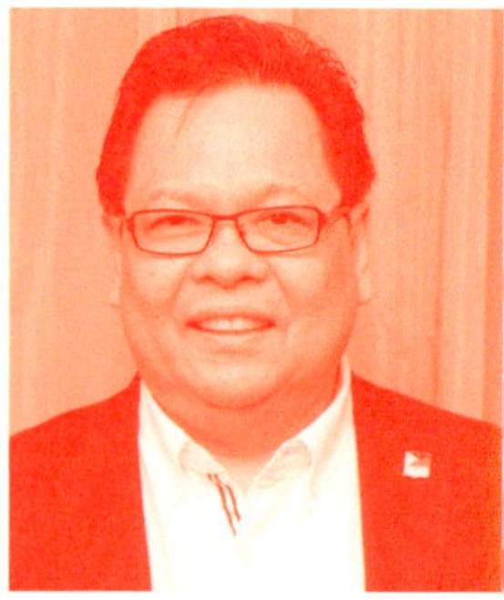

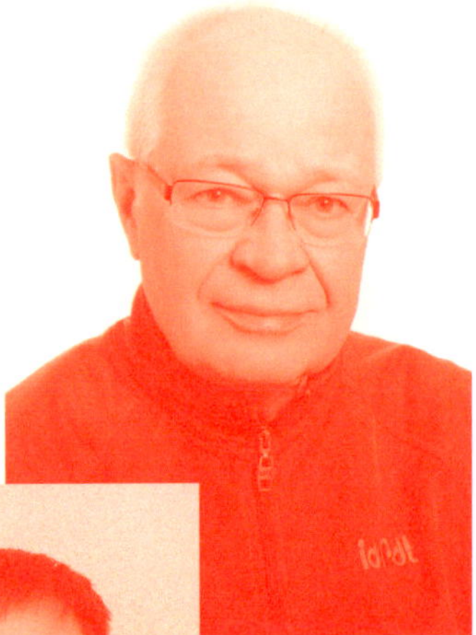

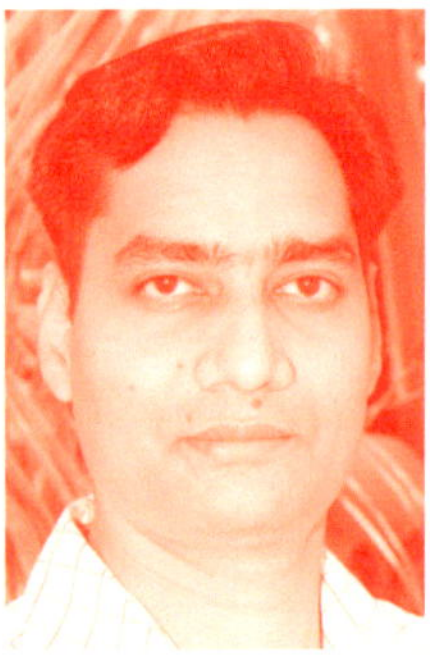

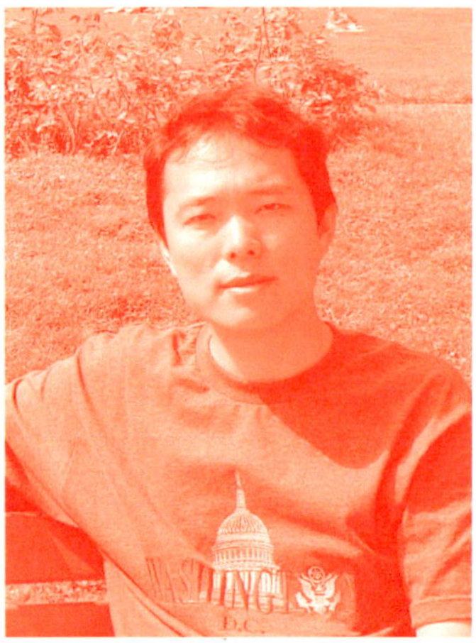

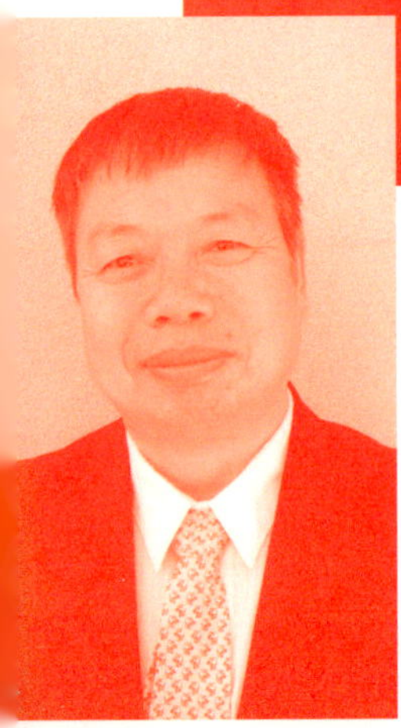

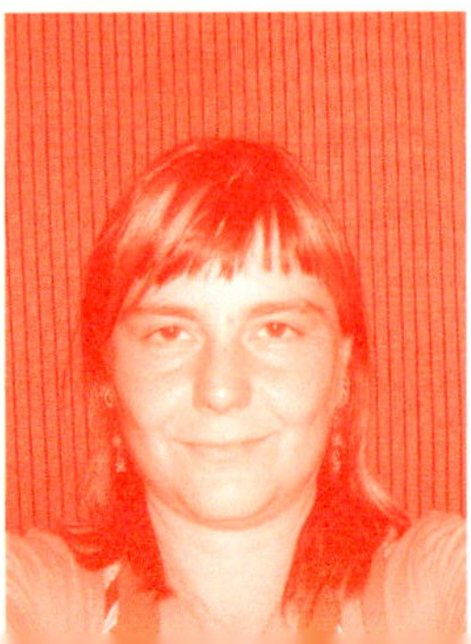

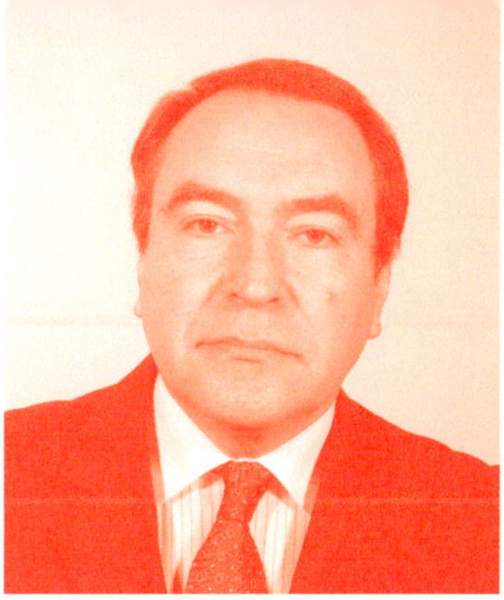
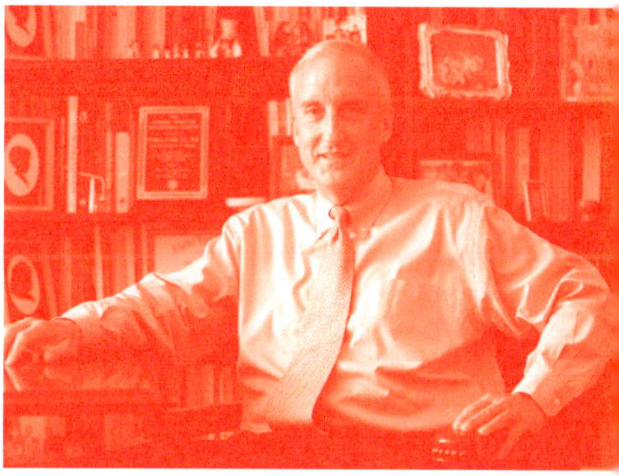
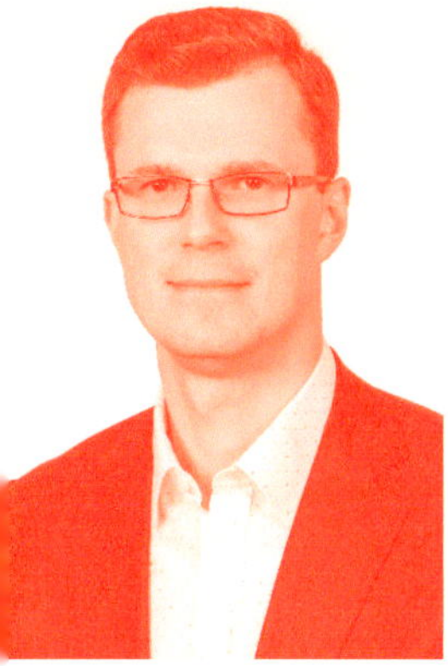
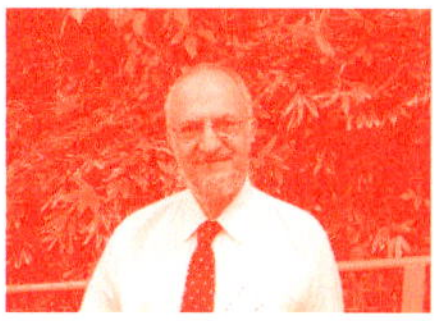
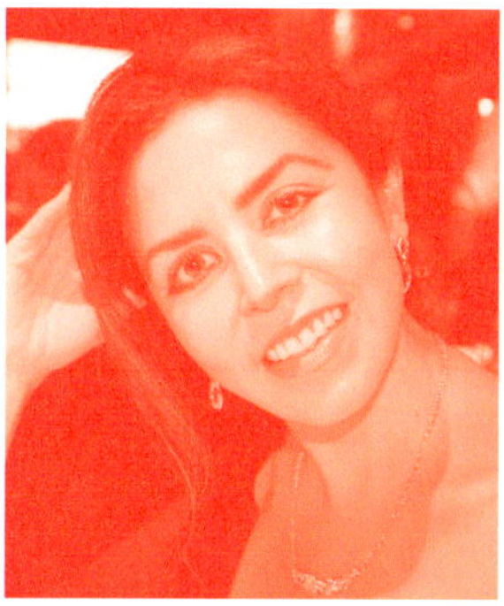

Supporting open minds since 2005

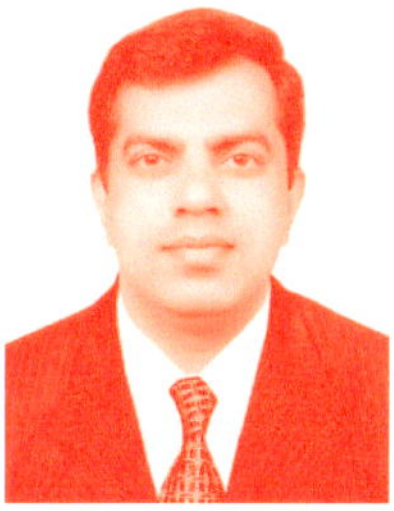
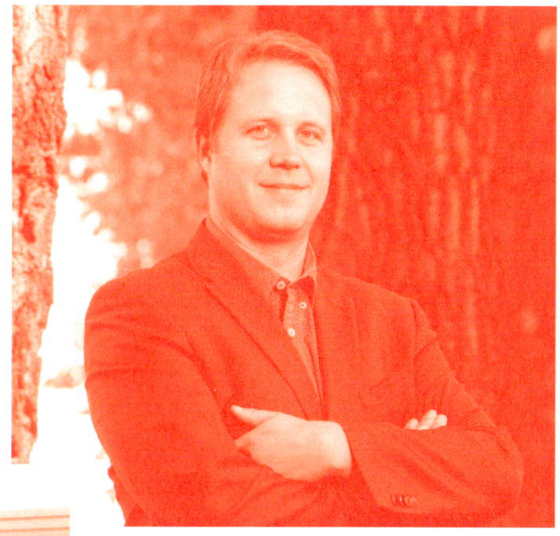
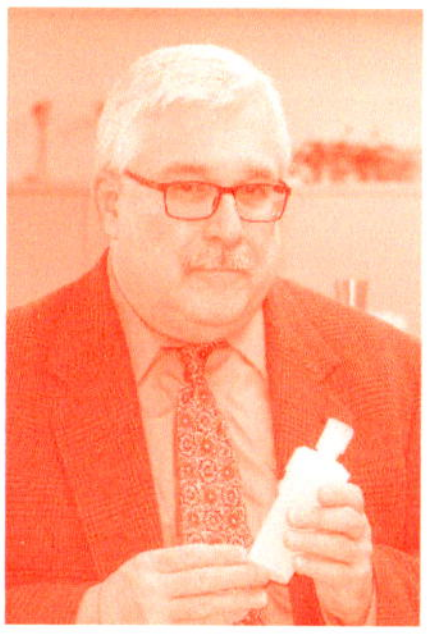
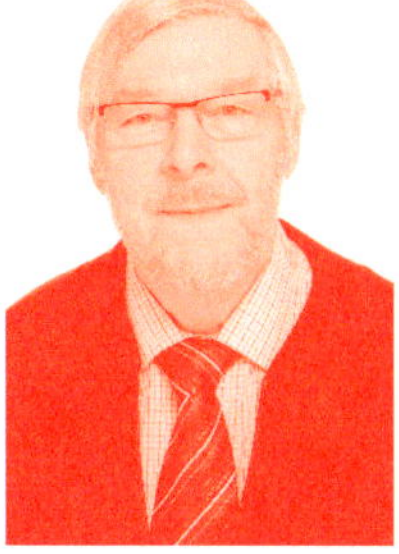
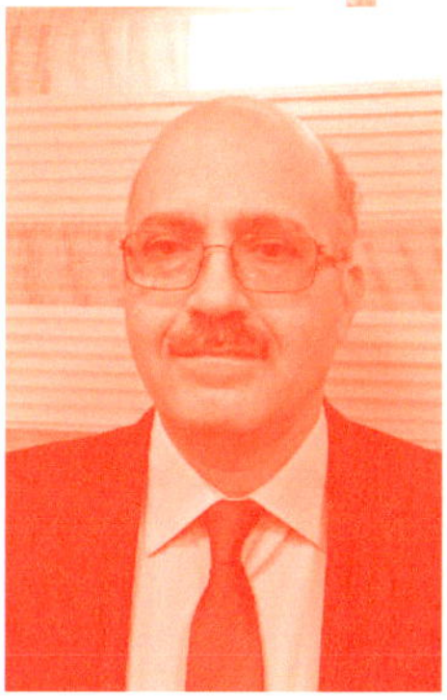
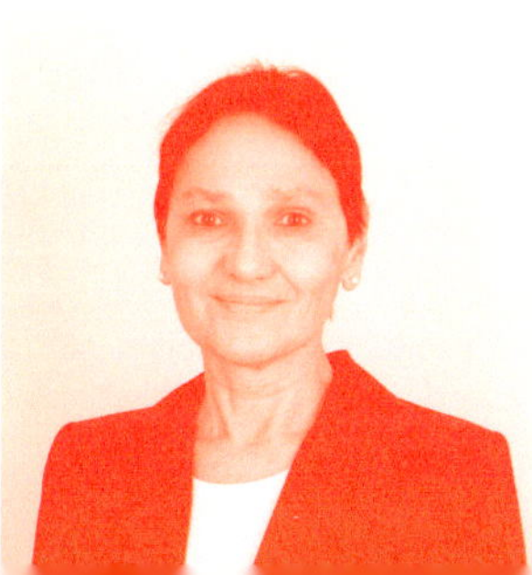
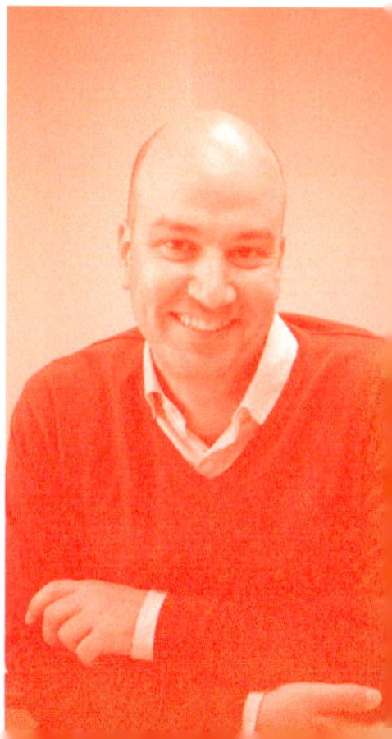

Environmental Health
http://dx.doi.org/10.5772/intechopen.91535
Edited by Takemi Otsuki

Contributors
Liz Kwo, Glen Cheng, Nischal Chennuru, Lucy Ngatia, Daniel Moriasi, Johnny M Grace Iii, Riqiang Fu, Cassel Gardner, Robert Taylor, Evens Emmanuel, Yolette Jérôme, Magline Alexis, Pascal Saffache, David Telcy, Ketty Balthazard-Accou, Max François Millien, Daphnée Michel, Gaston Jean, Alexandra Emmanuel, Hafiz Ishfaq Ahmad, Muhammad Bilal Bin Majeed, Abdul Jabbar, Ruqia Arif, Abudu Ballu Duwiejuah, Ammal Abukari, Ziblim Abukari Imoro, Abubakari Zarouk Imoro, Dhananjay Tripathi, Karuna Singh, Myriam El Ati-Hellal, Fayçal Hellal, Dharmeswar Barhoi, Sweety Nath Barbhuiya, Sarbani Giri, Ochuko Orakpoghenor, Talatu Patience Markus, Meshack Inotu Osagie, Paul Terkende Hambesha, Şevket Süleyman İrtem, Daphenide St. Louis, Ammcise Apply, Gulnaz Afzal

First published in London, United Kingdom, 2021 by IntechOpen
IntechOpen is the global imprint of INTECHOPEN LIMITED, registered in England and Wales, registration number: 11086078, 5 Princes Gate Court, London, SW7 2QJ, United Kingdom
Printed in Croatia

British Library Cataloguing-in-Publication Data
A catalogue record for this book is available from the British Library

Additional hard and PDF copies can be obtained from orders@intechopen.com

Environmental Health
Edited by Takemi Otsuki
p. cm.
Print ISBN 978-1-83968-720-4
Online ISBN 978-1-83968-721-1
eBook (PDF) ISBN 978-1-83968-722-8

For EU product safety concerns:
IN TECH d.o.o., Prolaz Marije Krucifikse Kozulić 3, 51000 Rijeka, Croatia, info@intechopen.com or visit our website at intechopen.com.

Meet the editor

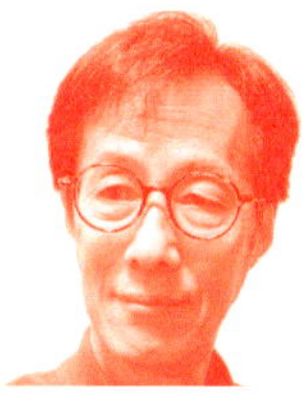

Honor. Prof. Takemi Otsuki graduated from Kawasaki Medical School (KMS), Kurashiki, Japan, in 1981. In 1986, at the Institutes of Medical Science, University of Tokyo, he was involved in clinical and experimental research in bone marrow transplantation. The theme of the post-doctoral school (1985–1989) was myeloma cell biology. After joining the Department of Hematology, University of Minnesota, USA, in 1992, Dr. Otsuki studied genes involved in chromosomal translocations of lymphomas in the Department of Hematopathology, US National Cancer Institute, National Institutes of Health. He returned to the Department of Hygiene, KMS, in 1996 and become a professor there in 2003. After retiring from KMS and obtaining an honorary professorship, Dr. Otsuki began working at the Shinjo Village National Health Insurance Clinic. Shinjo village has a small population of fewer than 900 people, and Dr. Otsuki is the sole medical doctor there.

Contents

Preface

Environmental Health discusses environmental effects on human health. It examines heavy metal pollution, biological effects of arsenic (on reproductive health, especially), effects of soil organic carbon, chemical pollution of drinking water, climate change and vector-borne diseases, marine fuels, particulate matter, and the United Nations Sustainable Development Goals (SDGs).

We must continue to consider all molecular and biological aspects of the environment and human health to ensure the wellbeing of the Earth, its inhabitants, and ecosystems.

Takemi Otsuki
Honorary Professor,
Kawasaki Medical School,
Kurashiki, Japan

Physician,
Shinjo Village National Health Insurance Clinic,
Shinjo Village, Japan

Section 1

Environmental and Human Health

Chapter 1

Land Use Change Affects Soil Organic Carbon: An Indicator of Soil Health

Lucy W. Ngatia, Daniel Moriasi, Johnny M. Grace III, Riqiang Fu, Cassel S. Gardner and Robert W. Taylor

Abstract

Soil organic carbon (SOC) is a major indicator of soil health. Globally, soil contains approximately 2344 Gt of organic carbon (OC), which is the largest terrestrial pool of OC. Through plant growth, soil health is connected with the health of humans, animals, and ecosystems. Provides ecosystem services which include climate regulation, water supplies and regulation, nutrient cycling, erosion protection and enhancement of biodiversity. Global increase in land use change from natural vegetation to agricultural land has been documented as a result of intensification of agricultural practices in response to an increasing human population. Consequently, these changes have resulted in depletion of SOC stock, thereby negatively affecting agricultural productivity and provision of ecosystem services. This necessitates the need to consider technological options that promote retention of SOC stocks. Options to enhance SOC include; no-tillage/conservation agriculture, irrigation, increasing below-ground inputs, organic amendments, and integrated, and diverse cropping/farming systems. In addition, land use conversion from cropland to its natural vegetation improves soil C stocks, highlighting the importance of increasing agricultural production per unit land instead of expanding agricultural land to natural areas.

Keywords: agriculture, land use change, organic carbon, soil health

1. Introduction

The basis and essence of life on earth depends on soil health, and its main indicator is soil organic carbon (SOC) content [1, 2]. Soil health has been defined as the capacity of a soil to support ecosystem functions and sustain environmental quality and biological productivity, while promoting plant and animal health [3]. Through plant growth, soil health is connected with the health of humans, animals, and ecosystems within its domain [4]. The SOC is an indicator of soil health and is an important component of the soil ecosystem [5, 6]. Deb et al. [7] indicate that the presence of organic carbon (OC) in soil is a key determinant for soil quality and productivity. In addition, organic matter is a key influencer on physical, chemical, and biological soil attributes [8]. The SOC stock exhibit the long-term balance between additions of OC from different sources and its losses through different pathways [9].

The term SOC is defined as C in soil derived from organic origins and soil organic matter (SOM) is generally considered to contain approximately 58% SOC.

Soil organic matter is a mixture of materials including particulate organics, humus, fine plant roots, living microbial biomass as well as charcoal [10]. Two words have commonly been used in reference to SOC; C sequestration and C storage. Carbon sequestration is the process of transferring carbon dioxide (CO_2) from the atmosphere into the soil which can be achieved through plants, plant residues and other organic amendments which are retained in the soil as part of SOM [10, 11]. Carbon sequestration in soil can range from short-term to long-term [12]. However, carbon storage in soil is defined as increase in SOC stocks over time, but it is not necessarily associated with a net removal of CO_2 from the atmosphere [12]. Soil storage of OC for longer time periods is preferable in terms of greenhouse gases mitigation, however, mineralization of SOC is important in terms of soil fertility [12, 13]. Soil health reflects the capacity of a soil to support both the agricultural production and provision of other ecosystem services [14]. Therefore, evaluation of soil health is essential because soil is a critically important component of the earth's biosphere whose, functionality is critical in the production of food and fiber as well as maintenance of environmental quality [15, 16].

In the soil profile, approximately 615 Gt of OC is stored in the top 20 cm, 1500 Gt of OC stored in the first meter, and 2344 Gt of OC is stored in the top three meters of soil [17, 18]. However, approximately 9 Gt C is anthropogenically released to the atmosphere annually from fossil fuel sources and ecosystem degradation [10]. Previous studies have illustrated that conversion of forest or natural vegetation to agriculture leads to an overall loss of SOC [5, 6, 19]. Through soil supply of plant macro and micronutrients, soil health, mediated by SOC dynamics is a major determinant of global food and nutritional security [4]. The projected increase of human population by 2050 will double food demand and put immense pressure on natural resources [20]. Therefore, one of the greatest challenges will be to increase food production by maintaining ecosystem services [21].

2. Importance of soil organic carbon

Soil organic C provides ecosystem services that are essential to human well-being for example climate regulation, water supplies and regulation, nutrient cycling, erosion protection and enhancement of biodiversity [2, 22–24]. In addition, SOC exerts an influence on many soil properties, for example water holding capacity, aggregate stability, total nitrogen, pH and cation exchange capacity [5, 6]. Increasing SOC can mitigate GHG emissions, benefit agricultural productivity through improvements in soil health, and improve environmental quality [25].

Under long-term management practices SOC pools influence soil quality, C sequestration pathways, and crop productivity [9]. It has been demonstrated that high SOC levels can enhance soil fertility and health, improve water infiltration, improve soil structure, enhance moisture retention and increased crop yield [26, 27]. A positive relationship has been reported between SOC content and soil nutrient status and crop yield [28, 29]. Since SOC content influences almost all soil functions and it is easily measurable, it can be a suitable indicator of the soil capacity to supply ecosystem services [22, 23].

3. Effects of climatic conditions on soil organic carbon

Generally, SOC stocks increase with decreasing mean annual temperature [30], whereby, cold, humid climatic regions exhibit C rich soils [31]. Decomposition releases to the atmosphere most of the C added to the soil through litter deposition, only a limited fraction becomes humus [10]. Both moisture and temperature influence the rate of litter decomposition through their effects on microbial activity [32]. In addition, both moisture and temperature also exhibit strong control of humus decomposition [10].

4. Land use change affect soil organic carbon and ecosystem services

Globally, there has been increased land use change from natural vegetation to agricultural land and urban areas as well as intensification of agricultural practices [33, 34]. These changes results in large increases in energy, water, and fertilizer consumption, as well as considerable losses of biodiversity [33]. The growing human population has driven both the land use change and land use intensification in order to meet global demand for food, water and energy [35]. However, conversion of forest or natural vegetation to agriculture leads to an overall loss of SOC [2, 5, 6, 19] (**Figure 1**), resulting in efforts to restore SOC in agricultural soils [36, 37]. Once soil is cultivated for agricultural production, SOM is rapidly decomposed as a result of modifications in conditions such as aeration, water content and temperature [38]. Land use change could affect soil functions that directly or indirectly relate to SOM, as a result of its capacity to retain water and nutrients as well as provide other ecosystem services [39, 40]. For example, changes in the SOC stock could result in significant impacts on the atmospheric C concentration [10]. Carbon dioxide is the main greenhouse gas responsible for global warming [41]. Soil organic C balances

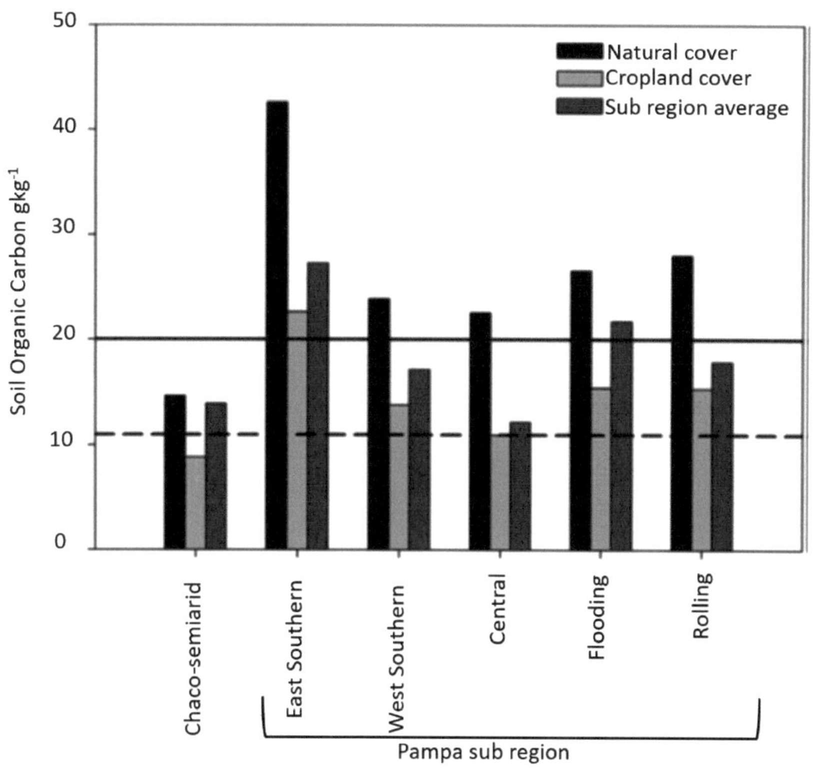

Figure 1.
Averages concentrations of soil organic carbon in semiarid Chaco and Pampa's sub-regions. Full line indicates critical thresholds proposed for temperate regions, and dashed line is for topical regions. Modified from [2].

are associated with CO_2 sequestration [36]. As a result, SOC stock is considered an intermediate ecosystem service that contributes to climate regulation [10].

Agricultural production can be increased by increasing cropland area or increasing productivity per unit area. When agricultural production increases as a result of land use change from natural cover areas to crop production agriculture, overall SOC mediated ecosystem services supply decreases [2] (**Figure 2A**). It was indicated that land use change from native forest to pasture (+8%), crop to pasture (+19%), crop to plantation (+18%), and crop to secondary forest (+53%) increased total C stocks, as well as SOC mediated ecosystem services (**Figure 2B** and **C**) whereas changes from pasture to plantation (−10%), native forest to plantation (−13%), native forest to crop (−42%), and pasture to crop (−59%) reduced total C stocks [17]. Generally, land use change from all other uses to cropping or monocultures result in losses of SOC [10]. In addition, Montgomery [42] indicated that accelerated soil erosion associated with conventional agriculture could occur at rates up to 100 times greater than the rate at which natural soil formation takes place. Additionally, peatlands have been drained for agricultural purposes [43]. Peatland store much more organic C in form of different C functional groups compared to upland. For example; in Apalachicola National Forest, the wetlands dominated by cypress (**Figure 3A**) and spikerush and water lily (**Figure 3B**) contain more alkyl, methoxyl, O-alkyl, aromatic, phenolic and carboxyl C compared to upland (**Figure 3C**). However, globally, peatland drainage causes carbon-rich peat to disappear at a rate 20 times greater than the rate at which the peat accumulated [44]. As a result, SOC affect both climate change and crop production in agricultural soils [9].

Soil management practices that sustain and enhance carbon stocks are crucial if we are to overcome near-term challenges and conserve this valuable resource for future generations. As a result of soil C loss during the past 25 years, one-quarter of the global land area has suffered a decline in productivity and the ability to provide

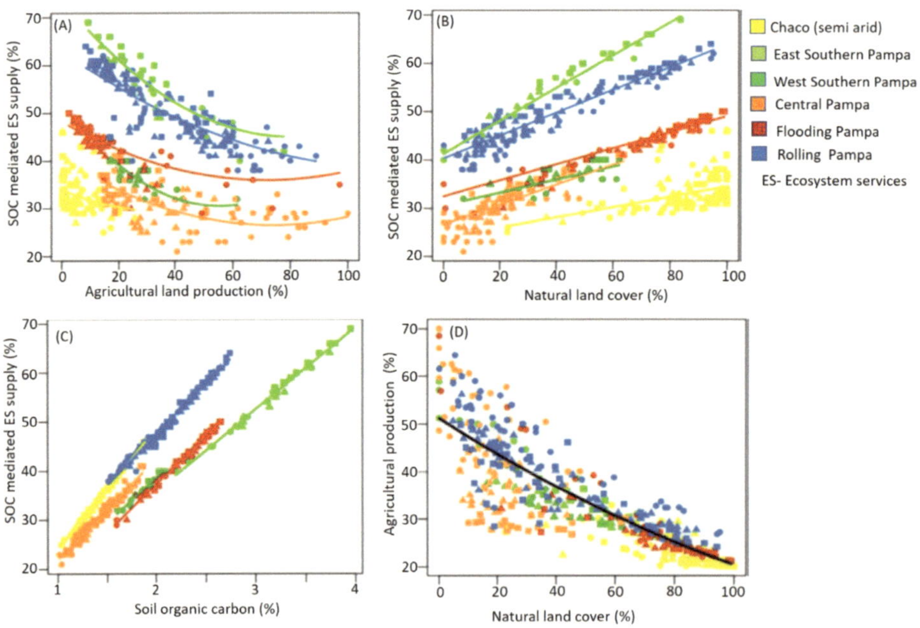

Figure 2.
Relations between ecosystem services mediated by SOC versus (A), agricultural production (B), natural cover (C), SOC and (D), relationship between agricultural production and natural cover. Modified from [2].

ecosystem services [39]. However, it has been observed that land use change from cropland to pasture or cropland to permanent forest results in the greatest gains of SOC [10] (**Table 1**). For example, Conant et al. [45] indicated that land use conversion from cropland to grassland improve soil carbon stocks. However, over time grassland area has been shrinking and arable land area expanding, indicating continued conversion of grassland to croplands [46]. In some cases where natural land cover has increased in expense of agricultural land cover, agricultural production

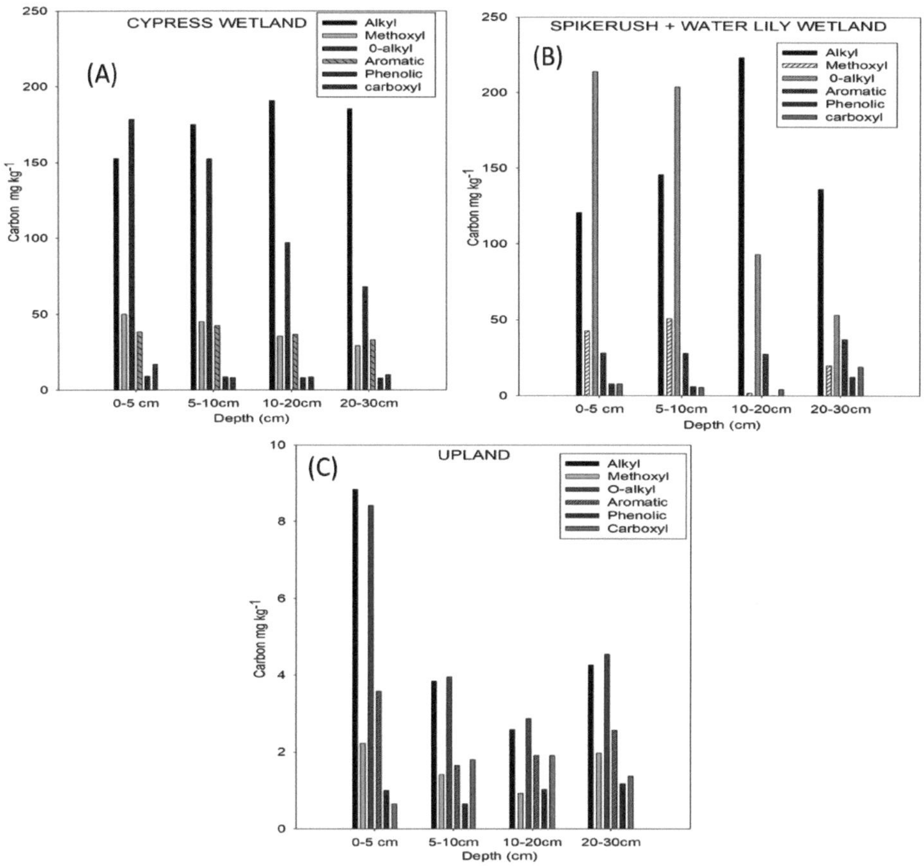

Figure 3.
Quantification of carbon functional groups in Apalachicola National Forest; which includes (A) cypress wetlands, (B) spikerush+water lily wetlands and (C) upland.

	Soil carbon change (%)		
Treatment	**Initial**	**Final**	**Change (%)**
Conversion: Cultivation to grass	0.97	1.35	39.2
Conversion: native to grass	2.97	2.55	−14
Fertilization	3.44	3.85	11.8
Grazing	2.62	2.89	9.99
Reclamation	8	15.9	98.8

Table 1.
Changes in soil carbon concentration presented by type of management change implemented. Modified from [45].

has been reported to decrease (**Figure 2D**). With increasing human population, this trend highlights the importance of increasing agricultural production by increasing crop yields per unit land area rather than expanding cropland and/or pasture over natural areas [2].

5. Increasing organic carbon stocks in agricultural soils

Agricultural systems are dependent on maintenance of four major functions; nutrients cycling, carbon transformations, soil structure maintenance, and regulation of pests and diseases [14]. Increasing SOM in agricultural soils contribute to food security and adaptation to climate change as well as mitigation of climate change [12]. SOM has a major role in soil fertility and water retention [47]. Therefore, SOM indirectly contributes to agricultural productivity and consequently to food security [12]. Management practices can influence SOC stocks by either decreasing SOC losses or increasing C inputs to soils. When OC input to a soil is larger than the OC outputs by mineralization or erosion, the SOC increases [12]. Below are technological options to manage SOC in agricultural ecosystem.

5.1 No-tillage and conservation agriculture

Soil organic matter is considered an important indicator of soil quality and health, which can be impacted by crop production practices such as tillage [48]. Tillage has the potential to increase the rate of C mineralization through breaking larger macro aggregates, mixing crop residues and exposing protected SOC in the aggregates to soil microorganisms [5, 6, 49, 50]. In general, tillage is considered to increase SOC mineralization as a result of mechanical and rain induced disruption of soil aggregates and the consequent release of CO_2. Hence, conservation tillage/no-tillage has been considered as a suitable practice to maintain or increase SOC stocks compared to conventional tillage [12, 51, 52]. Conservation tillage practices such as no till can enhance assimilation of SOC by decreasing soil disturbance and increasing crop residue accumulation in comparison to conventional tillage [12, 25, 48, 53]. For example; Blanco-Canqui and Lal [54] indicated an increase in SOC with increasing crop residue retention, whereby 16.0 t C ha^{-1} of SOC was reported without straw additions, 25.3 t SOC ha^{-1} with 8 t ha^{-1} of straw added and 104.9 t C ha^{-1} with 16 t ha^{-1} of straw added.

Global meta-analyses and reviews have recently confirmed that SOC stock increases in the upper soil layers (0–15 or 0–20 cm) under no tillage, but generally has low to non-significant effects on SOC stocks over 30 cm depth or deeper [51, 55–58] (**Figure 4**). In addition to carbon sequestration, conservation tillage can reduce CO_2 emissions [60]. Accumulation of SOC exhibit a positive correlation with the sequestration of atmospheric CO_2, while oxidation of SOC, as a result of practices such as tillage, can contribute to CO_2 emission from agricultural fields [48]. For example, CO_2 emission in conventional tillage was 29% greater than in no till in a loamy soil as reported by Bista et al. [61].

5.2 Irrigation

Irrigation may have similar effects on SOC decomposition in varying scenarios, but, its effects on primary production are likely to be much higher in arid and semi-arid areas compared to humid regions with dry summers [62]. It is reported that irrigation exhibited strong positive effects on SOC stocks in desert soils, positive effects in semi-arid areas, but no consistent trend was observed in humid areas [12, 62]. Further, it is emphasized that SOC stocks are dependent on climate and initial SOC content [62].

5.3 Increasing below-ground inputs

Below ground OC inputs, which includes roots and associated inputs, contribute more to SOC compared with above ground inputs [59, 63, 64] (**Figure 5**). For example, Kätterer et al., [63] reported long-term experimental results which indicated that root derived C was 2.3 times higher than that derived from above ground plant residue. Rasse et al. [64] estimated that mean residence time in soils of root derived C is 2.4 times compared with that of shoot derived C, indicating that root C has a longer residence time in soil compared to the shoot C.

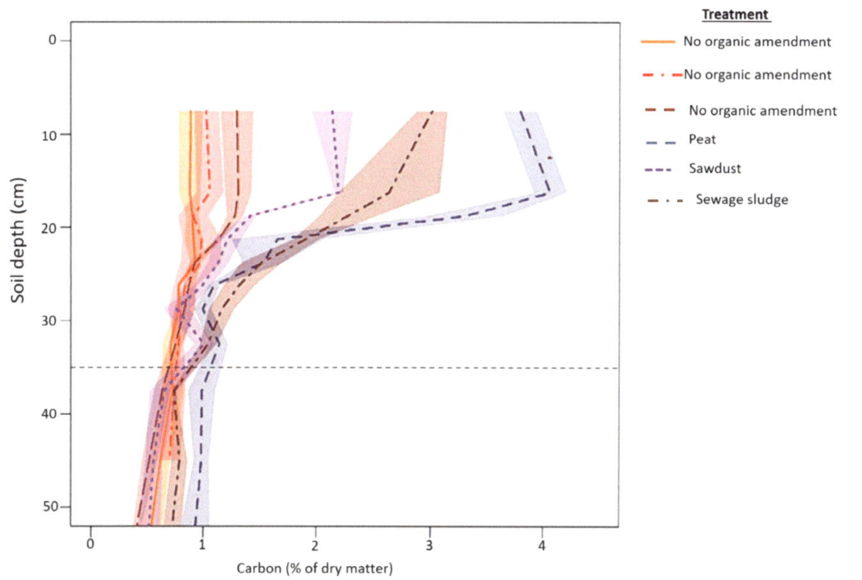

Figure 4.
Soil carbon content with depth. Shaded areas represent standard error of the mean. Data from long-term field experiment in Ultuna. Modified from [59].

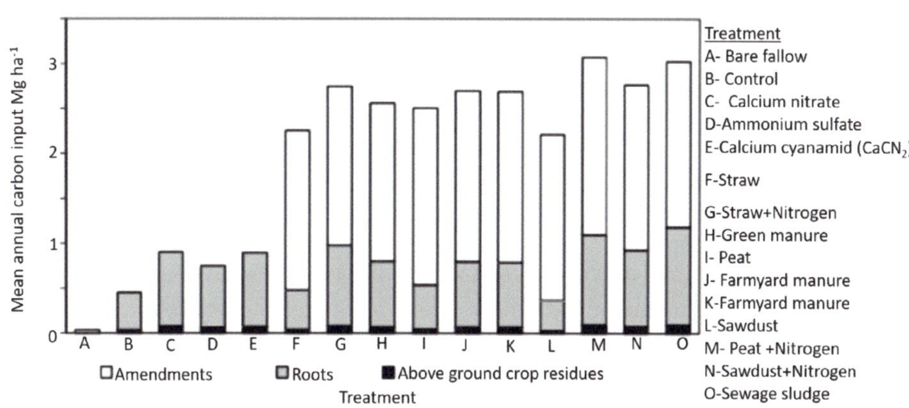

Figure 5.
Mean annual carbon inputs through above-ground crop residues, roots including rhizodeposition to equivalent topsoil depth (1957–2008), and organic amendments (1956–2008). Modified from [63].

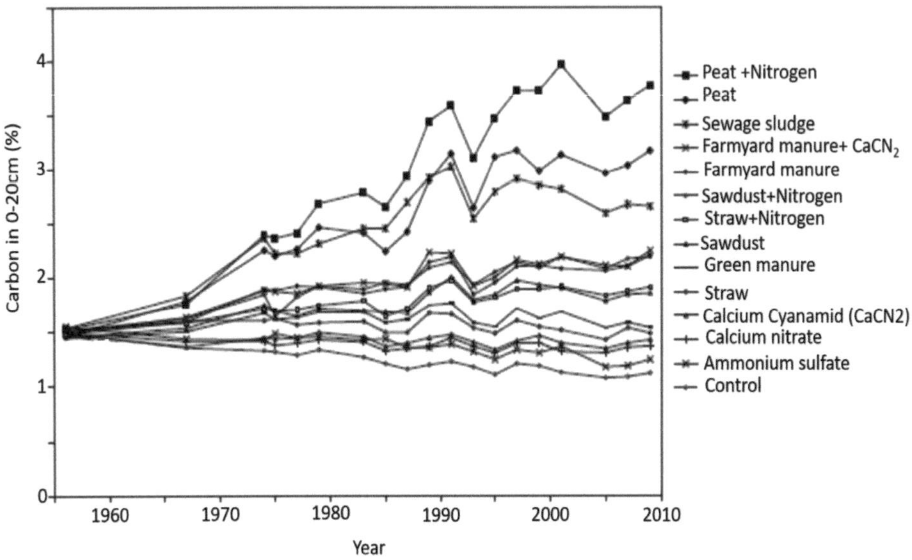

Figure 6.
Topsoil carbon concentrations over time in the Ultuna long-term soil organic matter experiment. Modified from [63].

5.4 Organic amendments

Organic amendment inputs can promote a buildup of SOM and hence SOC [65] (**Figure 6**). Menichetti et al. [59] reported that application of organic amendments affected SOC in the topsoil resulting in fourfold increases in C stock. Organic residues and wastes can be applied to soil, as fresh organic matter, after composting, methanisation, or pyrolysis [12]. However, the effects of residue quality on long term SOC is still a matter of debate [12]. Previous studies have indicated that the most labile and easily degradable compounds contribute more to SOM in the long term than recalcitrant materials such as lignin, this is especially common in clayey soil [66]. There are three explanations to this finding, which include: 1) long lasting SOM are mainly derived from microbial materials [67, 68]; 2) substrates that are easily degradable are processed with a high microbial C use efficiency [69], and 3) soluble compounds could be protected between mineral surfaces [12].

5.5 Integrated, and diverse cropping/farming systems

Compared with monoculture, introduction of crop diversity increases SOC which improves soil health [70]. Whereby, a combination of diversification within a cropping system and no-till soil management can help to improve SOC [71]. Increased plant diversity can enhance positive soil feedbacks on residue decomposition and soil SOM stabilization and may contribute to C accumulation in soils with rotated crops [72]. Further, Maiga et al. [71] demonstrated that use of diverse 4-year crop rotations for longer duration (>24 years) enhanced SOC, overall C and nitrogen fractions, and soil aggregation in comparison with those under 2-year corn–soybean rotations.

6. Conclusion

Soil organic C is an important indicator of soil health. Soil health is a major component of one health, which encompasses human, animal, and environmental health [73].

Soil organic C promotes land productivity and provides ecosystem services. Since SOC content influences almost all soil functions and is easily measurable, it can be a suitable indicator of the soil capacity to supply ecosystem services. This hypothesis reinforces the suitability of SOC as an appropriate indicator for soil management decisions, land use planning, and regulation. However, the rapidly increasing global human population is exerting enormous pressure on natural resources, as a result of the need to provide food and fiber to supply demands from this growing population. Consequently, there has been conversion of natural land areas to agricultural land globally in pursuit of meeting the human demand for food and fiber. This land use change has resulted in losses of SOC, which negatively affects productivity and diminish ecosystem services. Previous work has demonstrated that conversion of agricultural land to its natural cover provides positive feedback in terms of increasing soil C stocks. This finding highlights the importance of increasing agricultural production by increasing crop yields per unit area rather than expanding cropland and/or pasture to natural areas for long-term sustainability. In addition, there is need to invest in technological options that enhance SOC stocks in agricultural land. These options include no-tillage/conservation agriculture, irrigation, increasing below-ground inputs, organic amendments and integrated, diverse cropping/farming systems.

Acknowledgements

This work was supported by USDA-Forest Service grant number 17-CA-11330140-027 and USDA-ARS grant number 58-3070-7-009. All NMR measurements were performed at the National High Magnetic Field Laboratory, which is supported by National Science Foundation Cooperative Agreement No. DMR-1644779 and the State of Florida.

Author details

Lucy W. Ngatia[1*], Daniel Moriasi[2], Johnny M. Grace III [3], Riqiang Fu[4], Cassel S. Gardner[1] and Robert W. Taylor[1]

1 College of Agriculture and Food Sciences, Florida A&M University, Tallahassee, FL, USA

2 USDA-ARS Grazinglands Research Laboratory, USA

3 USDA-Forest Service, Southern Research Station, USA

4 National High Magnetic Field Laboratory, Florida State University, Tallahassee, FL, USA

*Address all correspondence to: lucy.ngatia@famu.edu

References

[1] Lal, R. 2014. Societal value of soil carbon. J. Soil Water Conserv. 69:186A–192A.

[2] Villarino, S. H., Studdert, G. A., and Laterra, P. 2019. How does soil organic carbon mediate trade-offs between ecosystem services and agricultural production? Ecological Indicators,103, 280-288. https://doi.org/10.1016/j.ecolind.2019.04.027

[3] Doran J.W., Safley M. 1997. Defining and assessing soil health and sustainable productivity, in: C.E. Pankhurst, B.M. Doube, V.V.S.R. Gupta (Eds.), Biological Indicators of Soil Health, CAB International, New York, 1997, pp. 1-28.

[4] Lal R. 2016. Soil health and carbon management. Food and Energy Security, 5(4):212-222

[5] Winowiecki, L., T.-G. Vågen, B. Massawe, N.A. Jelinski, C. Lyamchai, G. Sayula, and E. Msoka. 2016a. Landscape-scale variability of soil health indicators: Effects of cultivation on soil organic carbon in the Usambara Mountains of Tanzania. Nutr. Cycling Agroecosyst. 105:263-274. doi:10.1007/s10705-015-9750-1

[6] Winowiecki, L., T.-G. Vågen, B. Massawe, N.A. Jelinski, C. Lyamchai, G. Sayula, and E. Msoka. 2016b. Landscape-scale variability of soil health indicators: Effects of cultivation on soil organic carbon in the Usambara Mountains of Tanzania. Nutr. Cycling Agroecosyst. 105:263-274. doi:10.1007/s10705-015-9750-1

[7] Deb S., Bhadoria P.B.S., Mandal B., Rakshit A., Singh H.B. 2015. Soil organic carbon: Towards better soil health, productivity and climate change mitigation. Climate Change and Environmental Sustainability, 3(1): 26-34

[8] Bini D., Santos C.A.D., do Carmo K.B., Kishino N, Andrade G., Zangaro W., Marco Nogueira M.A. 2013. Effects of land use on soil organic carbon and microbial processes associated with soil health in southern Brazil. European Journal of Soil Biology 55:117-123

[9] Majumder, B., Mandal, B., Bandyopadhyay, P.K., Gangopadhyay, A., Mani, P.K. and Kundu, A.L., Mazumdar, D. 2008. Organic Amendments Influence Soil Organic Carbon Pools and Rice–Wheat Productivity. Soil Sci. Soc. Am. J. 72:775-785

[10] Stockmann, U., Adams, M.A., Crawford, J.W., Field, D.J., Henakaarchchi, N., Jenkins, M., Minasny, B., McBratney, A.B., de Courcelles, V.D., Singh, K., Wheeler, I., Abbott, L., Angers, D.A., Baldock, J., Bird, M., Brookes, P.C., Chenu, C., Jastrowh, J.D., Lal, R., Lehmann, J., O'Donnell, A.G., Parton, W.J., Whitehead, D., Zimmermann, M., 2013. The knowns, known unknowns and unknowns of sequestration of soil organic carbon. Agric. Ecosyst. Environ. 164, 80-99.

[11] Olson, K.R., Al-Kaisi, M.M., Lal, R., Lowery, B., 2014. Experimental consideration, treatments, and methods in determining soil organic carbon sequestration rates. Soil Sci. Soc. Am. J. 78, 348.

[12] Chenu, C., Angers, D. A., Barré, P., Derrien, D., Arrouays, D., and Balesdent, J. 2019. Increasing organic stocks in agricultural soils: Knowledge gaps and potential innovations. Soil and Tillage Research, 188, 41-52. https://doi.org/10.1016/j.still.2018.04.011

[13] Angers, D.A., Mehuys, G.R., 1989. Effects of cropping on carbohydrate content and water stable aggregation of a clay soil. Can. J. Soil Sci. 69, 373-380.

[14] Kibblewhite, M.G., Ritz, K., Swift, M.J. 2007. Soil health in agricultural systems. Philosophical Transactions of the Royal Society Series B, 363, 685-701.

[15] Doran, J. W., and M. R. Zeiss. 2000. Soil health and sustainability: managing the biotic component of soil quality. Appl. Soil Ecol. 15:3-11.

[16] Glanz, J.T., 1995. Saving Our Soil: Solutions for Sustaining Earth's Vital Resource. Johnson Books, Boulder, CO, USA.

[17] Guo, L.B., Gifford, R.M., 2002. Soil carbon stocks and land use change. Global Change Biol. 8, 345-360.

[18] Jobbágy, E.G., Jackson, R.B., 2000. The vertical distribution of soil organic carbon and its relation to climate and vegetation. Ecol. Appl. 10, 423-436.

[19] Don A., Schumacher J., Freibauer A. 2011. Impact of tropical land-use change on soil organic carbon stocks—a metaanalysis. *Glob Change Biol* 17:1658-1670. doi:10.1111/j.1365-2486.2010.02336.x

[20] Foley, J.A., 2011. Can we feed the world & sustain the planet? Scientific Am. 305, 60-65.

[21] Balmford, A., Green, R., Phalan, B., 2012. What conservationists need to know about farming. *Proc. R. Soc./Biol.* Sci. 279, 2714-2724.

[22] Lorenz, K., Lal, R., 2016. Soil organic carbon: an appropriate indicator to monitor trends of land and soil degradation within the SDG framework. Dessau-Roßlau, Germany (available at: http://www.umweltbundesamt.de/sites/default/files/medien/1968/publikationen/2016-11-30_soil_organic_carbon_ as_indicator_final. pdf).

[23] Powlson, D.S., Gregory, P.J., Whalley, W.R., Quinton, J.N., Hopkins, D.W., Whitmore, A.P., Hirsch, P.R., Goulding, K.W.T., 2011. Soil management in relation to sustainable agriculture and ecosystem services. Food Policy 36, S72–S87.

[24] Victoria, R., Banwart, S., Black H. et al., 2012. Benefits of soil carbon. UNEP yearbook. United Nations Environmental Programme, New York, 33 p

[25] Hati, K. M., Biswas, A. K., Somasundaram, J., Mohanty, M., Singh, R. K., Sinha, N. K., & Chaudhary, R. S. 2020. Soil organic carbon dynamics and carbon sequestration under conservation tillage in tropical vertisols. In P.K Ghosh S.K Mahanta D. Mandal B. Mandal and R Srinivasan (Eds.), Carbon management in tropical and sub-tropical terrestrial systems (pp. 201-212). Singapore City, Singapore: Springer.

[26] Fan, Y., Hou, X., Shi, H., and Shi, S. 2013. Effects of grazing and fencing on carbon and nitrogen reserves in plants and soils of alpine meadow in the three headwater resource regions. Russian *Journal of Ecology*, 44, 80-88. https://doi.org/10.1134/S1067 41361 2050165

[27] Xu, E., Zhang, H., and Xu, Y. 2020. Exploring land reclamation history: Soil organic carbon sequestration due to dramatic oasis agriculture expansion in arid region of Northwest China. Ecological Indicators, 108, 105746. https://doi.org/10.1016/j.ecolind.2019.105746

[28] Hashimi, R., Komatsuzaki, M., Mineta, T., Kaneda, S., and Kaneko, N. 2019. Potential for no-tillage and clipped-weed mulching to improve soil quality and yield in organic eggplant production. *Biological Agriculture and Horticulture*, 35, 158-171. https://doi.org/10.1080/01448 765.2019.1577757

[29] Xu, J., Han, H., Ning, T., Li, Z., and Lal, R. 2019. Long-term effects of tillage and straw management on soil

organic carbon, crop yield, and yield stability in a wheat-maize system. Field Crops Research, 233, 33-40. https://doi.org/10.1016/j.fcr.2018.12.016

[30] Post, W.M., Emanuel, W.R., Zinke, P.J., Stangenberger, A.G., 1982. Soil carbon pools and world life zones. Nature 298, 156-159.

[31] Hobbie, S.E., Schimel, J.P., Trumbore, S.E., Randerson, J.R., 2000. Controls over carbon storage and turnover in high-latitude soils. Global Change Biol. 6, 196-210.

[32] Meentemeyer, V., 1978. Macroclimate the lignin control of litter decomposition rates. Ecology 59, 465-472.

[33] Foley J.A., DeFries R., Asner G.P., et al. 2005. Global consequences of land use. Science, 309:(5734): 570-574.

[34] Vanwalleghem, T., Gómez, J.A., Infante, Amate J., González de Molina, M., Vanderlinden, K., Guzmán G., Laguna A., Giráldez J.V. 2017. Impact of historical land use and soil management change on soil erosion and agricultural sustainability during the Anthropocene. *Anthropocene* 17:13-29. https://doi.org/10.1016/j.ancene.2017.01.002.

[35] Foresight 2011. The Future of Food and Farming: Challenges and choices for global sustainability. Final Project Report. The Government Office for Science, London.

[36] Lal, R., 2004. Soil carbon sequestration impacts on global climate change and food security. Science 304, 1623-1627.

[37] Tittonell P., Giller K.E. 2013. When yield gaps are poverty traps: the paradigm of ecological intensification in African smallholder agriculture. Field Crops Res 143:76-90. doi:10.1016/j.fcr.2012.10.007

[38] Ashagrie, Y., Zech, W., Guggenberger, G., Mamo, T., 2007. Soil aggregation and total and particulate organic matter following conversion of native forests to continuous cultivation in Ethiopia. Soil and Tillage Research 94: 101-108.

[39] Bai, Z.G., Dent, D.L., Olsson, L. and Schaepman, M.E. 2008. Proxy global assessment of land degradation. Soil Use and Management, 24, 223-234

[40] Guimarães, D. V., Gonzaga, M. I. S., da Silva, T. O., da Silva, T. L., da Silva Dias, N., and Matias, M. I. S. 2013. Soil organic matter pools and carbon fractions in soil under different land uses. Soil and Tillage Research, 126:177-182. https://doi.org/10.1016/j.still.2012.07.010

[41] IPCC, 2013. Climate Change 2013: The Physical Science Basis. Contribution of Working Group I to the Fifth Assessment Report of the Intergovernmental Panel on Climate Change. Cambridge University Press, Cambridge, United Kingdom and New York, NY, USA.

[42] Montgomery, D.R. 2007. Soil erosion and agricultural sustainability. Proceedings of the National Academy of Sciences, 104, 13268-13272

[43] Ojanen P. and Minkkinen K., 2020. Rewetting Offers Rapid Climate Benefits for Tropical and Agricultural Peatlands But Not for Forestry-Drained Peatlands. *Global Biogeochemical Cycles*, 34, e2019GB006503. https://doi.org/10.1029/2019GB006503

[44] Joosten, H. 2009. The Global Peatland CO_2 Picture. Peatland status and drainage associated emissions in all countries of the World. Wetlands International, Ede, the Netherlands

[45] Conant, R.T., Cerri, C., Osborne, B., Paustian, K., 2017. Grassland management impacts on soil carbon

stocks: a new synthesis. Ecol. Appl. 9, 73-76.

[46] FAO. 2015. FAO STAT Statistical Database 2013. Food and Agriculture Organization of the United Nations, Rome, Italy. Follett, R. F., J. M. Kimble, and R. Lal. 2001. The potential of US grazing lands to sequester carbon and mitigate the green-house effect. CRC Press, Chelsea, Michigan, USA.

[47] Lal, R., 2008. Carbon sequestration. Philos. Trans. R. Soc. Lond. B Biol. Sci. 363, 815-830.

[48] Govindasamy, P., Liu, R., Provin, T., Rajan, N., Hons, F., Mowrer, J., Bagavathiannan, M. 2020. Soil carbon improvement under long-term (36 years) no-till sorghum production in a sub-tropical environment. Soil Use Manage. 2020;00:1-12.

[49] Kan, Z.-R., Ma, S.-T., Liu, Q.-Y., Liu, B.-Y., Virk, A. L., Qi, J.-Y., Zhang, H.-L. 2020. Carbon sequestration and mineralization in soil aggregates under long-term conservation tillage in the North China Plain. *Catena*, 188, 104428. https://doi.org/10.1016/j.catena.2019.104428

[50] Singh, S., Nouri, A., Singh, S., Anapalli, S., Lee, J., Arelli, P., and Jagadamma, S. 2020. Soil organic carbon and aggregation in response to thirty-nine years of tillage management in the southeastern US. Soil and Tillage Research, 197, 104523. https://doi.org/10.1016/j.still.2019.104523

[51] Haddaway, N.R., Hedlund, K., Jackson, L.E., Kätterer, T., Lugato, E., Thomsen, I.K., Jørgensen, H.B., Isberg, P.-E., 2017. How does tillage intensity affect soil organic carbon? A systematic review. Environ. Evid. 6, 2-48.

[52] VandenBygaart, A. J., Gregorich, E. G. and Angers, D. A. 2003. Influence of agricultural management on soil organic carbon: A compendium and analysis of Canadian studies. Can. J. Soil Sci. 83: 363-380.

[53] Jha, P., Hati, K. M., Dalal, R. C., Dang, Y. P., Kopittke, P. M., & Menzies, N. W. 2020. Soil carbon and nitrogen dynamics in a vertisol following 50 years of no-tillage, crop stubble retention and nitrogen fertilization. Geoderma, 358, 113996.

[54] Blanco-Canqui, H., and Lal, R. 2007. Soil structure and organic carbon relationships following 10 years of wheat straw management in no-till. *Soil and Tillage Research*, 95, 240-254. https://doi. org/10.1016/j.still.2007.01.004

[55] Luo, Z.K., Wang, E.L., Sun, O.J., 2010. Can no-tillage stimulate carbon sequestration in agricultural soils? A meta-analysis of paired experiments. Agric. Ecosyst. Environ. 139, 224-231.

[56] Meurer, K.H.E., Haddaway, N.R., Bolinder, M.A., Kätterer, T., 2018. Tillage intensity affects total SOC stocks in boreo-temperate regions only in the topsoil—A systematic review using an ESM approach. Earth Sci. Rev. 177, 613-622.

[57] Powlson, D.S., Stirling, C.M., Jat, M.L., Gerard, B.G., Palm, Ca., Sanchez, Pa., Cassman, K.G., 2014. Limited potential of no-till agriculture for climate change mitigation. Nat. Clim. Change 4, 678-683.

[58] Powlson, D.S., Stirling, C.M., Thierfelder, C., White, R.P., Jat, M.L., 2016. Does conservation agriculture deliver climate change mitigation through soil carbon sequestration in tropical agro-ecosystems? Agric. Ecosyst. Environ. 220, 164-174.

[59] Menichetti, L., Ekblad, A., Kätterer, T., 2015. Contribution of roots and amendments to soil carbon

accumulation within the soil profile in a long-term field experiment in Sweden. Agric. Ecosyst. Environ. 200, 79-87.

[60] Hernanz, J. L., Sánchez-Girón, V., and Navarrete, L. 2009. Soil carbon sequestration and stratification in a cereal/leguminous crop rotation with three tillage systems in semiarid conditions. *Agriculture, Ecosystems and Environment*, 133, 114-122. https:// doi.org/10.1016/j.agee.2009.05.009

[61] Bista, P., Norton, U., Ghimire, R., & Norton, J. B. 2017. Effects of tillage system on greenhouse gas fluxes and soil mineral nitrogen in wheat (Triticum aestivum, L.) -fallow during drought. Journal of Arid Environment, 147, 103-113. https://doi.org/10.1016/j.jaridenv.2017.09.002

[62] Trost, B., Prochnow, A., Drastig, K., Meyer-Aurich, A., Ellmer, F., Baumecker, M., 2013. Irrigation, soil organic carbon and N2O emissions. A review. Agron. Sustain. Dev. 33, 733-749.

[63] Kätterer, T., Bolinder, M.A., Andrén, O., Kirchmann, H., Menichetti, L., 2011. Roots contribute more to refractory soil organic matter than above-ground crop residues, as revealed by a long-term field experiment. Agric. Ecosyst. Environ. 141, 184-192.

[64] Rasse, D.P., Rumpel, C., Dignac, M.F., 2005. Is soil carbon mostly root carbon? Mechanisms for a specific stabilisation. Plant Soil 269, 341-356.

[65] Follett, R.F., 2001. Soil management concepts and carbon sequestration in cropland soils. Soil and Tillage Research 61: 77-92.

[66] Cotrufo, M.F., Wallenstein, M.D., Boot, C.M., Denef, K., Paul, E., 2013. The Microbial Efficiency-Matrix Stabilization (MEMS) framework integrates plant litter decomposition with soil organic matter stabilization: do labile plant inputs form stable soil organic matter? Glob. Change Biol. 19, 988-995.

[67] Kallenbach, C.M., Grandy, A.S., Frey, S.D., Diefendorf, A.F., 2015. Microbial physiology and necromass regulate agricultural soil carbon accumulation. Soil Biol. Biochem. 91, 279-290.

[68] Miltner, A., Bombach, P., Schmidt-Brücken, B., Kästner, M., 2012. SOM genesis: microbial biomass as a significant source. Biogeochemistry 111, 41-55.

[69] Wieder, W.R., Grandy, A.S., Kallenbach, C.M., Bonan, G.B., 2014. Integrating microbial physiology and physio-chemical principles in soils with the MIcrobial-Mineral Carbon Stabilization (MIMICS) model. Biogeosciences 11, 3899-3917.

[70] McDaniel M., Grandy A., Tiemann L., Weintraub M. 2016. Eleven years of crop diversification alters decomposition dynamics of litter mixtures incubated with soil. Ecosphere 7, e01426. doi:10.1002/ecs2.1426

[71] Maiga, A., Alhameid, A., Singh, S., Polat, A., Singh, J., Kumar, S., and Osborne, S. 2019. Responses of soil organic carbon, aggregate stability, carbon and nitrogen fractions to 15 and 24years of no-till diversified crop rotations. Soil Research,57, 149-157

[72] McDaniel, M. D., L. K. Tiemann, and A. S. Grandy. 2014. Does agricultural crop diversity enhance soil microbial biomass and organic matter dynamics? A meta-analysis. Ecological Applications 24:560-570.

[73] Mackenzie J.S. and Jeggo M., 2019. The One Health Approach—Why Is It So Important? Tropical medicine and infectious disease. *Trop. Med. Infect. Dis*.4:88; doi:10.3390/tropicalmed4020088

Chapter 2

Evaluating the Clinical and Cost Effectiveness of Musculoskeletal Digital Health Solutions

Glen Cheng, Nischal Chennuru and Liz Kwo

Abstract

This chapter will introduce the clinician to the quickly expanding field of musculoskeletal-focused digital apps (MDA), with an eye towards helping the clinician select and recommend MDAs for optimal patient care. MDAs are increasingly being used for physical therapy and rehabilitation, telehealth, pain management, behavioral health, and remote patient monitoring. The COVID-19 pandemic has vastly accelerated the adoption of telehealth and digital health apps by patients and clinicians, and the digital health field will only continue to expand as developers increasingly harness artificial intelligence (AI) and machine learning (ML) capabilities, coupled with precision medicine capabilities that integrate personal health data tracking and genomics insights. Here we begin with an overview of several types of MDA, before discussing the epidemiology of musculoskeletal conditions and injuries, clinical considerations in selecting a digital health solution, payor reimbursement for digital apps, and regulatory oversight of digital health apps.

Keywords: digital health, telemedicine, physical therapy, musculoskeletal, artificial intelligence

1. Introduction

Digital health is a rapidly growing field. As of early 2019, there were over 318,000 mobile health applications in different app stores--and that number itself doubled since 2015 as consumers increasingly used mobile apps to manage their health [1]. Popular mobile health apps include AI-powered health symptom checkers, clinical records management apps, remote patient monitoring tools, patient self-monitoring tools, rehabilitation programs, and apps for medical condition education and management. In fact, healthcare applications constitute the most popular smartphone activity. Currently, 90% of physicians use smartphone applications for medical records, communication with their teams and for clinical content like UptoDate [2]. Over 75% of the largest health systems now offer mobile applications focused on patient engagement [3]. The global mobile health market is growing and is expected to reach $111 billion by 2025 with fitness constituting $50B in the US health market. The current COVID-19 Pandemic will accelerate the adoption and will further increase the adoption and growth [4].

An American Medical Association survey found that physicians' use of technology to provide televisits or virtual visits doubled from 2016 to February 2020, with nearly 30% of doctors adopting digital health technology [5]. And since the start of

Application	Category	Physical and Mental Exercises	Relaxation Practices	Learning Modules	Effective for Low Back Pain	No Hardware Required	Online Mentors	In-Person Mentors	Best for Large Businesses
Kaia Health	Multimodal Pain Therapy	Yes	Yes	Yes	Yes	Yes	Yes	No	N/A
Wellness Coaches	Onsite Personalized Therapy	Yes	Yes	Yes	N/A	Yes	No	Yes	N/A
HBD International	Solutions To Reduce Client (Company) Injuries	Yes (Employee Morale Boost)	N/A	Yes	N/A	N/A	Yes	N/A	Yes
Movement RX	Mind-Body Connection Improvement	Yes	Yes	Yes	N/A	Yes	Yes	N/A	Yes
PHZIO Media	Early Prevention and Intervention (Thru PT)	N/A	N/A	N/A	N/A	N/A	Yes	N/A	Yes
Airrosti	Prevention, Recovery, and Education	N/A	N/A	Yes	N/A	Yes	Yes	N/A	Yes
SimpleTherapy	Personalized Pain Recovery	Yes	N/A	No	N/A	No	Yes	N/A	N/A
Hinge Health	Sensor-Guided Exercise Therapy	Yes	N/A	Yes	N/A	No	Yes	N/A	Yes

Table 1.
Digital Health Apps for Managing Musculoskeletal Pain and Functional Limitations [9].

the COVID-19 pandemic, physician use of telemedicine has increased exponentially as digital technologies have become increasingly adopted by both physicians and consumers. Physical therapist and physiotherapist adoption of musculoskeletal-focused digital apps (MDA) has likewise expanded exponentially [6]. Consumer adoption of telehealth increased from 11% of care visits in 2019 to 46% in May 2020, as providers scaled the offerings and are seeing 50 to 175 times the number of patients via telehealth compared to before. In 2019, the annual revenue of US telehealth vendors was $3 Billion with a big focus on the virtual urgent care segment. With new Centers for Medicare and Medicaid Services (CMS) policies being implemented during the crisis to expand the use of virtual care, up to $250 Billion of current US healthcare spend could potentially be virtualized [7]. Primary care and behavioral health have led in the number of virtual visits. The services/clinical models that have the greatest potential for virtual care include on demand virtual urgent care, office visits, home health services and home medication administration services [8].

In particular, the number of mobile medical apps for musculoskeletal conditions and injury management is increasing exponentially as organizational health and wellness initiatives increasingly focus on pain management and holistic care. **Table 1** provides an overview of features present in several MDAs on the market as of August 2020. The general purpose of these different musculoskeletal apps is to provide therapy on a large sale for patients with musculoskeletal disorders. The MDAs surveyed in this table have physical or mental exercise programs, and some have behavioral interventions such as mindfulness practice. Most apps also have learning modules to teach organizations and individuals how to stay safe and protect themselves from further issues.

The MDAs surveyed differ in their targeted goals and their approach to achieving their goals. For example, Kaia Health concentrates on using multiple approaches to minimize pain, whereas Movement RX focuses on strengthening the mind-body connection to reduce pain. Wellness Coaches places emphasis on a very personalized and face to face therapy program. And while many apps do not have physical hardware, SimpleTherapy and Hinge Health use sensors that can be placed over joints to track progress and pain.

Moreover, most of the surveyed MDAs can be effectively used to improve population health, injury prevention and rehabilitation in large organizations and companies. The MDAs focus on individual health and progress, while also addressing how to prevent organizational ergonomic issues and manage musculoskeletal injury recovery.

2. Epidemiology of Musculoskeletal Conditions and Injuries

Musculoskeletal conditions continue to increase in incidence and prevalence, especially as the geriatric population grows, and organizations continue to have unremedied ergonomics issues. Musculoskeletal disorders are highly prevalent, yet frequently mismanaged and costly. Musculoskeletal injuries are also a top cost driver for employers, as no other chronic health condition causes more lost workdays and more healthcare spend than musculoskeletal injuries [10]. Musculoskeletal lower back injury is the leading cause of disability both globally and in the U.S., and the number one reason for missing work [11]. In the U.S. alone, musculoskeletal lower back injuries result in more than 260 million lost workdays each year as well as significant healthcare and disability insurance costs [12]. 1 in 2 adults in the U.S. were diagnosed with musculoskeletal conditions in 2012. Despite the high prevalence of musculoskeletal conditions, 80% of patients do not receive evidence-based care [13]. As detailed below, musculoskeletal pain continues to be frequently mismanaged with opioid analgesics, and unnecessary surgery is frequently performed when physical therapy and rehabilitation would be more appropriate. Medical costs for imaging, diagnosis and treatment of musculoskeletal injuries and conditions continue to rise [14].

Musculoskeletal joint pain has significant impact on patient function and future health. Joint pain reduces physical activity, increases opioid use, impacts productivity, and leads to obesity [15]. Obesity in turn increases the risk for diabetes, heart disease, depression, and cancer [16].

Yet Musculoskeletal pain is frequently mismanaged with opioid analgesics. Even as warnings of an opioid crisis in the US have increased provider and patient awareness of the dangers of opioid analgesics, opioids remain a commonly prescribed treatment for lower back musculoskeletal pain. The dangers of opioid analgesics are well known and include dependence, dangerous side effects including respiratory depression, fatality from drug overdose, and high incidence of concomitant illicit drug use [17]. Moreover, when used to treat new diagnoses of lower back pain, opioid analgesics result in longer recovery times, increased serious adverse events, and greater healthcare utilization (emergency room visits and hospitalizations) compared to non-opioid analgesics [18].

Likewise, patients frequently receive inappropriate surgery for musculoskeletal conditions. Studies have shown that approximately 66% of surgeries are avoidable [19]. Inappropriate surgery for musculoskeletal conditions comes with significant recovery times, lengthening the treatment period, increasing cost of care, and yielding poorer pain and functional outcomes relative to conservative management and physical therapy [20].

Musculoskeletal issues will continue to rise, especially as the geriatric population grows, ergonomic work situations are not well controlled in factories and warehouses, and medical costs for imaging, diagnosis and treatment continue to rise. Studies predict that by 2030, there will be a 500% increase in total knee replacements [21], and a 200% increase in total hip replacements in 45- to 64-year-olds [22]. Likewise, studies project a 28% increase in spine surgeries by 2024 [23].

3. Critically Assessing Musculoskeletal Digital Apps

With increasing adoption of telehealth and digital solutions comes increasing demands on clinicians to recommend and use MDAs appropriately, while avoiding dangers and pitfalls. Here, we detail methods to assess the clinical effectiveness, the functionality, and the reliability of digital health solutions.

The landscape of digital health solutions on the Internet and app stores has been likened to the Wild West, given the inability of regulators to keep up with the explosive growth of medical apps. A significant pitfall to avoid is apps that falsely claim to diagnose, prevent, or treat a disease or medical condition. Such claims require FDA review and approval prior to marketing, and digital apps have been pulled off the market for making false claims. For example, in 2011, an app developer claimed that the app could use the blue light emitted from a mobile device to cure acne. The Federal Trade Commission (FTC) intervened to prohibit marketing of the app, and the app was removed from app stores for failure to obtain regulatory approval [24]. For digital health apps that do not make diagnostic, prevention, or treatment claims, however, regulatory approval is not required. Absent fraud, such apps will not be removed from the digital marketplace. It is thus important for clinicians to be able to assess the utility of digital health solutions.

Two well-known entities that evaluate Internet resources are the Health on the Net Foundation (HON) and the Agency for Healthcare Research and Quality

(AHRQ). HON published a HON Code of Conduct (HONcode) in 1996 that includes 8 principles for certifying information on health and medical websites. The 8 principles include Authority, Complementarity, Confidentiality, Attribution, Justifiability, Transparency, Financial Disclosure, and Advertising [25]. AHRQ proposed similar criteria, including credibility, content, disclosure, links, design, interactivity, and caveats [26]. Hanrahan et al. recommend applying similar criteria to the evaluation of digital health apps [27].

In assessing the clinical effectiveness of an intervention, the clinician will want to consider the types of study designs used to generate evidence of effectiveness [28]. Traditionally, randomized controlled trials are considered the gold standard in evidence assessment [29], followed by observational studies such as cohort, cross-sectional, and case-control studies, and ending with descriptive studies such as surveillance, surveys, and case reports [30]. However, a nuanced that takes into account the size of the study and the rigor of the study design, recognizes that large, well-designed observational studies can yield among the highest-quality clinical evidence. Moreover, observational studies offer evidence of clinical effectiveness under real-world conditions, in contrast with randomized trials, which may have restrictive inclusion and exclusion criteria and lack generalizability beyond the highly controlled experimental study settings [31]. A commonly used system of assessing the quality of evidence generated by medical studies is The Cochrane Collaboration's GRADE approach [32].

MDAs vary widely with regard to functionality. By being aware of the different functions offered by different MDAs, the clinician can tailor recommendations to patients with different musculoskeletal monitoring or rehabilitation needs. As detailed in **Table 1**, some apps are more focused on pain management, while others are focused on restoring and improving physical function. Some apps include hardware, such as EKG and heart rate sensors and sensors over joints to track movement. Other apps focus on behavioral interventions to address pain and help patients stay on track with physical therapy plans to address musculoskeletal injuries.

Evidence based exercise-therapy is another function offered by a number of digital vendors. From gathering detailed information on movement and activity and leveraging artificial Intelligence, digital apps can deliver personalized advice and exercise programs that adapt according to the progress made by the individual. Some apps focus on preventing the development of conditions and maintaining musculoskeletal health, including access to a comprehensive library of preventative exercise programs, including Pilates, yoga, stretching and strengthening options. TrackActive is a digital application that specializes in rehabilitation of musculoskeletal conditions and acts as virtual physio enabling people to assess and self-manage injuries and common conditions from home [33]. Based on the member profile, this application tracks members activities using different surveillance techniques and provides personalized recommendations. Telehealth apps that facilitate virtual second opinions for different musculoskeletal conditions are also increasingly being utilized [34].

Many digital apps now focus on musculoskeletal injury prevention in occupational settings. Musculoskeletal injuries are the largest single category of workplace injury and account for 28% of all occupational injuries [35]. Occupational health focused digital apps thus aim to reduce muscle, joint, tendon, ligament and nerve injuries/illnesses across the workforce to improve availability and productivity [36].

With 40% of all mobile apps related to healthcare, verifying accuracy of clinical content and validating apps for intended clinical uses is critical. While assessing the clinical benefit of MDA functions, it is important to review the available evidence. For example, one randomized controlled trial (n=215) concluded that an MDA that included behavioral interventions such as medication reminders, daily surveys of symptoms and potential adverse effects, fared no better than usual care in reducing pain scores [37].

Mobile health apps for monitoring postoperative pain are another promising frontier for MDAs. Such digital apps can provide real time monitoring and symptom management and can help improve self-management skills with post-operative pain. To alleviate pain, digital apps can provide appropriate distraction, relaxation, and guided imagery techniques. However, a critical review of digital apps focused on self-management of pain showed very limited involvement of healthcare specialists and limited evidence based self-learning content. Lalloo et al. found that of 10 mobile applications meeting inclusion criteria, none provided social support, goal setting criteria, or had scientific evaluation or end users in their development [38]. Only 50% of the apps included a provider specialist in the development. There is accordingly a need to build comprehensive pain self-management, evidence based, personalized, AI-driven mobile applications.

When assessing an MDA's functionality, the clinician will want to assess the MDA's ability to not only improve subjective pain scores, but also to improve objectively quantifiable measures of disability function. The MDAs with highest likelihood of yielding clinical benefit are those whose efficacy on objective measures have been established in peer-reviewed studies [39]. For example, two smaller randomized controlled trials demonstrated efficacy of MDAs with respect to improving both knee and back pain and disability function [40, 41]. These beneficial impacts on both chronic musculoskeletal pain and disability function were subsequently confirmed in a large 10,000 participant longitudinal cohort [42].

Moreover, some MDAs offer population health surveillance features that can be useful to health officers in organizations tracking the health of their workforce. While such features can be very useful in workforce injury surveillance and prevention, it is important to be aware of privacy issues when deploying such solutions in an organizational or work setting. In particular, the ability to leverage Artificial Intelligence (AI) focused digital health apps for population health surveillance have garnered critical attention during the COVID19 pandemic. Tools that track disease activity in real time include contact tracing applications that identify and track individuals who might have come in contact with an infected person. User consent is essential for the adoption and sustained growth of such digital health applications [43, 44].

Finally, in evaluating the utility of digital health apps, clinicians should also recognize app performance issues such as functionality, stability/reliability, and stage of development, which affect the usability of the app and the benefit to patients. The proliferation of digital health applications has led app developers to focus on functionality, stability, security, privacy, usability, reliability, and data accuracy. In evaluating performance of mobile apps, it is advisable to utilize a framework that evaluates each dimension of the application. We recommend a framework consisting of rating domains and criteria for each domain. The domains are (1) Usability, which includes functionality, visualization, ease of install and use, multi-language support and ability to customize; (2) Content (Technical), which includes performance, stability, interoperability, portability, bandwidth and application size; (3) Content (Health), which includes quality, presentation and validation of the information, literacy level, measurement and interpretation of the information and potential for harm; (4) Security/privacy/compliance, which includes data authentication, protection, tokenization, authentication and pro-active breach signaling; and (5) Transparency, which includes member consent, cost of the app and accuracy of the description in the app stores [45].

4. Employer and Payor Reimbursement

The COVID-19 pandemic fueled rapid healthcare provider adoption of telehealth, as social distancing measures were implemented and government and commercial payors relaxed regulations and reimbursement requirements [46]. The transformation of care delivery in turn enabled consumers and providers to connect via virtual healthcare visits and associated modalities. The widespread adoption of telehealth has led both employers and payers to accelerate and look for innovative ways to reimburse for different digital health apps. For example, the recent $37 Billion merger of telehealth leader Teladoc and digital chronic disease management company Livingo has set the precedent for rapid change in adoption of digital applications with payers and employers ready for embracing them as part of mainstream providers [47]. In the fragmented U.S. market, potential barriers remain in terms of who will pay, but payers are starting to cover digital apps.

The Decision Resources Group found that across healthcare executives in integrated health networks (IDNs), Medicaid managed care organizations (MCOs), and pharmacy benefits managers (PBMs), 25% said their organization provides coverage for digital therapeutics, and an additional 45% expressed interest in providing coverage. In a 2019 survey, the National Business Group on Health found that 25% of large self-funded employers are considering creating orthopedic centers of excellence by 2021 [48]. Moreover, 45% of orthopedic COE contracts are structured as bundled payments. Given the potential for clinical benefit and cost savings, employers and health insurance payors are increasingly reimbursing use of digital health apps.

5. FDA Regulation of Digital Health Apps

Products intended to diagnose, prevent, or treat disease must be approved by the FDA prior to marketing. FDA regulation of medical devices balances two competing goals: [1] promoting innovation and improvement in medical devices; and [2] ensuring that medical devices are safe and effective [49]. Accordingly, FDA classifies medical devices according to potential risk. Class I devices are low risk and subject to general controls, and examples include bandages and sunglasses. Class II devices are intermediate risk and are often approved subject to the abbreviated 510(k) pathway, if the devices are able to rely on the prior approval of a similar device. Examples include pregnancy test kits, hearing aids, and powered wheelchairs. Class III devices require a premarket approval application (PMA) and are subject to full FDA review of safety and efficacy. Only 10% of medical devices fall in this category, and examples include implantable pacemakers, and high-frequency ventilators.

FDA has historically struggled to fit medical software and apps into the traditional medical device classification. In recent years, however, FDA has issued more detailed guidance informing app developers when digital health products will need to undergo regulatory review, and the requirements for regulatory approval [50]. FDA takes a risk-based approach to medical software and app regulation, focusing on devices that could pose a risk to a patient's safety if the device were not to function as intended. For example, software functions that transform the mobile platform into a regulated medical device by using attachments, display screens, or sensors—such as motion tracking sensors or EKG functionality—will be subject to regulation as a medical device [51]. Apps that perform patient-specific analysis and provide patient-specific diagnosis, or treatment recommendations, such as image-processing software and radiation therapy treatment planning software, will also be subject to close regulatory scrutiny. On the other hand, FDA intends to exercise its discretion not to enforce regulations for lower risk apps that automate simple tasks for health care providers or help patients self-manage their disease without providing specific treatment suggestions. For example, FDA will not enforce its regulations on software functions that provide physicians easy access to the latest treatment guidelines, or software that coaches patients on the basics of conditions such as obesity or arthritis and provide strategies for weight reduction. Indeed, most digital health apps are not reviewed and cleared by FDA. In November 2013, only 100 of over 10,000 medical apps available on the marketplace were cleared by FDA [52].

To evaluate the clinical effectiveness and safety of software as a medical device, FDA will assess the following questions: [1] Is there a valid clinical association between the software output and the targeted clinical condition?; [2] Does the software correctly process input data to generate accurate, reliable, and precise output data?; and [3] Does use of the software's accurate, reliable, and precise output data achieve the intended purpose in the target population in the context of clinical care? [53]

Because medical-grade digital health solutions intended to diagnose, treat, or prevent a medical condition are subject to FDA scrutiny, the stamp of FDA approval is an important designation on which clinicians and organizations can rely in deciding whether to recommend or adopt digital health solutions. Conversely, lower risk consumer facing apps that do not make treatment recommendations are not subject to FDA enforcement. Thus, clinicians can use these principles, considering patient preferences, in recommending digital health apps to their patients.

6. Conclusion

Consumer driven health care is here to stay, and the digital health landscape is rapidly evolving to become increasingly consumer facing [54]. Payors are increasingly reimbursing for digital health solutions, especially medical apps that have proven effectiveness and that have obtained FDA approval. However, the functionality and clinical effectiveness of musculoskeletal digital health solutions varies widely. It is thus essential for healthcare providers to assess the available evidence supporting effectiveness claims in digital apps. By understanding the MDA landscape, healthcare providers can leverage digital health tools to provide optimal clinical care to individual patients, and to help manage and prevent musculoskeletal injuries on an organizational scale.

Author details

Glen Cheng[1]*, Nischal Chennuru[2] and Liz Kwo[1]

1 Harvard Medical School, Boston, MA, United States

2 Columbus Academy, Columbus, OH, United States

*Address all correspondence to: glenccheng@gmail.com

References

[1] Home - Mobius MD. Mobius. Md. https://www.mobius.md/blog/2019/03/11-mobile-health-statistics. Accessed September 5, 2020.

[2] Mearian L. Smartphones becoming primary device for physician and patient communications. Computerworld.com. https://www.computerworld.com/article/3268055. Published April 4, 2018. Accessed September 5, 2020.

[3] The rise of mHealth apps: A market snapshot - liquid state. Liquid-state.com. https://liquid-state.com/mhealth-apps-market-snapshot/. Published March 26, 2018. Accessed September 5, 2020.

[4] The digital healthcare timeline :: A heritage partners - RSA group project. Digitalhealthcaretimeline.com. http://Digitalhealthcaretimeline.com. Accessed September 5, 2020.

[5] Am. Med. Assoc., Why physicians' use of digital health is on the rise, February 2020, https://www.ama-assn.org/practice-management/digital/why-physicians-use-digital-health-rise

[6] McDonald K. Telehealth in the time of coronavirus. 2020. https://www.pulseitmagazine.com.au/blog/5399-telehealth-in-the-time-of-coronavirus. Retrieved Apr 28, 2020.

[7] Reuter E. CMS shares specifics on sweeping Medicare telehealth expansion. March 17, 2020. https://medcitynews.com/2020/03/cms-shares-specifics-on-sweeping-medicare-telehealth-expansion/?rf=1. Retrieved Oct. 25, 2020.

[8] Bestsennyy O, Gilbert G, Harris A, Rost J. Telehealth: A quarter-trillion-dollar post-COVID-19 reality? Mckinsey.com. https://www.mckinsey.com/industries/healthcare-systems-and-services/our-insights/telehealth-a-quarter-trillion-dollar-post-covid-19-reality. Published May 28, 2020. Accessed September 5, 2020.

[9] Adapted from List of Corporate Musculoskeletal Programs | top 15 Ergonomics in the Workplace Jul. '20. Myshortlister.com. https://www.myshortlister.com/corporate-musculoskeletal-programs/vendor-list. Accessed September 5, 2020.

[10] 2017 - D Magazine. Dmagazine.com. https://www.dmagazine.com/publications/d-ceo/2017/... Accessed September 5, 2020.

[11] Musculoskeletal health: A real pain in the back | virgin pulse. Virginpulse.com. https://www.virginpulse.com/blog-post/musculoskeletal-health-improve-lower-back-pain/. Published November 27, 2019. Accessed September 5, 2020.

[12] National Health Interview Survey (NHIS), www.cdc.gov/nchs/nhis/nhis_2012_data_release.htm

[13] Nih.gov. https://www.ncbi.nlm.nih.gov/pmc/articles/PMC4562413. Accessed September 5, 2020.

[14] The Cost of Musculoskeletal Disorders (MSDs) [Infographic]. Ergo-plus.com. https://ergo-plus.com/cost-of-musculoskeletal-disorders-infographic. Published July 24, 2015. Accessed September 5, 2020.

[15] Okifuji A, Hare BD. The association between chronic pain and obesity. *J Pain Res*. 2015;8:399-408.

[16] Obesity Symptoms, Complications and Comorbidities. Healthcentral.com. http://www.healthcentral.com/condition/complications-of-obesity. Accessed September 5, 2020.

[17] Ashaye T, Opioid prescribing for chronic musculoskeletal pain in UK

primary care: results from a cohort analysis of the COPERS trial, BMJ Open. 2018 Jun 6;8(6):e019491. doi: 10.1136/bmjopen-2017-019491.

[18] Wang DT et al., Complications in Musculoskeletal Intervention: Important Considerations, Semin Intervent Radiol. 2015 Jun; 32(2): 163-173.

[19] Mdedge.com. https://www.mdedge.com/.../musculoskeletal-procedures-predominate-top-20. Accessed September 5, 2020.

[20] Klokkari D, Mamais I. Effectiveness of surgical versus conservative treatment for carpal tunnel syndrome: A systematic review, meta-analysis and qualitative analysis. *Hong Kong Physiother J*. 2018;38(2):91-114.

[21] Statistical Brief #171. Healthcare Cost and Utilization Project (HCUP). January 2014. Agency for Healthcare Research and Quality, Rockville, MD. www.hcup-uss.ahrq.gov/reports/statbriefs/sb171-Operation-Room-Procedure-Trends.jsp

[22] Future Young Patient Demand for Primary and Revision Joint Replacement: National Projections from 2010 to 2030, Kurtz et al.

[23] The Global Market for Spine Surgery Products – Forecast to 2024 (published September 2018).

[24] “Acne Cure” mobile app marketers will drop baseless claims under FTC settlements [Internet]. Washington (DC): Federal Trade Commission; 2011 Sept 8 [cited 2014 Jan 28]. http://www.ftc.gov/news-events/press-releases/2011/09/acne-curemobile-app-marketers-will-drop-baseless-claims-under.

[25] HONcode [Internet]. Switzerland: Health on the Net Foundation; [updated 2013 Jun 13; cited 2014 Jan 28]. http://www.hon.ch/HONcode/Pro/Visitor/visitor.html

[26] Assessing the quality of Internet health information: summary [Internet]. Rockville, MD: Agency for Healthcare Research and Quality; 1999 June [cited 2014 Jan 28]. http://www.ahrq.gov/research/data/infoqual.html.

[27] Conor Hanrahan et al., Evaluating Mobile Medical Applications, American Society of Health-System Pharmacists eReports (2014).

[28] World Health Organization, Monitoring and Evaluating Digital Health Interventions (2016).

[29] Califf RM, Hernandez AF, Landray M. Weighing the Benefits and Risks of Proliferating Observational Treatment Assessments: Observational Cacophony, Randomized Harmony. JAMA. Published online July 31, 2020. doi:10.1001/jama.2020.13319.

[30] Gordis L. Epidemiology, fifth edition. Elsevier; 2014 (http://store.elsevier.com/Epidemiology/Leon-Gordis/isbn-9781455737338/, accessed 29 April 2016).

[31] Pundi K, PerinoAC,HarringtonRA,KrumholzHM, Turakhia MP. Characteristics and Strength of Evidence of COVID-19 Studies Registered on ClinicalTrials.gov. JAMA Intern Med. Published online July 27, 2020. doi:10.1001/jamainternmed.2020.2904.

[32] The Cochrane Collaboration, Cochrane Handbook for Systematic Reviews of Interventions, Version 6 (2019), https://training.cochrane.org/handbook/current.

[33] TrackActive Pro - exercise prescription software with outcome measures. Trackactive.co. https://www.trackactive.co. Accessed September 5, 2020.

[34] Bestsennyy O, Gilbert G, Harris A, Rost J. Telehealth: A quarter-trillion-dollar post-COVID-19 reality? Mckinsey.com. https://www.mckinsey.com/industries/healthcare-systems-and-services/our-insights/telehealth-a-quarter-trillion-dollar-post-covid-19-reality. Published May 28, 2020. Accessed September 5, 2020.

[35] Prevention weekly from ergonomics plus, issue 242 | ErgoPlus. Ergo-plus.com. https://ergo-plus.com/prevention-weekly-242. Published May 13, 2016. Accessed September 5, 2020.

[36] Researchgate.net. https://www.researchgate.net/publication/223872444_Occupatiou_risks_factors. Accessed September 5, 2020.

[37] Kravitz RL, Schmid CH, Marois M, et al. Effect of Mobile Device–Supported Single-Patient Multi-crossover Trials on Treatment of Chronic Musculoskeletal Pain: A Randomized Clinical Trial. JAMA Intern Med. 2018;178(10):1368-1377. doi:10.1001/jamainternmed.2018.3981.

[38] Lalloo C, Shah U, Birnie KA, et al. Commercially available smartphone apps to support postoperative pain self-management: Scoping review. *JMIR MHealth UHealth*. 2017;5(10):e162.0/

[39] Cottrell MA, Russell TG. Telehealth for musculoskeletal physiotherapy. Musculoskelet Sci Pract. 2020;48:102193. doi:10.1016/j.msksp.2020.102193.

[40] Mecklenburg G, Smittenaar P, Erhart-Hledik JC, Perez DA, Hunter S, Effects of a 12-Week Digital Care Program for Chronic Knee Pain on Pain, Mobility, and Surgery Risk: Randomized Controlled Trial. J Med Internet Res. 2018 Apr 25; 20(4):e156.

[41] Shebib R, Bailey JF, Smittenaar P, Perez DA, Mecklenburg G, Hunter S, Randomized controlled trial of a 12-week digital care program in improving low back pain. NPJ Digit Med. 2019; 2():1.

[42] Bailey JF, Agarwal V, Zheng P, et al. Digital Care for Chronic Musculoskeletal Pain: 10,000 Participant Longitudinal Cohort Study. J Med Internet Res. 2020;22(5):e18250. Published 2020 May 11. doi:10.2196/18250.

[43] Whitelaw S, Mamas MA, Topol E, Van Spall HGC. Applications of digital technology in COVID-19 pandemic planning and response. Lancet Digit Health. 2020;2(8):e435-e440. doi:10.1016/S2589-7500(20)30142-4.

[44] COVID-19 is clearly demonstrating how digital health solutions, like TrackActive, can make a difference | gen re. Genre.com. https://www.genre.com/knowledge/blog/covid-19-is-clearly-demonstrating-how-digital-health-solutions-like-trackactive-can-make-a-difference-en.html. Accessed September 5, 2020.

[45] Levine DM, Co Z, Newmark LP, et al. Design and testing of a mobile health application rating tool. *NPJ Digit Med*. 2020;3(1):74.

[46] AIS, COVID-19 RESOURCES. AIS COVID-19. Aischannel.com. https://covid19.aischannel.com/featured/posts/... Accessed September 5, 2020.

[47] Plato Data Intelligence, Plato Vertical Search. Zephyrnet.com. https://zephyrnet.com/teladoc-and-livongo-merge. Accessed September 5, 2020.

[48] National Business Group on Health, 2019 Large Employers' Health Care Strategy and Plan Design Survey.

[49] Xirui Zhang et al., The Interplay Between the FDA Regulatory Process for Medical Devices and Patent Law – FDA Premarket Review of Medical

Devices, Finnegan IP FDA Blog, https://www.finnegan.com/en/insights/blogs/ip-fda-blog/the-interplay-between-the-fda-regulatory-process-for-medical-devices-and-patent-law-fda-premarket-review-of-medical-devices.html

[50] FDA, Digital Health Guidance, https://www.fda.gov/medical-devices/digital-health/guidances-digital-health-content

[51] FDA, Policy for Device Software Functions and Mobile Medical Applications, Guidance for Industry and FDA Staff (Sept. 27, 2019).

[52] Dolan B. Analysis: 103 FDA regulated mobile medical apps [Internet]. MobiHealthNews; 2013 Nov 26 [cited 2014 Jan 28]. http://mobihealthnews.com/27645/analysis-103-fda-regulated-mobile-medical-apps/.

[53] FDA, Software as a Medical Device: Clinical Evaluation, Guidance for Industry and FDA Staff (Dec. 8, 2017).

[54] David Rook, The Pros and Cons of Consumer-Driven Healthcare (Nov. 6, 2015), https://www.griffinbenefits.com/blog/consumer-driven-healthcare-cdhc-cdhp

Chapter 3

Particulate Matter and Human Health

Karuna Singh and Dhananjay Tripathi

Abstract

This chapter provides an introduction to particulate matter by discussing various ways of categorisation, characterisation and their health effects. The natural and anthropogenic sources of atmospheric particulate matter are discussed. The chapter also introduces qualitatively some aerosol concepts, such as their chemical composition and size distribution. Some examples are provided to illustrate how particulate matter, despite being microscopic particles, can manifest themselves in the atmosphere. Finally, the various pathways by which particulate matter impacts the health system are reviewed along with their interactions to understand concept behind the PM-associated health effects.

Keywords: Aerosol, PM, Health effects, Chemical constituents, Heavy metals

1. Introduction

Air pollution has become a major environmental and health concern worldwide. Even though, the effect of air pollution has been recognised since classical times yet the studies correlating human health and air pollution came into existence in near twentieth century. According to WHO, air pollution refers to contamination/or changes in the natural environment by physical, chemical or biological agent (pollutants), which may be contributed by natural or anthropogenic sources. In reality, some of these pollutants are naturally present but are of least concern because of their lower levels. Once, their level cross prescribed levels they are harmful for humans including other living organisms and natural environment. National Ambient Air Quality Standards (NAAQS), sets limits for six criteria air pollutants viz. carbon monoxide (CO), lead (Pb), nitrogen dioxide (NO_2), ozone (O_3), particulate matter (PM) and sulphur dioxide (SO_2).

Particulate matter refers to a complex mixture of solid particles and liquid droplets (EPA). In general, they may vary in size and composition depending upon its location and time of its source e.g., PM emitted from mining activities will have metal contaminants associated with them whereas sea aerosols will mainly contain organic contaminants. Depending on these it might contain nitrates, sulphates, elemental and organic carbon, organic compounds (PAH), biological compounds (endotoxin, cell fragments) and heavy metals (Fe, Ca, Ni, Zn etc.). PM are becoming increasingly ubiquitous but the disease burden related to PM pollution is quite high in low- or middle-income nations as compared to developed countries. According to WHO every nine out of ten people breathe polluted air worldwide. The State of Global Air Report in 2020 reported that more than 90% of the world's population were exposed to $PM_{2.5}$ level that exceeds WHO guideline limits, with

IntechOpen

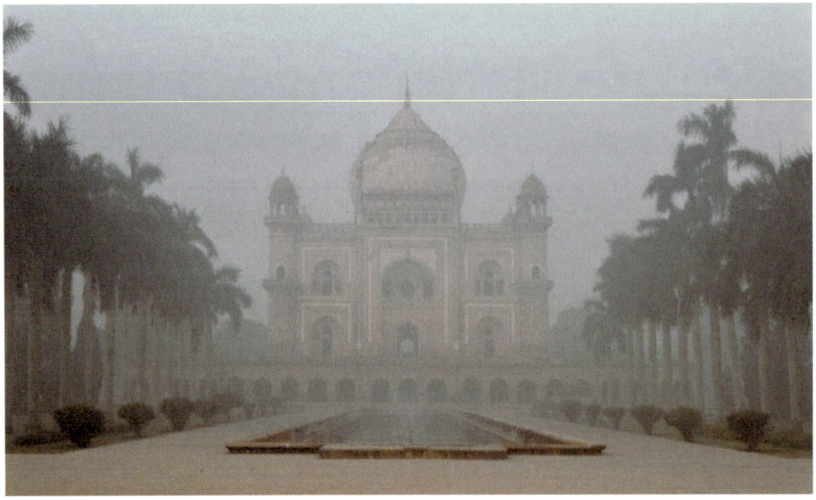

Figure 1.
Dust event at Safdarjung Tomb Delhi, India (Image Courtesy: Shubham).

developing countries more at risk. Also, studies on particulate matter exposure have explained the various health associated problems including heart attacks, asthma, decreased lung capacity, respiratory symptoms such as irritation of airways, difficulty in breathing and premature death (**Figure 1**) [1–4].

The size of PM can be related to their sources, due to the physical processes that form these particles and the atmospheric processes that control the fate and evolution of particle size distributions in the ambient atmosphere. PM_{10} (particles with aerodynamic diameters less than or equal to 10 μm) is generated largely by physical processes, including resuspension of soil and road dust, sea spray, agricultural tilling, vehicular abrasion (i.e. tyre and brake wear), and fugitive dust emission from industrial sources (**Figure 1**). $PM_{2.5}$ (particles with aerodynamic diameters less than or equal to 2.5 μm) comprise predominantly the condensation of secondary inorganic and organic compounds and $PM_{0.1}$ (particles with aerodynamic diameters less than or equal to 0.1 μm) particles comprise predominantly secondary sulphate and bisulphate ion, secondary nitrate ion, secondary ammonium ion, and carbonaceous PM from primary and secondary sources, but also include some crustal materials. The origin of $PM_{0.1}$ is attributed to combustion sources and atmospheric nucleation. They have short atmospheric lifespan as they grow to form accumulation particles. They get enriched in carbonaceous aerosols and metals from combustion of oil and other fuel, also from high temperature processing of metals. However, smaller particles can affect and damage the body organs to the greater extent; although the impact is variable depending upon the concentration and composition of particulate matter. For example, heavy metals like lead, arsenic and cadmium are well known to cause toxicity in the human body, whereas sulphur aerosols which form sulphuric acid are corrosive and can damage the tissues; PAHs are potent carcinogens and can cause cancer (**Table 1**).

1.1 Air quality standards

Air pollution levels in most of the urban areas have been a matter of concern. To improve air quality, WHO is working with different countries to understand the problem related with air pollution. It has revised guidelines for key air pollutants in the ambient environment: particulate matter, nitrogen dioxide, sulphur dioxide,

Category	Size range (μm)	Respiratory system permeability
Smog/Atmospheric dust/Tobacco smoke	0.01–1	Alveolar penetration/ Bronchial penetration
Fly ash/cement dust	1–100	Nostril to Bronchial area
Pollen/Household dust	0.1–100	Nostril to Alveolar area
Bacteria/Bacterial spores	0.7–10	From larynx to bronchial area
Viruses	0.01–1	Alveolar penetration/ Bronchial penetration

Table 1.
Particulate matter (PM); size attribution and penetration to human respiratory system [5–7].

Sl no.	Pollutant	Time weighted average	Ambient air quality standards for the European Union	Guideline values prescribed by WHO (2005)
1	Particulate matter (size less than 10 μm) μg/m^3	Annual Avg	40	20
		24 hours	50	50
2	Particulate matter (size less than 2.5 μm) μg/m^3	Annual Avg	25	10
		24 hours	—	25
3	Sulphur Dioxide(SO2) μg/m^3	24 hours	125	20
4	Oxides of Nitrogen as NO2 μg/m^3	Annual Avg	40	40
		hours	200	200
5	Ozone μg/m^3	8 hours	120	100

Table 2.
Air quality standards.

carbon monoxide and ozone. The concentration limits for these air pollutants along with prescribed European Union Ambient Air Quality Standards are given in **Table 2**.

2. PM: sources and classification

Depending on their origin, aerosols may be natural or anthropogenic. The main sources of anthropogenic particulate matter in the atmosphere lie in urban and industrial areas, e.g., vehicular exhaust emission, wear and tear mechanism on roadways, industrial emissions, construction sites and household emissions. On the other hand, main source of particulate matter in rural areas is dominated by agricultural activities and biomass burning.

Aerosol sources are classified into primary and secondary types on the basis of their origin. Primary particulate matter are those emitted into the atmosphere directly, whereas secondary particulate matter are formed in the atmosphere from pre-existing precursors. Thus it is clear that sea salt, mineral dust and soot particles are primary particulate matter, whereas organic particles formed from the oxidation of volatile organic compound and sulphates from the oxidation of SO_2 or other sulphur containing gases are secondary particulate matter. It is also noted that there is distinct zone, called as "grey zone" between primary and secondary particulate matter formed in case of some low volatile organic compounds that

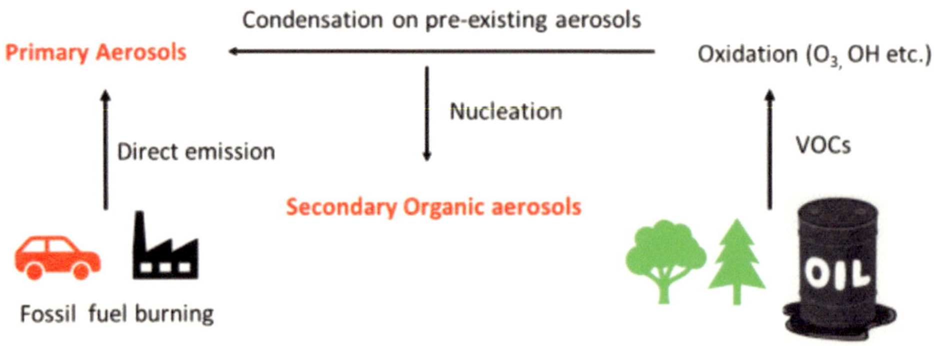

Figure 2.
Sources and formation process of PM.

condense onto particulate matter but not directly within emitting sources, such as some hydrocarbons in vehicular exhaust. In general, secondary particulate matter formation involves chemical transformation from volatile precursors (**Figure 2**) [8].

2.1 Primary natural sources of PM

Significant natural sources of primary particulate matter are dominating in nature due to the mass emissions of sea salt, which is the biggest contributor [7, 8]. Other natural sources of primary particulate matter is soil dust or rock debris generated through physical action, emission of smoke from biomass burning and debris from volcanic eruptions. Primary biogenic PM consists of pollen, spores and plant waxes.

2.2 Secondary natural sources of PM

Major source of natural secondary particulate matter are sulphates and nitrates. They are formed in atmosphere due to gas to particle conversion processes. The major chemical species responsible for this conversion process, involving the natural gaseous compound are nitrogen, sulphur, carbonaceous and organic molecules. Although, various organic substances derived from plants can add larger contribution to the total PM mass. The major generation of particulate matter occurs via condensation of sulphates and nitrogen containing gases. The amount of particulate matter generated by gas to particle conversion process is usually same as PM generated through direct emission of natural particulate matter and greater amount of PM is generated via this process in comparison to direct emission from anthropogenic action [9].

2.3 Primary anthropogenic sources of PM

A significant amount of atmospheric PM is contributed through the anthropogenic activities. It consists of both primary and secondary particulate matter. The primary particulate matter are sourced mainly from the fossil fuel burning, industrial activities, transportation activities and other nonindustrial activities. These particulate matter contains sulphate, nitrate, ammonium, trace elements, carbonaceous matter and water vapour. The carbonaceous portion of this particulate matter consists of elemental carbon and organic carbon and sourced from the combustion process and from condensation process.

2.4 Secondary anthropogenic sources of PM

Secondary anthropogenic PM is formed in the atmosphere by the chemical reactions of gaseous precursors such as sulphur dioxide, nitrogen oxides and ammonia during the transport process. During night, primary oxides of sulphur and nitrogen may get converted to secondary PM in the presence of nitrate radicals. Their origin and growth occur from pre-existing particles, that may grow via matter condensation and thereby leading to new particles formation through homogeneous nucleation. These processes regulate the mass transfer from the gas phase to the particulate phase which is being controlled by sulphur, nitrogen or organic and carbonaceous species.

3. Chemical constituents of PM

3.1 Sulphur containing species

The most sulphate particles in atmosphere are secondary and formed through nucleation and condensation processes due to the oxidation of its gaseous precursor (sulphur dioxide and dimethyl sulphide). Major portion of sulphate particles are contributed by emission from combustion process and found to be in the size range of 0.1 μm to 2 μm. The formation of sulphate are attributed to several mechanisms such as liquid-phase reactions within cloud droplets or oxidation of sulphur dioxide with hydroxide in gaseous phase reactions [10]. SO_2 is emitted to the atmosphere from both anthropogenic and natural sources, although it has been estimated that more than 70% of SO_2 global emissions are released by anthropogenic sources [11], and fossil fuel combustion is responsible for the majority of these emissions. Other SO_2 sources are biomass burning, shipping, metal smelting, agricultural waste burning, pulp and paper processing, and a modest volcanic source [12, 13]. While considering the historic point of view, sulphur dioxide emission from anthropogenic sources have soared from approximately 7.2 fold from 1890 to 2000 [14]. Anthropogenic emission of sulphur dioxide was maximum in early 1970s and decreased until 2000. However, there has been rapid increase in their emissions due to the developmental activities in the under-developed countries [12, 15, 16]. Study indicates the growing importance of international transport as a major factor in the increase of sulphur dioxide emissions [13].

3.2 Nitrogen containing species

As in the case of sulphates, nitrogen compounds are mainly of secondary origin and mainly arise from the reaction of natural and anthropogenic gaseous precursors. These aerosols generally have diameters smaller than 2.5 μm [17, 18]. Nitrate ion and ammonium ion are the two main nitrogen containing compounds in particulate matter. The major precursor gases released by natural and anthropogenic activities are NO, NO_2, N_2O and NH_3. Moreover, nitric acid is the main product generated by oxidation in the atmosphere.

The major anthropogenic addition of secondary nitrate precursor gases is mainly due to power generation and other combustion processes producing high temperature, such as those occurring in the vehicular motors and in biomass burning [19]. On the other hand, agricultural activities such as land fertilising are the main source of atmospheric NH_3, although it is emitted by other sources as well, including waste collection, vehicles and a number of production processes [20]. Natural nitrogen compounds come mainly from soil emissions (nitrification, N_2O), wildfires (NO_2, NO), electrical discharges (NO) and biogenic emissions (NH_3).

The production of secondary nitrate is heavily dependent on the amount of gaseous NH_3 and HNO_3 and of particulate SO_4, as well as on temperature and humidity [21]. Homogeneous (gas-phase reaction of NO_2 + OH) and heterogeneous (hydrolysis of N_2O_5 on aerosol surfaces) reactions are involved in the formation of nitric acid during the daytime and night time, respectively. In normal conditions, the gaseous nitric acid dissolved in liquid microparticles reacts with the ammonia in the atmosphere forming particulate ammonium nitrate [22]. Sometimes larger particles of sodium nitrate and calcium carbonate are formed due to high concentration of sodium and calcium ion, sourced from sea salt and mineral dust and due to acidic environment. These particles are larger than the particles of ammonium nitrate [23].

3.3 Carbonaceous particles

Carbonaceous particle are in a significant fraction of atmospheric particulate matter and constitutes a wide range of compounds. It has been estimated that carbonaceous fraction contributes 20–50% of the $PM_{2.5}$ mass fraction in urban and rural areas depending on source and 70% of the PM_1 mass fraction [24, 25]. The carbon fraction of particulate matter could be categorised into three main groups: carbonates, organic carbon and elemental carbon or black carbon.

The carbon found in the form of carbonates (mainly $CaCO_3$ and $MgCO_3$) occurs usually as super micrometric particles resuspended from the ground. This fraction is neglected because of the size and also, there is no straight forward technique for determining it (it is usually identified by acidifying the sample and determining CO_2). Organic carbon constitutes the non-absorptive fraction of the carbonaceous particles that may be of either primary or secondary origin. Sources of organic carbon are not well known, especially those formed by secondary atmospheric processes [26]. Studies related to the organic carbon formation have suggested that a significant fraction is formed by water soluble compounds. This is a crucial finding as it may responsible for the radiative balance of the atmosphere and influence the hydrological cycle [27]. Black carbon is the most refractory and polymerised part of the particulate matter, is generated mainly by fossil-fuel combustion and biomass burning [28]. Black carbon particles have diameter in the range of 10–100 nm and the mass ratio (H/C) of around 0.1 [29]. Black carbon fraction contributes less to overall particulate matter but absorbs incoming and outgoing radiation very actively [30, 31].

3.4 Elemental components

The main elemental components associated with PM are described in accordance of particle sizes measured. For $PM_{2.5}$ and PM_1 there are many components that are

Composition	Particulate matter diameter range (μm)		
	10–2.5	2.5–1.0	< 1.0
Elemental Components	Na, Mg, Al, Si, S, Cl, K, Ca, Fe, Zn, Pb, Cr, V, Ni, Cu,	Na, Mg, Al, Si, S, Cl, K, Ca, Fe, Zn, Pb, Cr, V, Ni, Cu,	Na, Mg, Al, Si, S, Cl, K, Ca, Fe, Zn, Pb, Cr, V, Ni, Cu,
Ionic Components	Cl^-, NO_3^-, SO_4^{--}, Na^+, K^+, Ca^{++}	NO_3^-, SO_4^{--}, NH_4^+, Na^+, K^+, Ca^{++}	Cl^-, NO_3^-, NO_2^- SO_4^{--}, NH_4^+
Origin	Terrestrial and sea salt	Secondary generated particles	Secondary generated particles

Table 3.
Size-resolved elemental composition of particulate matter [32–34].

thought to contain secondary generated particles. There are several elements that are identified by researchers [32–34] based on locations and it is considered that the atmospheric PM elemental compositions are source based, **Table 3** (viz. Na, Mg, Al, Si, P, S, Cl, K, Ca, Ti, Cr, Mn, Fe, Co, Ni, Cu, Zn, Cd, Se, Br, As, Rb, Sr., Y, Nb, Mo, Hg, Pb etc.). Also, it is noted that hydrogen ion is obviously included in PM components.

4. PM associated human health

4.1 Health impacts resulting from PM and its constituents

Growing number of studies in the last few years provided evidence linking disease and adverse effects to extremely low levels of PM and its toxic components. Many components for instance organics such as PAHs, inorganics such as heavy metals are known carcinogens and are responsible for numerous adverse health effects in humans. Apart from this, exposure to PM has been linked to increased hospital admissions, carcinogenicity, developmental disorders, nervous system effects, respiratory symptoms, cardiovascular diseases, decreased lung function and premature mortality [35–40]. Recent finding showed the presence of nanoparticles on the foetal side of the placenta indicating that the placenta barrier can be easily penetrated by the PM resulting in exposure to foetus [41]. This indicates that the extent of toxicity of PM is not only limited to the adults but also to the foetus as well. Moreover, long term exposure to PM pollution renders a population more vulnerable to COVID-19, increased hospitalisations of patients with predisposed asthma or other respiratory ailments were also reported. Hence, the impact and toxicity of PM and its components depend on various factors

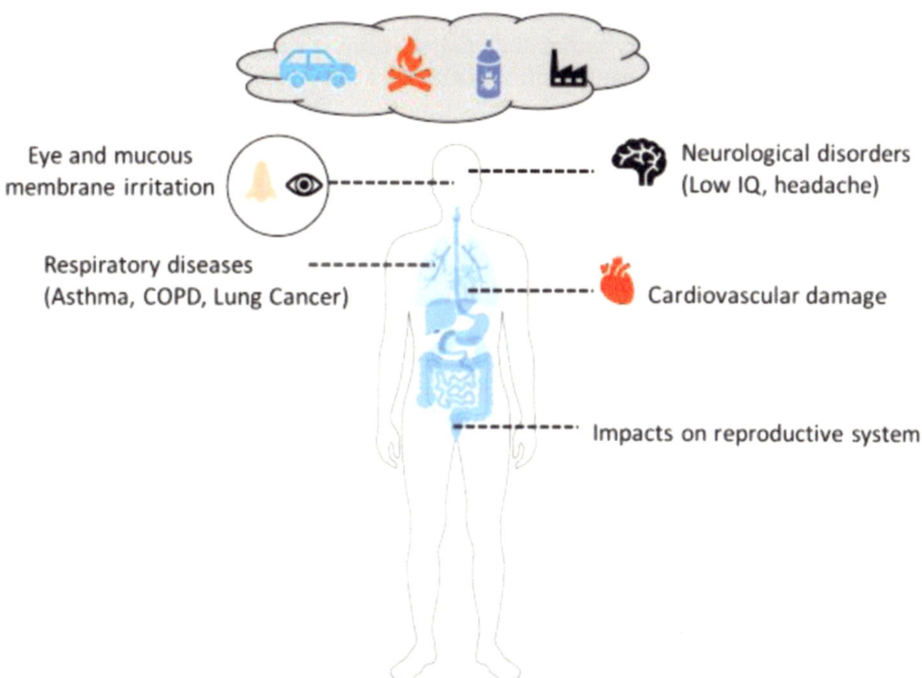

Figure 3.
PM and human health impacts.

Components	Health effects
Heavy metals	Respiratory infections, Neurological effects, Carcinogenicity, Renal disorders
PAH	Decreased immune function, carcinogenic effects, lung function abnormalities

Table 4.
PM component and its health effect.

including their solubility in water, residence time, elemental composition, particle size and chemical reactivity; local environmental conditions- season, wind speed, topography etc.

At present, research studies based on population data do not provide enough evidence to identify differences in the effects of particulate matter with different chemical constituents [37]. However it should be noted that the evidence for hazardous nature of particulate matter generated through the combustion process, from mobile and stationary sources, are more consistent than that from other sources [38]. The black carbon fraction of $PM_{2.5}$ that is resulted from incomplete combustion has great concern towards their contribution to detrimental effects on human health as well as on climate. Other constituents of particulate matter attached to black carbon are seen as responsible for various health effects, such as PAHs that are well known carcinogens and toxic to the cells, also metals and inorganic salts. It has to be noted that diesel engines exhaust, consisting mostly particulate matter, has been classified as carcinogen (Group 1) to humans by the International Agency for Research on Cancer [39]. This also includes some PAHs as well as some solid fuels used in household (**Figure 3** and **Table 4**) [40, 42].

4.2 Respiratory effects

Respiratory system is mainly affected by all types of air pollutants. High levels of sulphur dioxide, nitrogen oxides and ozone are linked to symptoms such as nose and throat irritation, cough, chest discomfort due to narrowing of airways, increased mucous production on the walls of upper airways following which inflammatory reactions may occur leading to asthma and more severe condition COPD [42, 43]. People with respiratory ailments are more sensitive to air pollution exposure.

The human health risks of PM are attributed to their deposition and transportation in the human body. The particles are deposited in the lungs by the process of impaction, interception, sedimentation and diffusion. In general, larger PM fractions (> $PM_{2.5}$) are mostly deposited in the upper respiratory tract by means of impaction. Smaller size PM (< $PM_{2.5}$) can deposit deeper into the lower airways and alveoli depending on the flow rates and diffusion, and may be transported to other tissues and organs via bloodstream. Several studies have also provided the evidence that exposure to smaller particles can result in serious health effects. Although, the impact is variable depending upon the composition (heavy metals, PAHs act as carcinogens), concentration and duration of exposure to the particles. Exposures to PM bound heavy metals (arsenic, nickel, lead etc.) are responsible for asthma, emphysema and even lung cancer [44].

Although in vitro studies on human health due to PM pollution are numerous, there are relatively few that focus on the epidemiological aspects. Studies are scarce regarding investigation focusing on the mechanism of PM toxicity at cellular and molecular levels (**Figure 4**).

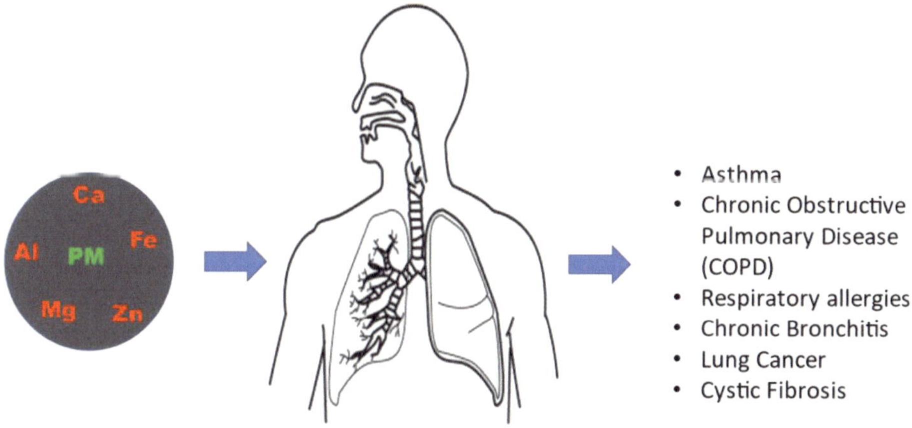

Figure 4.
PM and associated respiratory effects.

4.3 Cardiovascular effects

In recent studies, multiple cardiovascular effects have been documented due to the exposure of air pollutants. According to Global Burden of Disease report, 2018 air pollution was responsible for 19% of cardiovascular deaths in 2015. It was also the cause of about 21% of deaths due to stroke and 24% of deaths from coronary heart disease.

Carbon monoxide has high affinity for haemoglobin and thus it displaces the oxygen and binds with haemoglobin to form carboxyhaemoglobin. It is a stable compound which cannot bind and deliver oxygen to tissues leading to tissue hypoxia (decrease oxygen carrying capacity). Increased risks of ischemic heart disease and myocardial infarction have been demonstrated among occupational groups exposed to gaseous emissions whereas short term exposure studies have reported changes in vasomotor function among healthy individuals as well as increase in prothrombogenic effects. Increased hospital admissions due to myocardial infarctions, increased congestive heart failure among the elderly population as a result of elevated PM concentration were also reported. Long term exposure to traffic emissions have been linked to coronary arteriosclerosis while, short term exposure is related to hypertension, stroke, myocardial infarctions and heart abnormalities [44, 45]. In vitro studies in experimental animals exposed to PM results in systematic inflammation and oxidative stress in the cardiovascular system and may enhance the progression of atherosclerosis in animals predisposed to this disease. In addition to this, chronic exposure to nitrogen oxide may result in ventricle hypertrophy [45].

4.4 Neurological effects

Exposure to heavy metals (e.g., lead, mercury) and dioxins have been corelated with several neurological effects in humans. Lead exposure occurs through inhalation, ingestion and dermal absorption. Conditions such as neurological damage (mimics Ca and disrupts Ca homeostasis), lower IQ and attention impairment of hand-eye co-ordination and encephalopathy has been associated with chronic exposure of lead [40]. It is well recognised teratogen can easily pass through placenta and can cross blood–brain barrier. Therefore, it can cause more harm to the foetus. Mercury (methyl mercury) is another heavy metal that effects the nervous system. Organic mercury is fat soluble and can be distributed in the central nervous system where it is oxidised to Hg^{2+} and causes neurological damage. Symptoms include

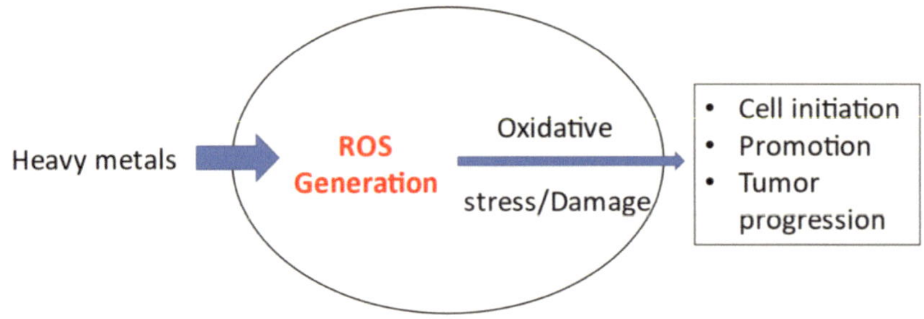

Figure 5.
Mechanism of toxicity of PM bound heavy metals.

memory loss, narrowing of vision, loss of muscle coordination and emotional instability [46].

4.5 Carcinogenicity

Presence of heavy metals, dioxins etc. have detrimental effect as they bioaccumulate and interfere with the normal functioning of the cell [40, 47]. Chemically, metals in their ionic form are more reactive and can interact with biological systems in different ways such as cadmium and mercury can readily attach to sulphur in proteins. Apart from this, they are known to mimic and replace essential metals, for instance cadmium can replace zinc and arsenic mimics phosphate. Furthermore, they are known to induce oxidative stress, producing oxidative modification of biomolecules; which might be a key step in the initiation of cancer cells (**Figure 5**) [47].

5. Conclusions

Particulate matter being the contributor for human health burden poses a major challenge globally. For comprehensive understanding and involved process and their interactions requires continuous investigation. The broad range study associated with atmospheric aerosols requires that integrate approaches be used for their investigation. As the impacts are high in developing countries as compared to developed nations where major cities are under development that poses major pollution burden. However, policies governing the same should be more stringent to control the menace of pollution burden.

Author details

Karuna Singh[1] and Dhananjay Tripathi[2*]

1 Department of Mining Engineering, NIT, Rourkela, India

2 Division of CBRN Defense, Institute of Nuclear Medicine and Allied Sciences, Delhi, India

*Address all correspondence to: dhatripathi@gmail.com

References

[1] Atkinson RW, Fuller GW, Anderson HR, Harrison RM, Armstrong B. Urban ambient particle metrics and health. A time series analysis. Epidemiology 2010;21:501-511.

[2] Meister K, Johansson C, Forsberg B. Estimated short-term effects of coarse particles on daily mortality in Stockholm, Sweden. Environ Health Perspect 2012;120:431-436

[3] Correia AW, Pope III CA, Dockery DW,Wang Y, Ezzati M, Dominici F. The effect of air pollution control on life expectancy in the United States: an analysis of 545 us counties for the period 2000 to 2007. Epidemiology 2013;24(1):23-31.

[4] Cadelis G, Tourres R, Molinie J. Short-term effects of the particulate pollutants contained in Saharan dust on the visits of children to the emergency department due to asthmatic conditions in Guadeloupe (French Archipelago of the Caribbean). PLoS ONE 2014;9(3): e91136.

[5] Kelishadi R, Poursafa P. Air pollution and non-respiratory health hazards for children. Archives of medical science: AMS. 2010 Aug 30; 6(4):483.

[6] Zhang L, Yang Y, Li Y, Qian ZM, Xiao W, Wang X, Rolling CA, Liu E, Xiao J, Zeng W, Liu T. Short-term and long-term effects of PM2. 5 on acute nasopharyngitis in 10 communities of Guangdong, China. Science of the Total Environment. 2019 Oct 20; 688: 136-142.

[7] Heal MR, Kumar P, Harrison RM. Particles, air quality, policy and health. Chemical Society Reviews. 2012; 41(19):6606-6630.

[8] Fuzzi, S., et al. "Critical assessment of the current state of scientific knowledge, terminology, and research needs concerning the role of organic aerosols in the atmosphere, climate, and global change." Atmospheric Chemistry and Physics 6.7 (2006): 2017-2038.

[9] Steinfeld JI. Atmospheric chemistry and physics: from air pollution to climate change. Environment: Science and Policy for Sustainable Development. 1998 Sep 1; 40(7):26.

[10] Penner, Joyce E., et al. "Aerosols, their direct and indirect effects." Climate Change 2001: The Scientific Basis. Contribution of Working Group I to the Third Assessment Report of the Intergovernmental Panel on Climate Change. Cambridge University Press, 2001. 289-348.

[11] Whelpdale, D. M., et al. "Atmospheric process." Global Acid Deposition Assessment, edited by: Whelpdale, DM and Kaiser, MS, World Meteorological Organization Global Atmosphere Watch, Report 106, 1996: 7-32.

[12] Andreae MO, Rosenfeld DJ. Aerosol–cloud–precipitation interactions. Part 1. The nature and sources of cloud-active aerosols. Earth-Science Reviews. 2008 Jul 1;89(1-2): 13-41.

[13] Smith SJ, Aardenne JV, Klimont Z, Andres RJ, Volke A, Delgado Arias S. Anthropogenic sulfur dioxide emissions: 1850-2005. Atmospheric Chemistry and Physics. 2011 Feb 9;11(3):1101-1116.

[14] Dentener F, Kinne S, Bond T, Boucher O, Cofala J, Generoso S, Ginoux P, Gong S, Hoelzemann JJ, Ito A, Marelli L. Emissions of primary aerosol and precursor gases in the years 2000 and 1750 prescribed data-sets for AeroCom. Atmospheric Chemistry and Physics. 2006 Sep 26;6(12):4321-4344.

[15] Stern DI. Reversal of the trend in global anthropogenic sulfur emissions.

Global Environmental Change. 2006 May 1;16(2):207-220.

[16] Lana A, Bell TG, Simo R, Vallina SM, Ballabrera-Poy J, Kettle AJ, Dachs J, Bopp L, Saltzman ES, Stefels JJ, Johnson JE. An updated climatology of surface dimethlysulfide concentrations and emission fluxes in the global ocean. Global Biogeochemical Cycles. 2011 Mar;25(1).

[17] Putaud JP, Van Dingenen R, Alastuey A, Bauer H, Birmili W, Cyrys J, Flentje H, Fuzzi S, Gehrig R, Hansson HC, Harrison RM. A European aerosol phenomenology–3: Physical and chemical characteristics of particulate matter from 60 rural, urban, and kerbside sites across Europe. Atmospheric Environment. 2010 Mar 1;44(10):1308-1320.

[18] Squizzato S, Masiol M, Brunelli A, Pistollato S, Tarabotti E, Rampazzo G, Pavoni B. Factors determining the formation of secondary inorganic aerosol: a case study in the Po Valley (Italy). Atmospheric chemistry and physics. 2013 Feb 19;13(4):1927-1939.

[19] Pinder RW, Davidson EA, Goodale CL, Greaver TL, Herrick JD, Liu L. Climate change impacts of US reactive nitrogen. Proceedings of the National Academy of Sciences. 2012 May 15;109(20):7671-7675.

[20] Battye W, Aneja VP, Roelle PA. Evaluation and improvement of ammonia emissions inventories. Atmospheric Environment. 2003 Sep 1;37(27):3873-3883.

[21] Bauer SE, Koch D, Unger N, Metzger SM, Shindell DT, Streets DG. Nitrate aerosols today and in 2030: a global simulation including aerosols and tropospheric ozone. Atmospheric Chemistry and Physics. 2007 Oct 2;7 (19):5043-5059.

[22] United States. Environmental Protection Agency. Office of Air Quality Planning. Review of the national ambient air quality standards for particulate matter: Policy assessment of scientific and technical information. DIANE Publishing, 1996.

[23] Querol X, Alastuey A, Rodriguez S, Plana F, Mantilla E, Ruiz CR. Monitoring of PM10 and PM2. 5 around primary particulate anthropogenic emission sources. Atmospheric Environment. 2001 Jan 1;35(5):845-858.

[24] Querol X, Alastuey A, Pey J, Cusack M, Pérez N, Mihalopoulos N, Theodosi C, Gerasopoulos E, Kubilay N, Koçak MU. Variability in regional background aerosols within the Mediterranean. Atmospheric Chemistry and Physics. 2009 Jul 16;9(14): 4575-4591.

[25] Zhang R, Shen Z, Cheng T, Zhang M, Liu Y. The elemental composition of atmospheric particles at Beijing during Asian dust events in spring 2004. Aerosol and Air Quality Research. 2010 Jan;10(1):67-75.

[26] Chen Y, Zhi G, Feng Y, Liu D, Zhang G, Li J, Sheng G, Fu J. Measurements of black and organic carbon emission factors for household coal combustion in China: implication for emission reduction. Environmental Science & Technology. 2009 Dec 15;43(24):9495-9500.

[27] Duarte RM, Santos EB, Pio CA, Duarte AC. Comparison of structural features of water-soluble organic matter from atmospheric aerosols with those of aquatic humic substances. Atmospheric Environment. 2007 Dec 1;41(37): 8100-8113.

[28] Bond TC, Bhardwaj E, Dong R, Jogani R, Jung S, Roden C, Streets DG, Trautmann NM. Historical emissions of black and organic carbon aerosol from energy-related combustion, 1850-2000. Global biogeochemical cycles. 2007 Jun;21(2).

[29] Venkataraman C, Habib G, Eiguren-Fernandez A, Miguel AH, Friedlander SK. Residential biofuels in South Asia: carbonaceous aerosol emissions and climate impacts. Science. 2005 Mar 4;307(5714):1454-1456.

[30] Quinn PK, Bates TS, Baum E, Doubleday N, Fiore AM, Flanner M, Fridlind A, Garrett TJ, Koch D, Menon S, Shindell D. Short-lived pollutants in the Arctic: their climate impact and possible mitigation strategies. Atmospheric Chemistry and Physics. 2008 Mar 25;8(6):1723-1735.

[31] Wang Q, Jacob DJ, Fisher JA, Mao J, Leibensperger EM, Carouge CC, Sager PL, Kondo Y, Jimenez JL, Cubison MJ, Doherty SJ. Sources of carbonaceous aerosols and deposited black carbon in the Arctic in winter-spring: implications for radiative forcing. Atmospheric Chemistry and Physics. 2011 Dec 13;11(23): 12453-12473.

[32] Saitoh K, Nakatsubo R, Hiraki T, Shima M, Yoda Y, Sera K. Chemical properties of significant Asian Dust particles observed at Himeji City from November 2009 to May 2012. International Journal of PIXE. 2017 Aug 7;27(01n02):71-85.

[33] Herner JD, Green PG, Kleeman MJ. Measuring the trace elemental composition of size-resolved airborne particles. Environmental science & technology. 2006 Mar 15;40(6):1925-1933.

[34] Valavanidis A, Fiotakis K, Vlachogianni T. Airborne particulate matter and human health: toxicological assessment and importance of size and composition of particles for oxidative damage and carcinogenic mechanisms. Journal of Environmental Science and Health, Part C. 2008 Dec 2;26(4): 339-362.

[35] State of Global Report, 2020

[36] Guaita R, Pichiule M, Maté T, Linares C, Díaz J. Short-term impact of particulate matter (PM2. 5) on respiratory mortality in Madrid. International journal of environmental health research. 2011 Aug 1;21(4): 260-274.

[37] Halonen JI, Lanki T, Yli-Tuomi T, Tiittanen P, Kulmala M, Pekkanen J. Particulate air pollution and acute cardiorespiratory hospital admissions and mortality among the elderly. Epidemiology. 2009 Jan 1:143-153.

[38] Samoli E, Peng R, Ramsay T, Pipikou M, Touloumi G, Dominici F, Burnett R, Cohen A, Krewski D, Samet J, Katsouyanni K. Acute effects of ambient particulate matter on mortality in Europe and North America: results from the APHENA study. Environmental health perspectives. 2008 Nov;116(11):1480-1486.

[39] Jiang XQ, Mei XD, Feng D. Air pollution and chronic airway diseases: what should people know and do?. Journal of thoracic disease. 2016 Jan;8(1):E31.

[40] Klaassen CD, editor. Casarett and Doull's toxicology: the basic science of poisons. New York: McGraw-Hill; 2013 Jun 19.

[41] Bové H, Bongaerts E, Slenders E, Bijnens EM, Saenen ND, Gyselaers W, Van Eyken P, Plusquin M, Roeffaers MB, Ameloot M, Nawrot TS. Ambient black carbon particles reach the fetal side of human placenta. Nature communications. 2019 Sep 17;10(1):1-7.

[42] Kurt OK, Zhang J, Pinkerton KE. Pulmonary health effects of air pollution. Current opinion in pulmonary medicine. 2016 Mar; 22(2):138.

[43] Guarnieri M, Balmes JR. Outdoor air pollution and asthma. The Lancet. 2014 May 3;383(9928):1581-1592.

[44] Brook RD. Cardiovascular effects of air pollution. Clinical science. 2008 Sep 1;115(6):175-187.

[45] Katholi RE, Couri DM. Left ventricular hypertrophy: major risk factor in patients with hypertension: update and practical clinical applications. International journal of hypertension. 2011 Oct;2011.

[46] Genc S, Zadeoglulari Z, Fuss SH, Genc K. The adverse effects of air pollution on the nervous system. Journal of toxicology. 2012 Oct;2012.

[47] Mandal PK. Dioxin: a review of its environmental effects and its aryl hydrocarbon receptor biology. Journal of Comparative Physiology B. 2005 May;175(4):221-230.

Section 2

Metals and Human Health

Chapter 4

Heavy Metals in the Environment and Health Impact

Myriam El Ati-Hellal and Fayçal Hellal

Abstract

Heavy metals are among the most harmful contaminants in the ecosystems due to their persistency, bioaccumulation and high toxicity. In this chapter, we presented the sources, distribution and pathways of heavy metals in soil, water and air. The physico-chemical properties, uses, toxicity and health hazards of the purely toxic heavy metals lead, cadmium and mercury were also described. Other essential heavy metals were briefly presented and the main health effects due to their deficiency or excess were displayed in this chapter. Finally, the various methods used for the removal of heavy metals from soil and aquatic environments were discussed with a focus on nanomaterials.

Keywords: Heavy metals, classification, properties, uses, health hazards, removal

1. Introduction

Environmental pollution has exposed humans to various contaminants such as pesticides, heavy metals or polycyclic aromatic hydrocarbons [1]. Unlike most organic pollutants, heavy metals are not removed from ecosystems by natural processes. They tend to accumulate in biotic and abiotic environments reaching toxic levels [2–4]. The introduction of heavy metals into the environment can result from natural events as volcanic eruptions, soil erosion and forest fires or anthropogenic activities including mining operations, industrial and domestic effluents and fertilizers application [3].

A number of heavy metals are considered essential for human health. They are important constituents of several key enzymes and play a crucial role in various biochemical reactions [5]. An insufficient supply of these elements leads to various deficiency syndromes. However, these micronutrients can become toxic from a threshold content in the body. Other elements are not beneficial for health and can be highly toxic even at very low levels. This is the case of lead, cadmium and mercury that are among the list of 10 chemicals of major public concern due to their high water solubility, toxicity, and carcinogenesis. Acute and chronic exposure to these elements affects human health and could cause incurable diseases leading to death [2, 3, 6, 7].

2. Classification of metals

Metals are elements with a good electric conductivity and whose electric resistivity is directly proportional to the absolute temperature. Several other physical

IntechOpen

properties such as high thermal conductivity, reflectivity, malleability and ductility are common to metals [4]. The term "heavy metals" has been widely used in the environmental literature and diverse definitions, based on density, atomic mass or atomic number and on chemical properties, have been proposed for this term [8, 9]. Usually, a heavy metal is an element with an atomic weight between 63.5 and 200.6 and a density greater than 5.0 [10]. Unlike organic contaminants, heavy metals are highly persistent and tend to accumulate in tissues of leaving organisms.

Metals can be classified according to their biological effect. They are considered as "essential" when deficiency symptoms are noted with depletion or removal and "nonessential" when they have no known beneficial role to play in biological function [4]. Essential metals include zinc, copper, iron, iodine, manganese, molybdenum, selenium and vanadium. Lead, cadmium and mercury are among nonessential elements that are highly toxic even at trace amounts. It is important to note that essential elements can become potentially toxic for living organisms if they are incorporated in amounts exceeding a certain threshold [9].

3. Heavy metals in the environment

3.1 Soil

Natural as well as anthropogenic sources of heavy metals including soil erosions, volcanic eruptions, forest fires, mining operations, industrial activities, fertilizers application as well as urban wastes may lead to the contamination of soils [3]. Heavy metals occur naturally in ores in different chemical forms such as sulfides or oxides. Industrial pollution results from various activities such as chemical manufacturing, oil refining, metal processing and plating, tanneries and plastics.

Wind, water and gravity are the principal factors controlling the heavy metals mobility in soils and landscapes. The distribution of metals between solid and solution phases depends on their chemical forms in each phase and on chemical factors such as pH, metal concentration or soil composition. The soil contamination by heavy metals may affect soil fertility by the reduction in populations of soil fauna [3].

3.2 Water

The outbreak of "Minamata disease" and "itai-itai-byo" or "ouch-ouch disease" in Japan during the 1940s and the 1950s drew the worldwide attention to the environmental hazards caused by aquatic heavy metal pollution. Minamata disease was due to the ingestion of fish and shellfish contaminated with highly toxic methylmercury, while ouch-ouch disease was caused by eating rice polluted with lethal amounts of cadmium [1].

Heavy metals enter the aquatic environment from both natural and anthropogenic sources. Entry may be due to direct discharges into both fresh and marine ecosystems or through indirect routes such as dry and wet deposition. Anthropogenic wastes, geochemical structure and mining effluents create potential sources of heavy metals pollution in the aquatic environment.

Once introduced into the aquatic environment, heavy metals are distributed among four interactive compartments (water, suspended matter, sediment and biota). Metals in the aquatic environment can exist in dissolved or particulate form. Sedimentation, adsorption/desorption, dilution and dispersion are the main processes governing the distribution of heavy metals in aqueous ecosystems. Adsorption could be the first step of metals removal from water. Both in marine environments and in fresh water, the permanent or temporary storage of metals takes place in sediments. Microbial activity and oxidative processes can alter the properties of sediments and influence the composition of pore water. Snooping organisms can also bring sediments to the surface, which will release a significant fraction of the metal [11]. The absorption of heavy metals by both fauna and flora could cause an increase in the concentration of the metals in the living organisms. If the evacuation phase is slow, it may result in a phenomenon of bioaccumulation, which could contaminate the aquatic food chain [11].

Unlike biosorption, bioaccumulation is an active process, whereby metals are integrated in the interior of cells [12]. Certain metals bind preferentially, either transiently or permanently, to the cell membrane and then cause structural and functional modifications, which are often fatal to the cell. A study by Dao and Beardall showed that increasing doses of lead administered to the algae *Chlorella sp.* were associated with a decrease in algal growth, as well as an inhibition of the photosynthetic function by the algae [13].

3.3 Air

Heavy metals occur in the atmosphere mainly in particulate form. Particulate matter refers to a mixture of solid and liquid particles that are dispersed in the air. It is composed of primary particles that are emitted directly into the atmosphere and secondary particulates formed through chemical transformation of gaseous pollutants [1]. Metals in the atmosphere result from natural processes (volcanic eruption, soil erosion, sand storms, dust re-suspension) and anthropogenic sources (mainly industrial, agricultural and vehicle emissions). Metal oxides constitute a major class of inorganic particles in the atmosphere. They result from the combustion of fuels containing metals.

Generally, the concentrations of atmospheric heavy metals are higher in winter than in summer. This is probably due to the high temperature, the strong diffusion capacity and the rainfall in summer season. Inversely, the atmospheric deposition of heavy metals tend to be higher in summer than in winter. According to Duan and Tan, the average atmospheric concentration of lead in China is 261.0 ± 275.7 ng m^{-3}, which falls below the guideline limit of the World Health Organization (WHO) of 500 ng m^{-3} [14]. The mean concentration of atmospheric cadmium in the same area is 12.9 ± 19.6 ng m^{-3}, which exceeds the WHO limit of 5 ng m^{-3}. The principal sources of atmospheric heavy metal pollution in China are coal burning, iron and steel industry and vehicle emissions [14].

4. Health impact of heavy metals

4.1 Lead

4.1.1 Physico-chemical properties

Lead (Pb) is one of the oldest heavy metals used in the past for hair dies, insecticides, and pottery glazes [15]. It is a naturally occurring bluish-gray metal, highly malleable and ductile and shiny when just cut. Lead is a dense metal, with a specific gravity of 11.35 and an atomic weight of 207.2 g mol^{-1}. It is present in many inorganic forms (acetates, nitrates, carbonates, sulphates and chlorides) especially in the earth's crust and ores [5]. Lead is also found in the environment as a result of radioactive decompositions because it is a natural product of the decay of uranium. Native lead is rare, it is currently extracted from ore associated with zinc (blende), silver and copper. The main mineral source of lead is galena (PbS) [5].

4.1.2 Uses

Despite its high toxicity, lead is still used in various anthropogenic activities such as storage batteries, fossil fuel combustion, PVC production, electricity generation, alloys, glass manufacture and nuclear industry. Due to environmental pressure, lead emissions from motor vehicle gasoline have decreased significantly over the last three decades. As a result, a great improvement in air quality was observed worldwide [1, 5]. In addition, the use of lead in paints and colorants was banned in most countries after children's intoxications from lead-based pigments.

4.1.3 Health hazards

The main routes of lead exposure include ingestion of contaminated food and drinking water as well as incidental ingestion of dust and soil. Another major exposure pathway is the lead-based paint in older homes. Once inside the body, lead is distributed in blood and soft tissues and accumulated in skeletal bones [1].

One of the major mechanisms of lead toxicity is its ability to interact with proteins and to inhibit enzyme activity by competing with essential metallic cations for binding sites [2, 16, 17]. Acute toxicity can cause fatigue, irritability, sleeplessness, headache, loss of appetite, dullness, hypertension and vertigo, while chronic toxicity can result in neurological disorders, cognitive impairments, premature birth, brain injury, kidney dysfunctions, reproductive pathologies, liver damage, paralysis and even death [16, 18, 19]. Lead poisoning affects particularly children leading to hyperactivity, behavioral problems, lowered intelligence quotient (IQ) and cognitive deficits [20]. In Chicago, after adjustment for all socio-demographic factors, it was reported that exposure to lead caused 13% of reading failure and 14.8% of math failure in children [21]. Adverse effects of lead toxicity are also found in contaminated ecosystems, including biodiversity losses, decreased growth in plants and animals and neurological damages in vertebrates [22].

4.2 Cadmium

4.2.1 Physico-chemical properties

Cadmium (Cd) is a soft, bluish-white metal with an atomic weight of 112.4 g mol^{-1} and a density of 8.65. It melts at 594 K. Cadmium was first discovered by Friedrich Stromeyer in Germany in 1817. It is a rare element that is not found as a pure state in nature and is commonly associated with zinc (one ton of zinc provides about 2.5–3 kg of cadmium. Cadmium is also present in lead and copper ores, as well as in natural phosphates (40 ppm for Tunisian phosphates, 26 ppm for Moroccan phosphates). In the latter case, various decadmination processes can be implemented [23]. Cadmium persists in the environment and has a biological half-life of 10 to 25 years [1].

4.2.2 Uses

Cadmium is used in various industrial processes including electronics, electricity, metallurgy, plastics, PVC manufacture, pigments and paints and pesticides [1, 24]. Significant quantities of cadmium are also found in discharges from industries processing crude phosphate [23]. Due to environmental restrictions, the use of cadmium in the manufacturing of nickel-cadmium batteries decreased and has been replaced by nickel-metal hydride and lithium-ion batteries. Recently, cadmium telluride was used in semiconducting solar panels and infrared optical windows [25].

4.2.3 Health hazards

Dietary intake is the most important pathway for cadmium exposure in humans. Tobacco smoke is another source of exposure containing appreciable amounts of the metal. As the absorption of cadmium from the lungs is much higher than from the gastrointestinal tract, smoking contributes significantly to the total body burden [1]. Cadmium is absorbed in the gut and the lungs, and transported to the liver by blood. Accumulation of cadmium in the body is done mainly in the liver and the kidneys [18]. Cadmium metallothionein is the form in which cadmium enters the kidneys. This complex has a protective role against cadmium toxicity through binding up to seven metal atoms per molecule. When the cadmium intake is too high, the metal is transported further to the kidneys and binds to other proteins [5, 17].

Adverse effects of cadmium toxicity include high blood pressure, reproductive disorders, fetal growth reduction, pregnancy loss, iron deficiency, gastrointestinal disorders, bone fracture, nephrotoxicity, renal dysfunction, neurological troubles, lung damage and lung cancer [1, 18, 24, 26]. In humans, blood, urine, hair and nails have been used as biomarkers of cadmium exposure and health risk evaluation [27]. Recently, Du et al. (2020) evaluated the environmental and human health hazards from cadmium exposure near an active lead-zinc mine and a copper smelter in China. They found that the cadmium concentration in hair and urine biomarkers in the mining and smelting areas were much higher than in the general population. Additionally, rice and vegetable ingestion were the two major pathways of cadmium exposure [28].

4.3 Mercury

4.3.1 Physico-chemical properties

Mercury (Hg) is a heavy metal with a density of 13.6 and an atomic weight of 200.6 g mol^{-1}. It is rare in the earth's crust and occurs in several forms of ore. *Cinnabar* HgS is the principal mercurial mineral [1, 5]. Mercury is a unique metal, as it is the only metal liquid at room temperature. In addition, it exists in nature in three forms (elemental, inorganic, and organic). In the atmosphere, most mercury is present in the form of elemental mercury vapor, while inorganic and organic species predominate in soil, water, plants and animals. Methylmercury, an organic compound of mercury, is formed as a result of the methylation of inorganic forms of mercury by microorganisms in soil and water [29].

4.3.2 Uses

Mercury is extensively used in various industries such as the production of caustic soda, the wood processing, the pulp and paper industry or the manufacture of batteries. Mercury is also employed as preservative of pharmaceutical products, as amalgams in dental industry, or as catalysts in chemical industry. Due to the linearity of its coefficient of expansion, mercury is used as a metal in thermometers. In addition, mercury is used in jewelry making, pesticides, barometers and incandescent lights [1, 5, 16, 30].

4.3.3 Health hazards

Fish consumption and dental amalgam are the major sources of mercury exposure in humans. Inhalation of mercury vapor is an other important pathway of exposure. Due to their high lipophilicity, elemental mercury and methylmercury are highly absorbed in the tissues. Inorganic mercury salts are not lipid soluble; therefore, they do not cross the placental and blood–brain barriers. Absorption of methylmercury from the gastrointestinal tract in humans exceeds 90%, whereas absorption of inorganic mercury salts is less than 10% [7]. Once absorbed in the body, the inhaled mercury vapor is quickly diffused into the blood and distributed into all of the organs [6]. Then it is accumulated in the brain and the kidney and excreted through urine and feces. As regards methylmercury, this organic compound is accumulated in the liver and kidney after consumption and slowly converted to inorganic mercury by microflora in the intestines [31].

The toxicity of mercury, especially methylmercury, derives from its ability to interact with nucleophiles due to its electrophilic nature. During interactions, the catalytic, binding, and transport functions of nucleophiles are impaired. One essential mechanism related to the toxicity of mercury is the damage to mitochondria that enhances the generation of free radicals [17]. The major clinical features of mercury acute and chronic exposures are insomnia, weight loss, vomiting, diarrhea, cough, dyspnea, fever, tremors, gingivitis, erythrism, delusions, hallucinations, acrodynia disease, congenital malformation, renal tubular dysfunction, neurologic disorders, paralysis and death [17, 32].

4.4 Other essential metals

Most essential metals act as catalysts for enzymes and can become toxic at high levels. In tissues and fluids, metals very often form complexes with organic compounds such as amino acids, proteins and peptides. **Table 1** displays the main health effects due to deficiency or excess of five essential metals (iron, zinc, copper, iodine and selenium) [33–38].

4.4.1 Iron

Iron (Fe) is a vital nutrient as it is a cofactor of a wide variety of cell functions. In the human body, iron is found as heme compounds (hemoglobin or myoglobin), heme enzymes, or nonheme compounds (flavin-iron enzymes, transferring, and ferritin). The body requires iron for oxygen transport, respiration, the tricarboxylic acid cycle, lipid metabolism, gene regulation and DNA synthesis [39, 40]. Inorganic iron and heme iron are the two forms of dietary iron. Good sources of heme iron include meat, poultry and fish whereas nonheme iron is obtained from cereals, pulses, legumes, fruits and vegetables. Iron absorption is enhanced by vitamin C, ascorbic acid and meat consumption, while phytates, calcium and some dietary fibres inhibit the nutrient absorption [41, 42].

4.4.2 Zinc

Zinc (Zn) is an essential nutrient found in all human tissue. It is a structural compound of nearly 300 enzymes, important for the metabolism of macromolecules and that of nucleic acids. It has been estimated that the adult human body contains approximately 2 g of zinc. Lean red meat is an important dietary source of zinc. In addition, its zinc is present in a highly available form. However, fats, oils, sugar and alcohol have a very low zinc level [34, 43].

4.4.3 Copper

Copper (Cu) is essential for the activity of several metalloproteins and enzymes. It plays a crucial role in the regulation of the gene expression. Copper is required for

Metal	Deficiency health effects	Toxicity health effects
Iron	• Anemia • Mental retardation • Brain damage • Behavioral impairment	• Liver and heart disease • Cancer • Neurodegenerative disorders • Diabetes • Hormonal abnormalities
Zinc	• Diarrhea • Growth retardation • Behavioral changes • Defects in the immune systems • *Acrodermatitis enteropathica* genetic disorder	• Nausea and vomiting • Diarrhea • Fever • Lethargy • Anemia • Copper deficiency
Copper	• Hypochromic anemia • Neutropenia • hypopigmentation • Osteoporosis • Vascular abnormalities • Neurologic disorders	• Wilson's disease • Hepatocellular degeneration • Necrosis • Brain damage • Death
Iodine	• Goiter • Congenital anomalies • Cretinism • Hypothyroidism • Impaired mental function • Hyperthyroidism	• Goiter • Hypothyroidism • Hyperhyroidism
Selenium	• Keshan disease • Kashin-Beck disease	• Gastrointestinal disturbances • Hair loss • Nail brittleness • Skin rash • Garlic breath odor • Fatigue • Irritability • Neurologic disorders

Table 1.
Main health effects of deficiency and excess of essential heavy metals.

growth, defense, strength, blood cell production, iron transport and metabolism. The total body content of copper has been estimated to be 80 mg, with a range of 50–120 mg. Dietary sources rich in copper include seafood, organ meats, legumes and nuts. Refined cereals, sugar and dairy products are poor in the nutrient [35, 44].

4.4.4 Iodine

Iodine (I) is needed for the synthesis of thyroid hormones which are involved in the growth, development and control of metabolic processes. Deficiency of iodine during early development of the brain and nervous system leads to cretinism, which is irreversible. At an older age, it leads to hypothyroidism and goiter, the first endemic disease that has been attributed to environmental factors. Marine fish and shellfish are foods particularly rich in iodine [37, 45].

4.4.5 Selenium

Selenium (Se) is a component of the amino acid selenocysteine. Enzymes that depend on selenium play a very important role in cells. They offer protection against oxidative damage, modulation of growth and development as well as defense against infection. In humans, selenium deficiency can cause endemic cardiomyopathy known as "Keshan disease", which mainly affects children and women of childbearing age. Liver, kidney and seafood are particularly rich in selenium [36, 46].

5. Removal of hazardous heavy metals

5.1 Methods of treatment

Due to their toxicity, non-biodegradability and persistency, heavy metals can exert adverse effects on the environment and other ecological receptors. Therefore, their removal from soil and aqueous environments has drawn tremendous attention. Various methods have been developed and used to decrease heavy metals concentrations in the ecosystems. These technologies can be categorized in physico-chemical processes such as ion exchange, reverse osmosis, membrane filtration, adsorption, precipitation, electrolytic removal and biological processes involving activated sludge and phytoremediation [12, 47, 48]. Adsorption is one of the most extensively used methods due to its low cost and simple preparation. It is based on mass transfer between the liquid phase and the solid phase called adsorbent. This process can run in reversible mode and the adsorbents will be regenerated by desorption. Some widely used adsorbents for removal of metal ions include clay minerals, activated carbon,, biomaterials, industrial solid wastes and zeolites [48]. Low cost adsorbents include natural material or certain waste from industrial or agricultural operation.

5.2 Nanomaterials for heavy metals removal

Over the past decades, nanomaterials have gained a lot of attention due to their high specific surface area, catalytic potential and chemical reactivity [49]. Various cost-effective and safe nanomaterials have been developed in treating wastewater solutions. Among them, nano metal oxides (NMO), nano zero-valent iron (nZVI) and hybrid magnetic nanoparticles (MNP) are particularly efficient in the improvement of water quality.

5.2.1 Nano metal oxides

Metal based nanomaterials are commonly oxides of iron, manganese, titanium, magnesium, copper and cerium. These metal oxides are low-cost materials and provide a high adsorption capacity and selectivity. However, NMO are prone to agglomeration due to their poor stability. Different techniques could be used for NMO synthesis such as hydrothermal techniques, chemical co-precipitation, thermal decomposition or chemical vapor condensation [50, 51]. Generally, highly stable, monodisperse and shape-controlled NMO are the result of efficient synthetic techniques. Luther et al. (2012) synthetized iron oxides nanoparticles for the removal of arsenic (III) or (V) from aqueous solutions. The adsorption followed the Langmuir Isotherm and capacities were determined for each nanomaterial and arsenic ions [52]. Optimum binding capacities reaching 20000 μg/g for arsenic (III) and 4904 μg/g for arsenic (V) were observed at pH =6, after 24 h of contact time at room temperature.

5.2.2 Nano zero-valent iron

Due to the reducing capacity of iron (0) and the high reactivity of ferric oxide, nZVI composite was extensively investigated as a novel adsorbent to remove heavy metals from wastewater [53]. Several methods have been developed to produce nZVI including abrasion, grinding, reduction with sodium borohydride, carbothermal reduction, ultrasound assisted method, electrolysis or biosynthesis [54]. In spite of their effectiveness in water treatment and remediation, some disadvantages mainly due to aggregation, difficult separation and lack of stability are encountered with the use of nZVI. To overcome these technical difficulties, modifications of nZVI could be applied such as doping the composite with noble metals, surface coating with polymers or anionic surfactants, emulsification or immobilization with silica, activated carbons or zeolites. Huang et al. (2015) applied modified nZVI with sodium dodecyl sulfate anionic surfactant for chromium (VI) removal [55]. They found an enhanced removal capacity and a great stability with nZVI modification. The adsorption followed the pseudo-second order kinetic model and the Freundlich Isotherm. The highest removal efficiency of chromium (VI) was obtained at pH 3.0 and 25°C, at the value of 98.919% after 120 min of contact time.

5.2.3 Hybrid magnetic nanoparticles

Hybrid magnetic nanostructures contain two or more nanometer-scale components with at least one component being magnetic [56]. These hybrid nanocomposites take the advantages of the magnetic nanoparticles such as their high surface area, their easy separation under external magnetic fields and their excellent recyclability after separation and prevent from their precipitation or aggregation due to their tendency to oxidation [57]. Up to date, different MNP have been researched by the scientific society. The investigated nanostructures include magnetite (Fe_3O_4), maghemite (γ-Fe_2O_3) and hematite (α-Fe_2O_3). They could be functionalized with different materials such as polymers, biomolecules, inorganics, organics or carbon nanotubes [57]. This surface functionalization improves the homogeneity, selectivity and adsorption capacity of magnetic nanoparticles leading to an effective removal of toxic pollutants. Asadi et al. (2020) synthetized the spinel ferrites nanoparticles $MnFe_2O_4$ and $CoFe_2O_4$ to investigate the zinc removal from aqueous solution. High respective adsorption capacities of 454.5 and 384.6 mg/g for $MnFe_2O_4$ and $CoFe_2O_4$ were obtained at optimum pH =6, by following the Langmuir Isotherm model [58].

Acknowledgements

The authors want to acknowledge professor Jalila El Ati, responsible of the laboratory SURVEN of the National Institute of Nutrition and Food Technology for her precious advice.

Author details

Myriam El Ati-Hellal[1]* and Fayçal Hellal[2]

1 IPEST (Preparatory Institute for Scientific and Technical Studies), Laboratory Materials Molecules and Applications, Tunis, Tunisia

2 INNTA (National Institute of Nutrition and Food Technology), SURVEN (Nutrition Surveillance and Epidemiology in Tunisia) Research Laboratory, Tunis, Tunisia

*Address all correspondence to: mfh22002@yahoo.fr

References

[1] Yu M-H, Tsunoda H, Tsunoda M. Environmental toxicology. Biological and Health Effects of Pollutants. Third Edition. Boca Raton, London, New York: Taylor & Francis Group, CRC Press; 2011.

[2] Tchounwou PB, Yedjou CG, Patlolla AK, Sutton DJ. Heavy metal toxicity and the environment. Exp Suppl. 2012;101:133-64.

[3] Tiller KG. Heavy Metals in Soils and Their Environmental Significance. In: B.A. S, editor. Advances in Soil Science. New York: Springer; 1989. p. 113-42.

[4] Forstner U, Wittmann GTW. Metal Pollution in the Aquatic Environment. Berlin, Heidelber, New York: Springer-Verlag; 1981.

[5] Enghag P. Encyclopedia of the Elements; Technical Data · History · Processing · Applications. Weinheim: WILEY-VCH Verlag GmbH & Co. KGaA; 2004.

[6] Park JD, Zheng W. Human exposure and health effects of inorganic and elemental mercury. J Prev Med Public Health. 2012;45(6):344-52.

[7] Valko M, Morris H, Cronin MT. Metals, toxicity and oxidative stress. Curr Med Chem. 2005;12(10):1161-208.

[8] Duffus JH. "HEAVY METALS"—A MEANINGLESS TERM? (IUPAC Technical Report). Pure and applied chemistry. 2002;74(5):793-807.

[9] Gadd GM. Metals and microorganisms: a problem of definition. FEMS Microbiol Lett. 1992;100(1-3):197-203.

[10] Srivastava NK, Majumder CB. Novel biofiltration methods for the treatment of heavy metals from industrial wastewater. J Hazard Mater. 2008;151(1):1-8.

[11] Calamari D, Naeve H. Revue de la pollution dans l'environnement aquatique africain. Document Technique du CPCA N°25. 1994:1-129.

[12] Mantzorou A, Navakoudis E, Paschalidis K, Ververidis F. Microalgae: a potential tool for remediating aquatic environments from toxic metals. International Journal of Environmental Science and Technology. 2018;15:1815-30.

[13] Dao LH, Beardall J. Effects of lead on growth, photosynthetic characteristics and production of reactive oxygen species of two freshwater green algae. Chemosphere. 2016;147:420-9.

[14] Duan J, Tan J. Atmospheric heavy metals and Arsenic in China: Situation, sources and control policies. Atmospheric Environment 2013;74:93-101.

[15] Ye X, Wong O. Lead exposure, lead poisoning, and lead regulatory standards in China, 1990-2005. Regul Toxicol Pharmacol. 2006;46(2):157-62.

[16] Jaishankar M, Tseten T, Anbalagan N, Mathew BB, Beeregowda KN. Toxicity, mechanism and health effects of some heavy metals. Interdiscip Toxicol. 2014;7(2):60-72.

[17] Wu X, Cobbina SJ, Mao G, Xu H, Zhang Z, Yang L. A review of toxicity and mechanisms of individual and mixtures of heavy metals in the environment. Environ Sci Pollut Res Int. 2016;23(9):8244-59.

[18] Briffa J, Sinagra E, Blundell R. Heavy metal pollution in the environment and their toxicological effects on humans. Heliyon. 2020;6(9):e04691.

[19] Jan AT, Azam M, Siddiqui K, Ali A, Choi I, Haq QM. Heavy Metals and

Human Health: Mechanistic Insight into Toxicity and Counter Defense System of Antioxidants. Int J Mol Sci. 2015;16(12):29592-630.

[20] Naranjo VI, Hendricks M, Jones KS. Lead Toxicity in Children: An Unremitting Public Health Problem. Pediatr Neurol. 2020;113:51-5.

[21] Evens A, Hryhorczuk D, Lanphear BP, Rankin KM, Lewis DA, Forst L, et al. The impact of low-level lead toxicity on school performance among children in the Chicago Public Schools: a population-based retrospective cohort study. Environ Health. 2015;14:21.

[22] Levin R, Zilli Vieira CL, Mordarski DC, Rosenbaum MH. Lead seasonality in humans, animals, and the natural environment. Environ Res. 2020;180:108797.

[23] Roberts TL. Cadmium and Phosphorous Fertilizers: The Issues and the Science. Procedia Engineering 2014;83:52-9.

[24] Genchi G, Sinicropi MS, Lauria G, Carocci A, Catalano A. The Effects of Cadmium Toxicity. Int J Environ Res Public Health. 2020;17(11).

[25] Maani T, Celik I, Heben MJ, Ellingson RJ, Apul D. Environmental impacts of recycling crystalline silicon (c-SI) and cadmium telluride (CDTE) solar panels. Sci Total Environ. 2020;735:138827.

[26] Geng HX, Wang L. Cadmium: Toxic effects on placental and embryonic development. Environ Toxicol Pharmacol. 2019;67:102-7.

[27] Waseem A, Arshad J. A review of Human Biomonitoring studies of trace elements in Pakistan. Chemosphere. 2016;163:153-76.

[28] Du B, Zhou J, Lu B, Zhang C, Li D, Zhou J, et al. Environmental and human health risks from cadmium exposure near an active lead-zinc mine and a copper smelter, China. Sci Total Environ. 2020;720:137585.

[29] Castoldi AF, Coccini T, Manzo L. Neurotoxic and molecular effects of methylmercury in humans. Rev Environ Health. 2003;18(1):19-31.

[30] Genchi G, Sinicropi MS, Carocci A, Lauria G, Catalano A. Mercury Exposure and Heart Diseases. Int J Environ Res Public Health. 2017;14(1).

[31] Díez S. Human Health Effects of Methylmercury Exposure. In: Whitacre DM, editor. Reviews of Environmental Contamination and Toxicology. 198. New York: Springer; 2008. p. 111-32.

[32] Duruibe JO, Ogwuegbu MOC, Egwurugwu JN. Heavy metal pollution and human biotoxic effects. International Journal of Physical Sciences Vol pp 2007; 2 (5):112-8.

[33] WHO. Vitamin and mineral requirements in human nutrition. Second edition. Geneva, Switzerland: World Health Organization; 2004. 341 p.

[34] WHO. Zinc. In: WHO, editor. Trace elements in human nutrition and health. Geneva, Switzerland: World Health Organization; 1996. p. 72-104.

[35] WHO. Copper. In: WHO, editor. Trace elements in human nutrition and health. Geneva, Switzerland: World Health Organization; 1996. p. 123-43.

[36] WHO. Selenium. In: WHO, editor. Trace elements in human nutrition and health. Geneva, Switzerland: World Health Organization; 1996. p. 105-1222.

[37] WHO. Iodine. In: WHO, editor. Trace elements in human nutrition and health. Geneva, Switzerland: World Health Organization; 1996. p. 49-71.

[38] Otten JJ, Pitzi Hellwig J., Meyers LD. Dietary Reference Intakes: The Essential Guide to Nutrient Requirements. Medicine Io, editor. Washington, DC: The National Academies Press; 2006. 1344 p.

[39] Cairo G, Bernuzzi F, Recalcati S. A precious metal: Iron, an essential nutrient for all cells. Genes Nutr. 2006;1(1):25-39.

[40] Abbaspour N, Hurrell R, Kelishadi R. Review on iron and its importance for human health. J Res Med Sci. 2014;19(2):164-74.

[41] Umbreit J. Iron deficiency: a concise review. Am J Hematol. 2005;78(3):225-31.

[42] WHO/FAO. Iron. In: WHO/FAO, editor. Vitamin and mineral requirement in human nutrition Second edition. Geneva, Switzerland: World Health Organization and Food and Agriculture Organization; 2004. p. 252-4.

[43] McCall KA, Huang C, Fierke CA. Function and mechanism of zinc metalloenzymes. J Nutr. 2000;130(5S Suppl):1437S-46S.

[44] Milne DB. Copper intake and assessment of copper status. Am J Clin Nutr. 1998;67(5 Suppl):1041S-5S.

[45] Doggui R, El Ati-Hellal M, Traissac P, Lahmar L, El Ati J. Adequacy Assessment of a Universal Salt Iodization Program Two Decades after Its Implementation: A National Cross-Sectional Study of Iodine Status among School-Age Children in Tunisia. Nutrients. 2016;9(1).

[46] Rayman MP. The importance of selenium to human health. Lancet. 2000;356(9225):233-41.

[47] Joseph L, Jun BM, Flora JRV, Park CM, Yoon Y. Removal of heavy metals from water sources in the developing world using low-cost materials: A review. Chemosphere. 2019;229:142-59.

[48] Lakherwal D. Adsorption of Heavy Metals: A Review. International Journal of Environmental Research and Development. 2014;4(1):41-8.

[49] Yadav VB, Gadi R, Kalra S. Clay based nanocomposites for removal of heavy metals from water: A review. J Environ Manage. 2019;232:803-17.

[50] Hua M, Zhang S, Pan B, Zhang W, Lv L, Zhang Q. Heavy metal removal from water/wastewater by nanosized metal oxides: a review. J Hazard Mater. 2012;211-212:317-31.

[51] Qu X, Alvarez PJ, Li Q. Applications of nanotechnology in water and wastewater treatment. Water Res. 2013;47(12):3931-46.

[52] Luther S, Borgfeld N, Kim J, Parsons JG. Removal of arsenic from aqueous solution: A study of the effects of pH and interfering ions using iron oxide nanomaterials. Microchemical Journal. 2012;101 30-6.

[53] Yang J, Hou B, Wang J, Tian B, Bi J, Wang N, et al. Nanomaterials for the Removal of Heavy Metals from Wastewater. Nanomaterials (Basel). 2019;9(3).

[54] Tasharrofi S, Sadegh Hassani S, Taghdisian H, Sobat Z. Environmentally friendly stabilized nZVI-composite for removal of heavy metals. In: C. MH, Kumar Mishra A, editors. New Polymer Nanocomposites for Environmental Remediation. Oxford, UK: Elsevier; 2018. p. 623-42.

[55] Huang D-L, Chen G-M, Zeng G-M, Xu P, Yan M, Lai C, et al. Synthesis and Application of Modified Zero-Valent Iron Nanoparticles for Removal of Hexavalent Chromium from Wastewater. Water Air Soil Pollut. 2015;226:375.

[56] Zeng H, Sun S. Syntheses, Properties, and Potential Applications of Multicomponent Magnetic Nanoparticles. Adv Funct Mater. 2008;18:391-400.

[57] Tahoon MA, Siddeeg SM, Salem Alsaiari N, Mnif W, Ben Rebah F. Effective Heavy Metals Removal fromWater Using Nanomaterials: A Review. processes. 2020;8:645.

[58] Asadi R, Abdollahi H, Gharabaghi M, Boroumand Z. Effective removal of Zn (II) ions from aqueous solution by the magnetic $MnFe_2O_4$ and $CoFe_2O_4$ spinel ferrite nanoparticles with focuses on synthesis, characterization, adsorption, and desorption. Advanced Powder Technology. 2020;31(4):1480-9.

Chapter 5

The Challenge of Water in the Sanitary Conditions of the Populations Living in the Slums of Port-au-Prince: The Case of Canaan

Yolette Jérôme, Magline Alexis, David Telcy, Pascal Saffache and Evens Emmanuel

Abstract

Haitian cities are more and more prone to demographic growth, which has a lasting effect on water distribution infrastructures, as well as those that make it possible to clean it up. They are in touch with the growing demand for water, but also with the management methods of this resource. Over the past 25 years, the enlarged agglomeration of Port-au-Prince, the largest agglomeration in the country, has experienced very strong urban expansion with the creation of new precarious spaces. The literature reports that Haiti is now more than 64% urban and 35% of its population lives in the metropolitan area of Port-au-Prince, in the West Department. Over the past decade, the footprint of the Port-au-Prince metropolitan area has grown by 35%. Recent observations on the formation and development of some slums highlight the country's vulnerability to land-based hazards, which support this form of urbanization through the emergence of environmental displaced persons. Canaan, a human settlement created following the earthquake of January 12, 2010 by presidential decree, and inhabited by the victims of this event, has a deficit in infrastructure and basic urban services. The results of our previous work on this territory lead to a much more in-depth reflection on the need to develop an index of vulnerability to environmental diseases for the population. In fact, most of the households that live there face very precarious situations. The health conditions associated with this context expose the population to increased risks of disease. The measures taken by families to treat water at home do not seem to limit their vulnerability to environmental diseases (infectious and chronic). Improving living conditions in Canaan with a view to sustainability therefore underlies major challenges. What avenues of intervention should be favored to facilitate a favorable development of the population, while taking into account the strong constraints that weigh on their daily lives? The objective of this study is precisely to analyze the vulnerability of the population to water-borne diseases.

Keywords: slums, vulnerability index, urban precariousness, water and sanitation quality, overpopulation, Canaan

1. Introduction

Ensuring a quality water supply to human communities in the North and South is an ongoing process [1]. Indeed, water is essential for sustaining life and a satisfactory supply of drinking water must be made available to all consumers [2]. According to the WHO (2003) [3], 80% of illnesses and deaths among children worldwide are due to unsafe drinking water. Kosek et al. [4] note that between 1992 and 2000, 2.5 million annual deaths in children under five were due to diarrhea. The main component of this disease burden being linked to water [5].

For more than four decades, the issue of access to water in quantity and quality has never ceased to be raised worldwide. The United Nations, academic institutions, NGOs and governments have shown, through the organization of several international conferences, their interest in the global crisis caused by the mismatch between available resources and the increase in human, economic and environmental, as well as pollution due to human actions and global changes. Indeed, the first international conference on water, held in Mar del Plata (Argentina) from March 14 to 25, 1977, had a major impact on dialog at the global level and on the development of United Nations programs. It led to the International Drinking Water Supply and Sanitation Decade (1981–1990), which, among other things, aimed to reduce the incidence of water-related diseases.

Many international events and initiatives have followed one another on the issue of water - a determinant of health - since the Mar del Plata conference in 1977, sometimes under the aegis of the United Nations, sometimes under that of international financial institutions, but also within the framework of ad hoc forums where multinationals and their supporters played a preponderant role [6]. In January 1992, the International Conference on Water and the Environment in Dublin made an alarming observation: the world water situation is in danger, fresh water is scarce and its use must be done with consideration [7]. This observation was taken up at the Rio Earth Summit in 1992 and was the subject of chapter 18 of Agenda 21 established at the time ("Protection of freshwater resources and their quality: application of integrated approaches to in value, management and use of water resources").

The adoption of the Millennium Development Goals (MDGs) from the United Nations Millennium Declaration [8] embraced a vision of the world in which developed and developing countries would fight together against poverty. At the signing of the said declaration, the number of people without access to safe drinking water and improved sanitation facilities around the world was alarming: 1.1 (or 17% of the world population) and 2.4 billion, respectively [9]. The majority reside in precarious neighborhoods, especially in countries without running water and adequate sanitation systems, and mainly use traditional methods for their provision [10–12].

Among the MDG goals, target 7 (c) aimed to halve, by 2015, the percentage of the population without access to safe drinking water and basic sanitation services. WHO/UNICEF [13] report that in 2010, the global MDG target for drinking water was reached in 2010. According to this report [13]: (i) 91% of the world population used 2010 improved water point; (ii) 96% of the world's urban population uses improved water points compared to 84% in rural areas; (iii) in 2015, 663 million people still do not have access to water points. Improved water supply; (iv) 2.4 billion people still do not have improved sanitation facilities.

The PNUD [14] reports "beyond the issue of water supply for personal and domestic use, the lack of safe water and sanitation infrastructure is also a leading causes of poverty and malnutrition, and insecure water supplies linked to climate change threaten to increase the number of people affected by malnutrition, which is expected to reach between 75 and 125 million by 2080". This analysis is of particular concern to the human settlement of CANAAN. This slum constitutes in itself a particular epidemiological environment, where the absence of collective collection of solid waste, of drainage of domestic wastewater and the consumption of water of non-guaranteed quality promotes the circulation of pathogenic germs which constitute risk factors for the health of the population and the environment [15]. The objective of this study is to study the challenge of water in the daily sanitary conditions of the populations living in the slums of Canaan. This work revolves around two main axes: (i) firstly, urbanization and sanitary conditions (water, sanitation and hygiene) in the slums of Port-au-Prince are addressed; (ii) the second axis traces the history of Canaan, a shanty town built in a drought-stricken area.

2. The sanitary conditions of the slums of Port-au-Prince in the face of morbidity due to water, sanitation and hygiene

2.1 Urban socio-spatial organization of Port-au-Prince

Port-au-Prince is the political and economic capital of the Republic of Haiti. It is, according to Millian and Tamru [16], "a town founded on an exceptional site, between sea and hill: the bay of Gonâve and the foothills of the Selle chain, surrounded by two fertile agricultural plains, that of Cul-de-sac and that of Léogâne. The map of the Republic of Haiti is presented in **Figure 1**. Despite these favorable geographical conditions, the city suffers from a degraded environment: few green spaces, urbanization of the hillsides, polluted coastline occupied by unsanitary neighborhoods, poor quality of the building, generalization of precarious housing". Port-au-Prince testified and still testifies today to the symptom of urban macrocephaly which characterizes certain under-urbanized countries. In the Haitian

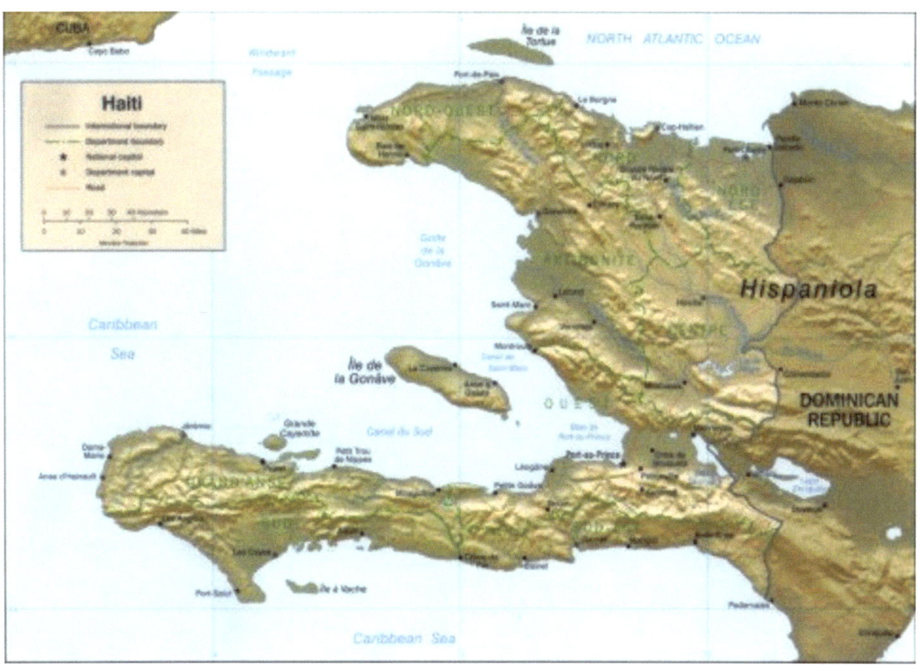

Figure 1.
Map of the Republic of Haiti - (map: Reprinting with permission of CNIGS-Haiti).

universe, this city has long been seen as an island of urban civilization, in a largely rural space [17]. There was Port-au-Prince and there was, as Barthélémy [18] put it, "the land outside".

Between 1950 and 1982, the population of the city of Port-au-Prince increased from 143,534 inhabitants to 719,517 inhabitants [18]. In fact, in order to attract foreign capital and promote the establishment of subcontracting industries, the Haitian State began during the second half of the decade 1970–1980, a process of liberalization of the economy [19]. Centralized largely in the Metropolitan Region of Port-au-Prince (RMPP), this process has, among other things, led to a significant displacement of the country's rural population to the urban space of Port-au-Prince [20]. If the census metropolitan area includes the following six cities: Port-au-Prince, Delmas, Cité Soleil, Tabarre, Carrefour and Pétion-Ville, public urban planning bodies speak more of eight Communes (adding Kenscoff and Croix- des-Bouquets to the previous six), when they deal with the metropolitan area of Port-au-Prince [21]. In 2015, the city's population was estimated at 987,310 inhabitants, with the metropolitan area estimated at 2,618,894 inhabitants [22]. At the turn of the new millennium, the Haitian capital spread out in all directions, without a comprehensive development policy, and its inhabitants are mostly poor or impoverished (workers and soldiers made redundant, pensioners without means) [16]. The evolution of the urban task of Port-au-Prince between 1980 and 2016 is presented in **Figure 2**.

The great attractiveness of the capital for rural populations causes deep urban changes (unprecedented spatial extension, densification and degradation of the existing urban fabric) and an aggravation of the problems facing the Haitian metropolis [23]. The socio-spatial modifications characterizing the urban organization of precarious neighborhoods in Port-au-Prince can be summed up perfectly in the definition of the five levels or dimensions of precariousness in the slums:

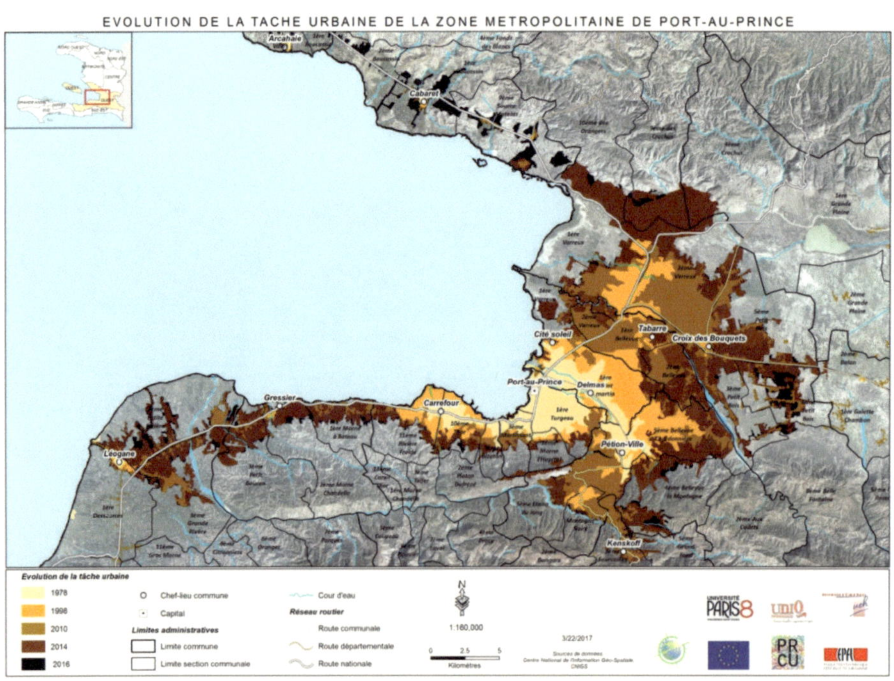

Figure 2.
The evolution of the urban task of Port-au-Prince between 1980 and 2016 [16] - (map: Reprinting with permission of authors).

"(i) physical precariousness, which highlights the environmental dangers due to the very location of the neighborhoods (presence of ravines, swamps, rubbish, etc. (ii) environmental precariousness, which results from the absence of basic services (drinking water, sanitation, elimination of excreta) and the resulting health risks. (iii) land insecurity, which highlights the invasion of land by populations who are not legally the owners. (iv) economic insecurity, because the level of poverty is generally very high. (v) social precariousness, insofar as the inhabitants of precarious neighborhoods are hardly recognized by the public authorities" [24].

2.2 Sustainable access to safe water supply and basic sanitation services

In the joint WHO/UNICEF [13] water and sanitation monitoring program, safe drinking water and basic sanitation are defined as follows: (a) drinking water means water used for domestic purposes, drinking, cooking and personal hygiene; (b) access to drinking water means that the source is located less than one kilometer from the place of its use and that it is possible to obtain regularly at least 20 liters of water per inhabitant and per day; (c) drinking water is water with microbial, chemical and physical characteristics that meet WHO guidelines or national standards for the quality of drinking water; (d) access to drinking water is indicated by the proportion of people using improved drinking water sources: home connection; public standpipes; sounding holes; protected wells; protected sources; rainwater; and (e) basic sanitation is the least expensive technology that ensures hygienic disposal of black and gray water, as well as a clean and healthy living environment both at home and in the vicinity of users. Access to basic sanitation services includes safety and privacy in the use of these services. The coverage shows the proportion of people using improved sanitation services: connection to a public sewer; connection to a septic tank; flush latrine; simple pit latrine; improved latrine with self-ventilated pit.

2.3 Access to water in the slums and the prevalence of water-borne diseases in Port-au-Prince

Dynamic, regional and global pressures, such as climate change, population growth and the degradation of urban infrastructure that cities are undergoing today, are causing water scarcity, making it difficult to manage water effectively. Resource [25]. This situation deprives the populations of the slums of this vital element. The increase in demand for water and the increase in pollution of aquatic ecosystems - two situations resulting from accelerated urbanization - make regional disparities, as well as socio-spatial inequalities more and more visible [26] and make access to water one of the major challenges for humanity [27]. Developing countries are the most affected by massive urbanization. Today, 1 billion people live in the slums, the most deprived are deprived of drinking water and sanitation, the cities then turning into "real health bombs" [28].

Cities are always born and develop near water, which is necessary for the biological and economic life of any community. However, for many years the countries of the North as well as those of the South have been confronted with an increasing speed of urbanization and a growing population, which leads to an increasingly important need for space [29]. In the cities of the South, the services in charge of water management are indeed faced with the challenge of accelerated urbanization of poverty: despite the fact that socio-economic inequalities and social polarization have increased, the heterogeneity of poor households has increased, including the increase in socio-economic inequalities and social polarization [30]. In Port-au-Prince, the water supply rate is less than 50% of the population [31]. The most disadvantaged categories of the population in the RMPP do not have access to water under satisfactory or sufficient conditions [32]. These findings allow us to suggest that water is no longer the driving force behind the creation of human settlements; it seems to become one of the factors of health risks and of crisis or of urban violence.

In Haiti, DINEPA, a public institution responsible for executing state policy in the drinking water and sanitation sector, is struggling to fulfill its role [33]. In fact, Haitian cities, more particularly Port-au-Prince, where the demand for water is already high, are increasingly exposed to demographic growth which considerably affects water and sanitation infrastructures [15]. The conditions of water supply and sanitation, which were already precarious, deteriorated with the earthquake of January 12, 2010 [34].

The assessments of the burden of disease associated with poor WASH (Water, Sanitation and Hygiene) are 90% dominated by mortality from diarrheal disease and acute morbidity [35]. By combining the multiple health effects, some researchers and research organizations in the health sciences estimate that unsafe WASH is responsible for nearly a tenth of the global burden of disease [36]. Indeed, beyond diseases of the fecal-oral cycle, the scientific literature reports several pathologies resulting from the chronic effect of exposure to poor-quality WASH [37], particularly diseases chronic associated with chemical contamination of water [38].

According to IHE and ICF [39], "73% of the Haitian population uses an improved source of water. Access to an improved source is much more common in urban areas than in rural areas (95% versus 60%). 33% of the population has improved unshared toilets, mainly cesspools with slabs (21%) and a sanitation system connected to a septic tank (9%). It is in urban areas that the proportion of the population with access to improved unshared toilets is highest (43% compared to 23% in rural areas)".

In Port-au-Prince, the risk of fecal contamination of the environment is particularly high. Clusters of fecal coliforms have been found in the water sources used to supply the population of the RMPP [40]. A more probable number (MPN) of 700 fecal coliforms per 100 ml was detected in the groundwater of the Cul-de-Sac plain [41]. This aquifer is the largest source of groundwater used by the population of the Port-au-Prince region to meet their water needs. These results highlight the existence of a bacteriological danger linked to these water resources for the health of consumers.

In addition, oocysts of *Cryptosporidium parvum*, a parasitic protozoan responsible for an infection called cryptosporidiosis, have been detected in surface water, in groundwater and in public water fountains [42]. During the cholera epidemic, declared in October 2010, Cryptosporidium oocysts ranging from 6 to 233 per 100 L of water were detected in water supply points in the RMPP [43]. Cryptosporidiosis is responsible in Haiti for 17% of acute diarrhea observed in children under 2 years of age and 30% of chronic diarrhea in patients infected with HIV [44]. Cryptosporidium oocysts are among the pathogens most resistant to conventional types of treatment such as chemical disinfection, for example [45]. The comparison of statistical data on *Cryptosporidium parvum* contamination of water resources in the City of Port-au-Prince, with those of two other cities (Cap-Haitien [43] and Cayes [46]) is presented in **Table 1**. These studies confirm the need for monitoring of the microbiological quality of water, with a view to reducing the morbidity of infections linked to the consumption of contaminated water.

In Haiti, the basement is primarily limestone [47]. **Figure 3** presents the general geology map of the country [48]. The northern watershed of the Massif de la Selle, the highest chain in the Republic of Haiti with an altitude of more than 2000 meters, is abundantly watered by rainwater [47, 49, 50].

City	Mean	Minimum	Maximum	Standard deviation	n	References
Cap-Haïtien	5053	3583	6088	1095	4	[43]
Cayes	28	3	63	25	5	[46]
Port-au-Prince	64	6	233	68	12	[43]

Table 1.
Statistical data on Cryptosporidium parvum *contamination of water resources in 3 large cities of Haiti.*

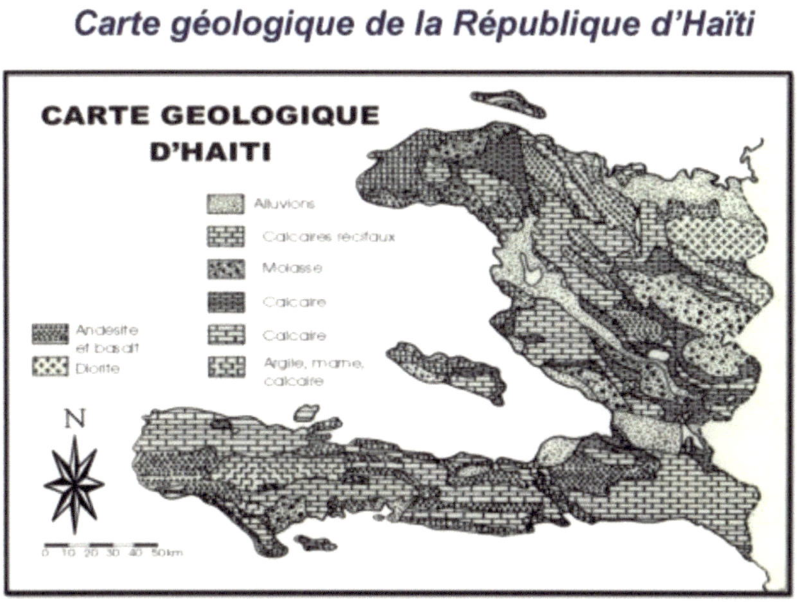

Figure 3.
Geological map of the Republic of Haiti [48] - (map: Reprinting with permission of authors).

This basin is of interest for the water resources of Port-au-Prince, it contains intensely fractured limestone, allowing the storage and circulation of underground water. It follows that this is a major aquifer, a real potential water tower for the RMPP [41]. The geological section of the northern watershed of the Massif de la Selle is shown in **Figure 4** [47]. The predominance of limestone in the geology of this aquifer increases the hardness of these water resources. The work carried out on the surface and underground water resources exploited, to supply the population of the Metropolitan Region of Port-au-Prince (RMPP), revealed a total hardness above 200 mg/L with concentrations in Mg^{2+} less than 7 mg/L [41, 51].

Studies on the health effects of hardness have shown that a total hardness concentration greater than 200 mg/L with a magnesium concentration less than 7 mg/L could affect various organs, including cardiovascular physiology [52]. At very high concentrations, calcium can negatively impact the absorption of other essential minerals for the body, in particular magnesium which is the agent of protection against the calcification of soft tissues due to myocytes [53]. The beneficial effects of water hardness in karst regions come from magnesium. Its deficiency could accelerate the development of atherosclerosis and the induction of platelet aggregation, thus promoting myocardial infarction and cerebrovascular pathologies [54]. The low Mg2+ concentration measured in the water resources of the RMPP may generate health risks for consumers exposed to the influence of

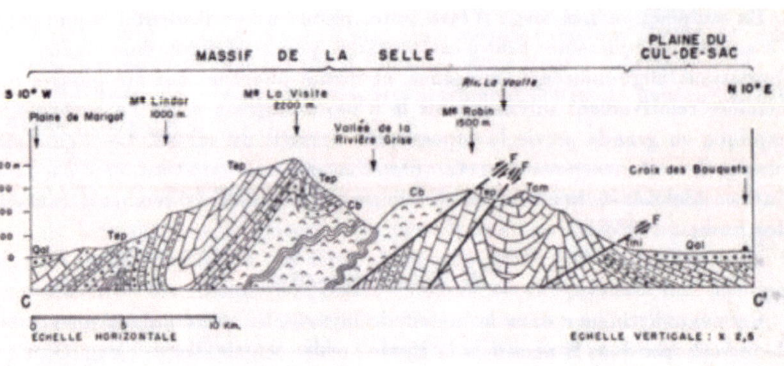

Figure 4.
Geological section of the massif de la Selle [47].

geological and environmental factors. In Haiti, cardiovascular diseases have been placed for several years among the ten (10) leading causes of morbidity in the country [55]. In 2016, 29% of registered deaths were due to cardiovascular diseases [56]; this percentage was 57% for 2018 [57].

Fluorine concentrations ranging from 0 to 1.92 mg/L were measured in the resources of the RMPP. This concentration is distributed up to 1 mg/L in carbonate aquifers and from 1.00 to 1.92 mg/L in sedimentary formations [58]. This variation in fluorine can cause health problems, such as tooth decay in people (especially children) living in areas dominated by carbonate aquifers and fluorosis in people living in areas dominated by sedimentary formations [58].

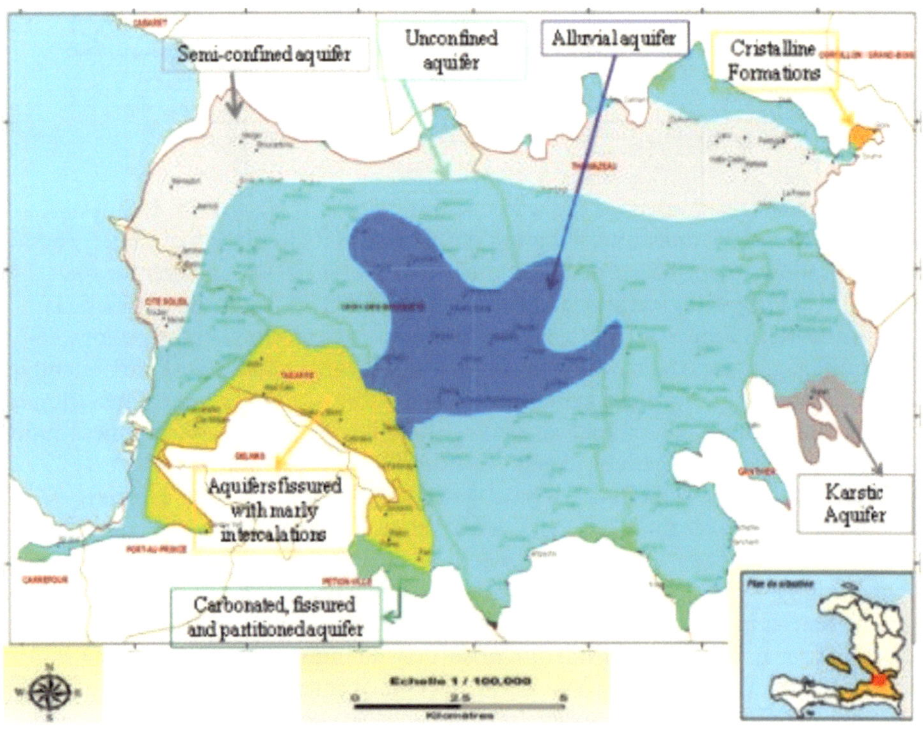

Figure 5.
Map of the Cul-de-sac plain [62] - (map: Reprinting with permission of authors).

The salt contamination of the coastal aquifer of the Plaine du Cul-de-Sac (**Figure 5**) was investigated. According to Gonfiantini and Simonot [59], the salinity of these groundwater is the result of seawater intrusion following intensive exploitation. Between 1988 and 1999, the salinity of these waters increased by 246% [60]. Saline contamination of groundwater is manifested by a high concentration of chlorides, which is associated with dissolved solids and conductivity values in groundwater [61]. At chloride levels greater than or equal to 700 mg/L, salinity can cause problems with pregnancy toxemia or preeclampsia in pregnant women and high blood pressure [2].

Studies have shown the impact of urban pollutants on the physico-chemical quality of groundwater in the Plaine du Cul-de-sac [62]. Lead (40 to 90 μg / L), nickel (15 to 250 μg / L) and Cr (18 to 470 μg/L) concentrations were measured in boreholes in the Plaine du Cul-de-Sac [41, 63]. These values are well above the thresholds recommended by the World Health Organization (WHO) for water intended for human consumption [2]. The behavior of heavy metals (Pb, Cu and Cd) during their transfer into the slick was studied. The conclusions made it possible to understand that cadmium poses many more problems than lead and copper, by comparing their affinity to soil ($Pb2+ > Cu2+ > Cd2+$) [64].

3. Canaan: a shanty town built in a drought-stricken area

3.1 Canaan: a new human settlement in the environmental and urban context of Haiti

The Republic of Haiti occupies the western part of the island of Hispaniola, the eastern part of which constitutes the Dominican Republic (**Figure 6**). It is located at the border of two tectonic plates, the North American plate and the Caribbean plate (**Figure 7**). The country is also on the path of tropical cyclones that originate in the Atlantic Ocean. Like the other territories of the Caribbean, the country is exposed to natural hazards and its history bears witness to these events. Between 1986 and 2016, Haiti recorded several major environmental events (floods, droughts, cyclones and the magnitude 7.2 earthquake on the Richter scale of January 2010).

The environmental and human damage generated by its natural disasters, more particularly that of the earthquake of January 12, 2010, has been the subject of several studies reported in the literature. Indeed, "in the history of urban disasters, the earthquake of January 12, 2010 occupies a special place. Not only in view of the

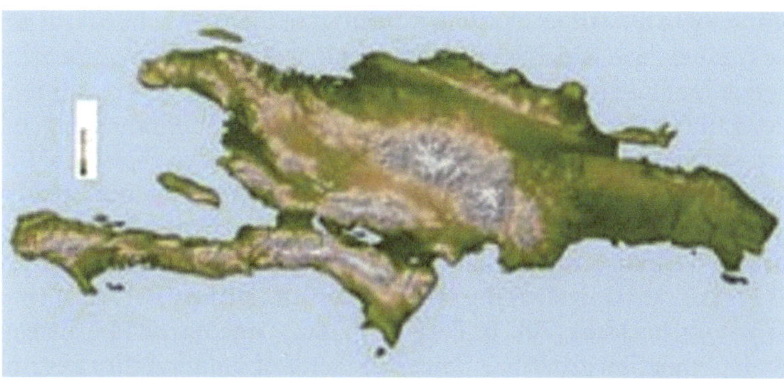

Figure 6.
Topographic map of the island of Hispaniola (Haiti and Dominican Republic). https://simple.wikipedia.org/wiki/Hispaniola.

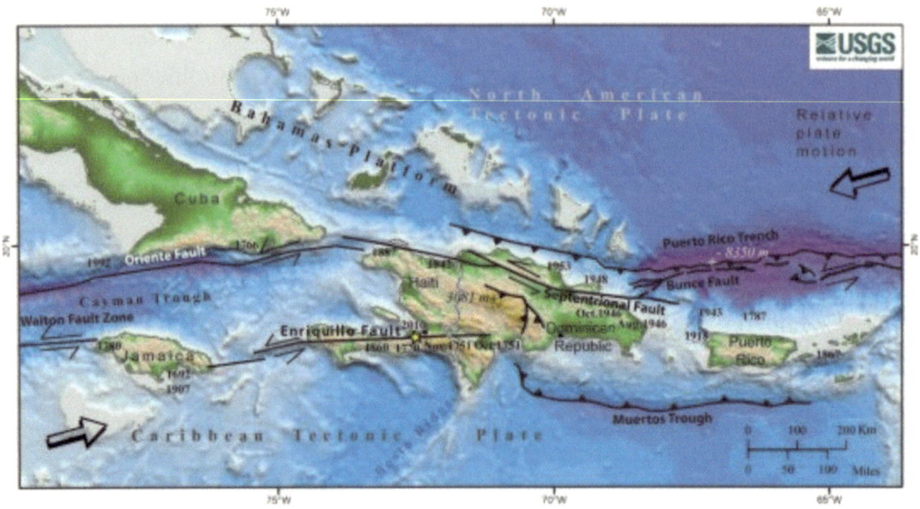

Figure 7.
Map of the north American - Caribbean tectonic plate boundary. https://www.usgs.gov/media/images/map-north-american-caribbean-tectonic-plate-boundary.

extent of the losses and damage caused, but also of the lessons that can be drawn from them in terms of spatial diagnosis and land use planning. Understanding what happened to guard against a bereavement as immense as that caused by the 300,000 deaths in 2010 is a civic duty and an obligation of the state" [65]. Ribordy et al. [66] argue, "the risks engendered by nature and by human activity have accompanied humanity since its origins. In addition to the direct impact of these events on the life of the population, it seems appropriate to retain the intangible impacts (which, in the current state of knowledge, are not translated into monetary terms) such as the degradation of natural environments. and the loss of irreplaceable goods such as heritage", but also the displacement and relocation of inhabitants as well as the increase in the process of urban sprawl [15]. Caught in the paradox of urbanization, the earthquake of January 12, 2010 raises many questions in the scientific community. Why are urban environments the most exposed today to the consequences of natural disasters? How can we understand that contemporary urbanization is intensifying despite the multiplication of disasters and the limits of management efforts [67]? How and why does the disaster produce new urban areas at risk or new vulnerable urban areas likely to contribute to new crises [68]? [...].

Answering these questions requires returning to the very concepts of urbanization, of the rural exodus which is one of the factors of slum development, as well as the function of land use planning in the structuring of human population in Haitian cities. Among the multiple causes of the rural exodus, the migrant's search for a better standard of living should be put in the forefront [69]. The absence of an urban planning and viable housing policy, as well as the non-implementation of land use plans, when they exist, gives free rein to the anarchic development of cities. In fact, in the growth of Haitian cities, precarious slum-type housing has always prevailed. For 11,700 hectares urbanized at the end of the 20th century, Port-au-Prince had 1,802 shanty-town hectares [70]. In Port-au-Prince, "uncontrolled urban sprawl is, along with population growth, a powerful factor of vulnerability to so-called natural hazards. He played a major role in the process of producing vulnerabilities that contributed to the transformation of the hazards of the 2000s in Haiti into real crises linked to major disasters. These catastrophes were crises within the crisis" [68].

According to Gubry [69], "urbanization is in a way a culmination of ongoing economic processes, both those which are part of a development logic, and those which result from the destructuring of rural societies. In addition, urbanization often causes an exacerbation of conflicts between the population and its environment. The importance of the subject will be noted, insofar as the strongest urban growth is to be expected in the countries which are probably the most deprived of the means to cope with it. The urban environment often deteriorates in developing countries as a result of the low standard of living of the population, itself linked to unemployment. Municipal resources are very insufficient to maintain the quality of life: lack of sewerage system, inadequate water supply and garbage collection system, resulting in groundwater pollution; proliferation of pests (rodents, insects, bacteria, etc.)" [69].

In the cities of the South, demographic growth causes heterogeneity of poor households to various forms of lumpenproletariat in addition to socioeconomic inequalities and increased social polarization [30]. Beyond these anthropogenic phenomena and their socioeconomic consequences, it seems appropriate, in the specific case of Haitian cities, to take into account the marked mode of disaster management, according to Desse et al. [68] by "the absence of good coordination between numerous actors within the framework of what we will call humanitarian supervision. Popular strategies of rehousing or access to housing then developed after the catastrophes, hence the pressure on the peri-urban belts. Indeed, all the imbalances suffered by Haitian cities come from their risky growth. The poor occupation of space and the environmental degradation it induces are at the basis of the production of vulnerabilities that have contributed to disasters".

It is in this environmental context characterized, among other things, by an absence of an urban development policy exposed by the earthquake of January 12, 2010 that the human settlement Canaan was founded. The first CANAAN occupants occupied the premises during the first months following the earthquake, ie February/March 2010 [70]. As of April 2010, Canaan lacked basic urban infrastructure such as water, sanitation, and electricity [15]. The situation of Canaan is, however, particularly critical because of the characteristics of the site and the circumstances which led to its rapid settlement.

3.2 Canaan: its creation and its history

The 2010 earthquake was the founding element of many camps established in the metropolitan region of Port-au-Prince while waiting for the issue of the homeless due to the destruction of numerous housing losses to be addressed, and for the right to living in a viable space is applied. The omnipresence of camps throughout the devastated region highlights an often hidden population in Haiti with a major component, that of the poorest. Inside the camps - places of waiting - there is a diversity of people among whom their houses had been destroyed, others coming from disadvantaged neighborhoods and who found in the camps of better living conditions [71].

Canaan is located in the far north of the Metropolitan Region of Port-au-Prince (RMPP), about 18 km from the city center, precisely on a house formerly called Corail Cesselesse, in the communal section of Varreux II, Municipality of the Croix-des-Bouquets. Before 2010, this vast virgin and arid space housed a few peasant families who practiced animal husbandry. For more than 250,000 people, this space has accommodated informally, outside of any urban planning. This dry and hot region with low rainfall (on average 900 mm/year) was declared a public utility area in 1971 with a view to tourist development [72]. Among others, private projects of great importance were considered as part of a master plan for the development of the North Pole. Canaan was the subject of another declaration of public utility published in the Official Journal le Moniteur of March 22, 2010 for the purpose of relocating the victims of the earthquake. This decision first appears to provide a solution to emergency needs following the numerous housing losses and under the weight of land pressure facing the metropolitan region of Port-au-Prince (RMPP). However, previous initiatives never went beyond the project framework for several reasons, including lack of political will for follow-up, lack of funding and the complexity of the land issue. Since then, this space has experienced rapid development with newcomers coming from all over, in search of better living conditions and land ownership [73] to constitute a vast informal habitat [71]. As a system of predatory land developed, "land speculators" saw the opportunity for cheap land to be valued [72]. However, the presidential decree declaring the zone of public utility in its article 2 - Monitor of March 22, 2010 - stipulates that "all construction work, road boring, subdivision or other exploitation of the land, as well as any transaction or real estate alienation"were prohibited there. But over time, the complexity of making it a public space given the high rate of compensation that this population would claim for their relocations would be far too costly. The geographic coordinates of Canaan are 18 ° 38 '46 "N, 72 ° 16' 23" W [74].

3.3 The territory of Canaan: morphology and modes of occupation

Bodson et al. [75] consider that "the recent settlement of the territory of Canaan in the communes of Croix des Bouquets, Thomazeau and Cabaret is part of a major trend which affects all areas near Port-au -Prince. On the other hand, it constitutes a unique phenomenon by the speed of its emergence and by its importance. At the beginning of 2010, the territory was almost unoccupied. The trigger for this meteoric expansion was the presidential decree of March 22, 2010. It followed a very rapid "spontaneous" occupation of the territory". **Figure 8** presents the map of Canaan [76].

The very dry climate and the very dispersed plant cover make the territory a semi-desert area. Along with the poor vegetation cover, the territory is exposed to three major natural environmental risks. Risks related to irregular surface water flows and the lack of availability of quality water have been identified, seismic risks and risks of landslide and surge of friable tailings [77].

In addition to the natural vulnerabilities of the territory, there were major deficiencies in the process of allocating plots and in the organization of services, which could not keep up with the accelerated pace of residential construction. When the post-earthquake emergency response organizations left, national and municipal public authorities did not take over. Besides, could they have done it in the face of the speed and enormity of the current phenomenon? In the absence of the involvement of national and municipal public authorities, the new inhabitants, in collaboration with numerous private initiatives, have organized themselves according to priority emergencies and limitations in the means available. Together with the increase in housing, a relatively dense network of streets and dirt roads (see map below) has thus developed under the control of "local solidarity" and has emerged with the help of private organizations (Protestant missions, Catholic organizations ...) a set of initiatives offering fragments of basic services. The result is a relatively large and complex urban fabric but private, despite the many partial achievements in progress, important basic services to the population, in particular as regards the availability of water for the daily needs of the population. and treatment of sewage and waste.

This situation is not unique to Canaan. It is found in various forms throughout the neighborhoods of the wider area of Port-au-Prince. It is nevertheless

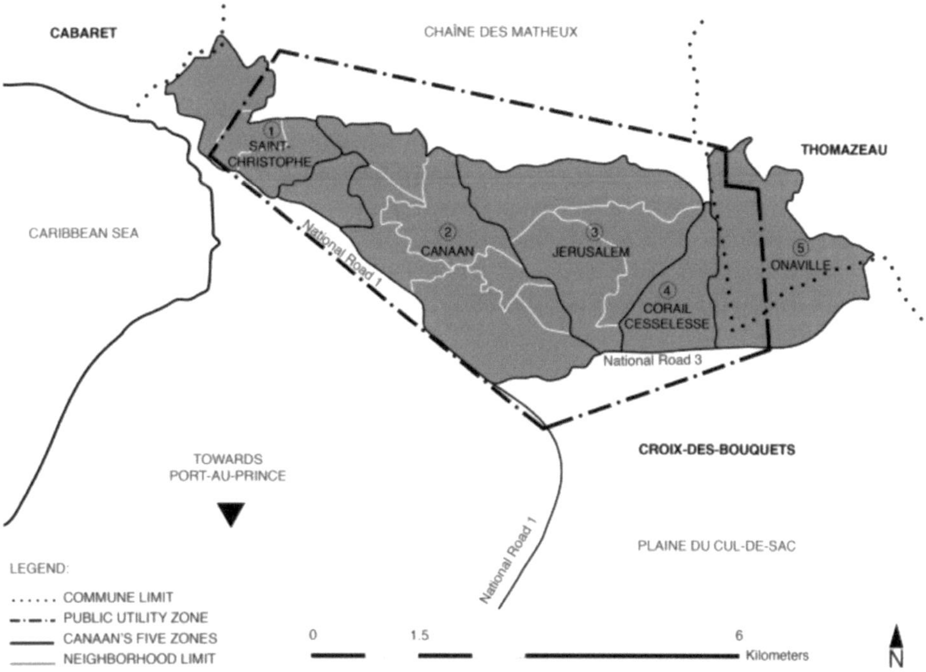

Figure 8.
Map of Canaan [76]- (map: Reprinting with permission of authors).

particularly acute there because of the characteristics of the site and the circumstances which led to its rapid settlement. Canaan is a very vulnerable epidemiological environment today. Little is known about living conditions there. It is in this perspective that we conducted a survey of a sample of 439 households [15]. Carried out within the framework of the research program "Water in the human settlements of the future", of the Center for Research and Support for Urban Policies (CRAPU) of the University of Quisqueya, this survey aimed to analyze the problems of availability and use of water for households located in Canaan and their possible link to the vulnerability of its population to water-borne diseases. Households were selected on the basis of a Simple Systematic Sampling (SSS) design. This plan had to adjust the sounding pitch to take into account the peculiarities of the terrain and as such must be considered non-standard. The selected households are spread over 6 territorial sections of Canaan (11.62% in Canaan 1, 18.68% in Canaan 2, 38.50% in Canaan 3, 5.01% in Canaan 4, 8.66% in Canaan 5, 17.54% in Jerusalem and Bellevue). These 6 sections do not cover the whole of the territory commonly referred to by Canaan, but include most of the nucleus behind the current expansion [15, 75].

3.3.1 Socio-economic characteristics of households

The households appearing in the sample present characteristics similar to those highlighted by the ECVMAS 2012 survey [78] for the metropolitan area, but some traits are modified due to the contribution massive migration that Canaan has experienced since the 2010 earthquake.

Heads of household are on average 42 years old. They are mostly men (60%). These figures contrast with the data from ECVMAS 2012 for the metropolitan area where the average age of heads of household is 46 and where the proportion of women heads of household is 49% [78]. Their level of education is generally slightly lower than that observed in the metropolitan area. The vast majority of heads of household (98%) live in the household. 72% of these are married or "placed".

4.56% of the households surveyed nevertheless have a dwelling provided by humanitarian aid. The homes are located in plots that are generally larger than those in precarious neighborhoods in the metropolitan area. The plots are not systematically contiguous. The result is a relatively dispersed residential space in contrast to the majority of urbanized spaces in the metropolitan area. Residential housing is systematically built on one level. The materials used reflect a very great precariousness.

These households have an average of 5.11 people. In the metropolitan area, this average is 4.5. There are many under 18 s in the households surveyed: 2.25 on average per household, which at least partially explains the difference observed compared to the metropolitan area. The household profile thus partially resembles the mononuclear family without however excluding the extended family profile. The size of the households leads to an overloading of inhabited spaces.

In addition to the overload of occupancy, there are major deficiencies in the services directly associated with homes. Toilets are systematically rudimentary or non-existent. Private toilets are nevertheless predominant (73%). These are very generally located near the inhabited structure or are contiguous to it. Access to electricity from city power is limited to 26.7% of the households surveyed.

Solid waste is treated in a very rudimentary manner. Evacuation by truck from the town hall is almost non-existent (0.5%). The majority of solid waste is incinerated, most often near the house, but dumping in the ravine or in vacant lots is also a common practice (16.6%). In addition, 5.3% of households do not specify what to do with their solid waste. In turn, wastewater receives virtually no specific treatment. For 87.2% of the households interviewed, wastewater is simply thrown outside. 3.2% nonetheless have a canal or ditch to facilitate the evacuation of wastewater, while the remaining 9.1% use another system without specifying the details.

3.3.2 Problems of water availability and use

How are the problems of availability and use of water addressed in this environment marked at the same time by semi-desert climatic conditions, by very rapid population growth, widespread poverty, rudimentary development of residential habitats and degradation? of the environment associated with it? In Canaan, easily accessible quality water resources are systematically lacking. The rains there are relatively infrequent and flow quickly to the surface in a torrential manner. The water in the first levels of the aquifer is salty.

237 water points had been identified, the vast majority of which are located in the 6 sectors of the area covered by the survey. For 166 selected households, an average of 16% of the household head's income is devoted to water. For 25% of households, the percentage of water weight in monthly income exceeds 24% [15].

3.3.3 Vulnerability to diseases associated with the environment

The vast majority of households settled in Canaan are confronted with extremely precarious situations which come from constraints from the natural environment, income limitations, installation conditions (land tenure, quality housing, lack of infrastructure) and the progressive degradation of the environment. The health conditions associated with this context have serious shortcomings and expose the population to increased risk of disease. The households contacted by the survey were affected in various ways by several diseases (diarrhea - 54%;

cholera - 3.6%; malaria - 28.9%; typhoid - 19.8%) associated with the modalities according to which health relations are managed at the environment.

The occurrences per household of the diseases mentioned were grouped together and calibrated into an "index of vulnerability to environmental diseases scaled from 0 to 10. The value 0 corresponds to the absence of any "environmental" disease in the household considered, taking into account the sector where it is located. The value 10 corresponds to a situation where all the households surveyed in a sector would have incurred all the diseases considered by the survey. Over the entire area covered by the survey, the vulnerability index to "environmental" diseases stands at 3.06. The vulnerability index is higher (3.10) in sectors 1, 2, 3 compared to sectors 4, 5 (2.97). On the other hand, this difference fades as certain social-demographic characteristics of households are taken into consideration, the quality of drinking water and water for other domestic uses, and the attitude towards - with regard to the various uses of water (whether or not to distinguish drinking water from other uses), supply systems, certain housing infrastructures, additional water treatment.

The vulnerability index to "environmental" diseases is positively correlated with the size of households (.16 **), with the proportion of young people under 18 in the household (.16 **), but more weakly with proportion of women in the household (.08). It is also negatively correlated in a very statistically very significant way with the quality of drinking water (−.25 **) and with the quality of water for other domestic uses (−.22 **). The explicit distinction by households between drinking water and water for other domestic uses seems to play an important role (F: 9.96, Sig. 002) on the level of vulnerability to environmental diseases. This index stands at 2.97 if the distinction is explicit, but rises to 3.32 otherwise. The choices of supply systems also seem to have a determining influence on the level of vulnerability to environmental diseases. If the drinking water supply is by gallon / sachet, the environmental disease vulnerability index is 2.98, but rises to 3.29 when using other water supply systems. The F-test (8.54) for the relationship between the two variables is statistically very significant (.004). The use of the truck-based supply system when it comes to water for other domestic uses also seems to have a beneficial, but statistically less precise, effect on vulnerability to environmental diseases (F: 3.61 Sig: .058). The environmental disease vulnerability index is 2.99 if the truck-based supply system is used, but rises to 3.17 if other supply systems are preferred.

Whether it is water for drinking or water for other household uses, a number of households resort to water treatment. Do these practices, which are both diverse and variable in their application, help reduce the vulnerability of households to "environmental" diseases? It should be noted first of all that these practices concern a limited percentage of households: 39.2% of households if it is water for drinking and 64.7% of households if it is water for other uses. Domestic workers.

With regard to drinking water, recourse to the Aquatab methods - sodium hypochlorite tablet - (2.95), water filter (2.91) and "Other" (2.59) seem to promote a reduction in vulnerability to environmental diseases. It is quite different if it comes to the use of sodium hypochlorite in liquid form. In this case, the Vulnerability Index increases (3.36) suggesting that this method, as used, makes the situation worse.

If it concerns water treatments for other domestic uses, the results of the statistical analysis are in the same direction as for the treatment of drinking water with regard to the System filter and Aquatab methods but are not statistically significant (F: 1.52, Sig: .20) for all the categories considered. In addition, the results are dominated by the more frequent use of sodium hypochlorite in liquid form, which appears to correspond to an increased vulnerability to "environmental" diseases.

Toilets and their use for the disposal of human excreta can be contaminating factors favoring the spread of environmental diseases. According to the survey data, the average differences in the index of vulnerability to environmental diseases after the methods of disposal of human excreta are not statistically significant. However, we should highlight the almost generalized use of private latrines (73% of households surveyed) and the higher average level of the index of vulnerability to environmental diseases associated with it (3.11), a situation which suggests poor conditions on the health plan in the organization and use of private toilets.

The various factors mentioned interact together on the level of vulnerability to environmental diseases. Their joint incidence was studied by multiple regression.

All the independent variables retained in the model give rise to statistically significant estimates that follow the same logic as that suggested by the bivariate analysis. The estimates highlight the vulnerability to environmental diseases of two categories of people: those under 18 and women. The quality of the water, whether it is drinking water or water for other household uses, contributes to reducing vulnerability to environmental diseases. Implicitly, this type of relationship concerns two major modes of water supply: the purchase of drinking water by gallon / sachet and the delivery of water by truck. These two supply methods are indeed decisive for the quality of the water. According to the estimates obtained, they also contribute directly to the reduction of vulnerability to environmental diseases.

4. Conclusion

Improving living conditions in a sustainable perspective in Canaan presents major challenges. What avenues of intervention should be encouraged or prioritized to facilitate favorable development for the population while taking into account the heavy constraints that weigh on their daily lives? Examination of the data collected by the survey opens up some avenues for reflection that could guide interventions in the field, including from a short-term perspective.

The methods of integrating households in Canaan compromise the quality of life in many aspects: WASH of questionable quality, poor housing, lack or deficiencies in infrastructure and / or basic services, lack of treatment of solid and liquid waste, serious deficiencies in health infrastructures and their functioning, profound degradation of the environment.

In practice, however, local community groups occupy an almost exclusive key position in responding to the basic service needs of the populations. A greater margin for improving the situation is nevertheless accessible from the involvement of these groups and the mobilization of the local population. However, it is a complex challenge to take up because it requires from the population, at the same time an awareness of the situation and of the current issues, sustained and systematic steps of consultation and decision-making. Organization, mastery of a varied range of skills and discipline to promote the best accessible development conditions while minimizing negative external repercussions on the community and the environment.

In the current context of scarce resources and the destitution of almost all households, many loopholes are likely to arise and remain in this community approach. Analysis of the survey data revealed several:

- The non-distinction on the part of many households between drinking water and water for other domestic uses,
- the ineffectiveness of home water treatments,

- the operation of private toilets,
- methods of disposal of wastewater, solid waste and human excreta.

To address these difficulties, targeted interventions to be implemented in consultation and with the participation of local communities would benefit from being considered.

This is particularly the case for water used by households. Measures taken by households to treat water seem unlikely at this stage to even reduce vulnerability to environmental diseases. Household training programs would no doubt be appropriate. But the problem could also be corrected at its source by means of systematic and controlled treatment of the water delivered by gallons and / or by truck.

Complementary to this systematic and controlled treatment, the density of water access points could be intensified. Well coordinated by community groups, this operation could also help reduce spatial disparities in water prices for households. This type of improvement would particularly help to reduce the percentage of households not distinguishing between drinking water and water for other domestic uses.

A support program for the functional establishment of private washrooms would also help reduce the risk of contamination and reduce vulnerability to environmental diseases.

It is also important that local health care organizations take into account the most vulnerable categories of the population, including young people and women.

In setting up these adjustments, consultation with local groups, their initiative and their involvement are essential conditions for success.

Acknowledgements

The authors are thankful to FOKAL-Open Society Foundation Haiti, the AOG (Association communautaire paysanne des Originaires de Grande Plaine) and the SCAC (Service de Coopération et d'Action Culturelle) of the France Ambassy in Haiti for their financial support.

Author details

Yolette Jérôme[1,2,3], Magline Alexis[3,4], David Telcy[4], Pascal Saffache[2] and Evens Emmanuel[5]*

1 Université Quisqueya, Centre de Recherche et d'Appui aux Politiques Urbaines (CRAPU), Port-au-Prince, Haïti

2 Université des Antilles, Faculté des Lettres et Sciences Humaines - Laboratoire de Recherche GEODE Caraïbe (EA 929), Schoelcher, Martinique

3 Association Haïtienne Femmes, Science et Technologie (AHFST), Port-au-Prince, Haïti

4 Université Quisqueya, Faculté des Sciences, de Génie et d'Architecture (FSGA), Programme de Maîtrise en Aménagement et Développement Urbains des Quartiers Précaires, Port-au-Prince, Haïti

5 Université Quisqueya – École doctorale "Société et Environnement" (EDSE), Port-au-Prince, Haïti

*Address all correspondence to: evens.emmanuel@gmail.com

References

[1] Tallon, P., Magajna, B., Lofranco, C., & Leung, K. T. (2005). Microbial indicators of faecal contamination in water: a current perspective. Water, air, and soil pollution, 166(1-4), 139-166.

[2] WHO. (2006). Guidelines for drinking water quality, First Adendum to third ed., Recommendations, vol. 1, 2006, Geneva, Switzerland.

[3] WHO. (2003). Assessing microbial safety of drinking water improving approaches and methods: Improving approaches and methods. OECD Publishing.

[4] Kosek M, Bern C, Guerrant R. The global burden of diarrhoeal disease, as estimated from studies published between 1992 and 2000. Bull. World Health Organ 2003;81(3):197-204.

[5] Copeland, C. C., Beers, B. B., Thompson, M. R., Fitzgerald, R. P., Barrett, L. J., Sevilleja, J. E., ... & Guerrant, R. L. (2009). Faecal contamination of drinking water in a Brazilian shanty town: importance of household storage and new human faecal marker testing. Journal of water and health, 7(2), 324-331.

[6] Petitjean, O. (2009). Gouvernance de l'eau : l'évolution des modèles au niveau international. De Mar del Plata à Istanbul, le rôle des grandes conférences. Débats et enjeux au niveau mondial. Partage des eaux. https://www.partagedeseaux.info/Gouvernance-de-l-eau-l-evolution-des-modeles-au-niveau-international

[7] IS@D (2014). 1992 Conférence èinternationale sur l'eau et l'environnement de Dublin. 26 Janvier - Principes de Dublin. Information sur le développement durable. (IS@D).https://ise.unige.ch/isdd/spip.php?article255

[8] Nations Unies (2000). Déclaration du Millénaire des Nations Unies. Résolution 55/2 de l'Assemblée générale. New York: Nations Unies.

[9] WHO/UNICEF. (2000). Global water supply and sanitation assessment 2000 report. Geneva:World Health Organization.

[10] Herischen, D., Ruwaida, M. S., & Blackburn, R. (2002). Répondre au défi urbain. Population Reports, Série M, 16, 23.

[11] UN-Water WWAP. (2006). L'eau : une responsabilité partagée. Résumé du 2ème rapport mondial des Nations Unies sur la mise en valeur des ressources en eau. Vol 2. 52 p.

[12] Diagne, A. (2009). Interactions entre l'Accès à l'eau Potable et les autres Objectifs du Millénaire pour le Développement: une Analyse à partir de Données sur les Banlieues de Dakar. https://media.africaportal.org/documents/Interactions_entre_l%C3%A1cces_a_leau_potable.pdf

[13] WHO/UNICEF Joint Water Supply, Sanitation Monitoring Programme, & World Health Organization. (2015). Progress on sanitation and drinking water: 2015 update and MDG assessment. World Health Organization.

[14] PNUD (2006). Rapport mondial sur le développement humain de 2006 : Au-delà de la pénurie : pouvoir, pauvreté et crise mondiale de l'eau. New York:PNUD.

[15] Jérôme, Y., Emmanuel, E., Roy, P.-M., Bodson, P. (2017). The issue of water in slums development in Haiti: the case study of Canaan. Aqua-LAC, Vol. 9 (1):87-97.

[16] Milian, J., & Tamru, B. (2018). Port-au-Prince, ville du risque? Un mythe au

prisme d'une urbanisation vulnérable. Études caribéennes, (39-40).

[17] Goulet, J. (2006). L'organisation des services urbains: réseaux et stratégies dans les bidonvilles de Port-au-Prince (Doctoral dissertation, Université du Québec à Montréal).

[18] Barthélémy, G. (1990). L 'univers rural haïtien: le pays en dehors. Paris: L'Harmattan, 189 p.

[19] Etienne S.P. Haïti, Misère de la Démocratie. CRESFED, Paris: l'Harmattan, 1999, 285p.

[20] Bras, A., Kern, A. L., Lucien, G. E., & Emmanuel, E. (2016). Poor Neighbourhood and Natural Disaster. In Learning from the Slums for the Development of Emerging Cities (pp. 81-91). Springer, Cham.

[21] Experco International/Daniel Arbour & Associés. (2003). Plan-Programme de Développement de la Zone métropolitaine de Port-au-Prince. Port-au-Prince, 95 p.

[22] IHSI. (2015). Population totale, de 18 ans et plus: Ménages et densités estimés en 2015. Port-au-Prince: IHSI (Institut Haïtien de Statistique et d'Informatique). 131p.

[23] Godard, H. (1985). Port-au-Prince (Haïti). Les «quartiers» et les mutations récentes du tissu urbain. Les Cahiers d'Outre-Mer, 38(149), 5-24.

[24] Blary,R., N'Guessan,S-M., ANDRÉ F. (2000). Urbanité et quartiers précaires. Revue canadienne d'études du développement, Volume XXI, No. 1, p. 55-87.

[25] Jérôme, Y. (2018). Cycle hydrosocial et la gestion de l'eau dans les bidonvilles du sud : étude de cas de Canaan. Communication orale – 20e rencontre international d'APERAU, 19 au 22 juin 2018, Lille, France.

Lefeuvre J-C., (1996). La pollution des eaux et des systèmes aquatiques. In : Douze questions d'actualité sur l'environnement. Ministère de l'Environnement. Nice : Z'Editions, p.11-16.

[26] Lefeuvre J-C., (1996). La pollution des eaux et des systèmes aquatiques. In : Douze questions d'actualité sur l'environnement. Ministère de l'Environnement Nice : Z'Editions, p.11-16.

[27] PNUE (2010). Un droit de l'eau plus vert : Gérerles ressources en eau douce pour les hommes et l'environnement. PNUE (Programme des Nations Unies pour l'Environnement) – Division du Droit de l'Environnement et des Conventions (DELC), ISBN : 978-92-807-3206-1, 120p.

[28] Les Agences de l'eau (2012). L'eau dans le monde. Disponible sur : http://www.lesagencesdeleau.fr/wp-content/uploads/2012/07/4-Fiche-eau-dans-le-monde_web.pdf. Consulté le 8 janvier 2017.

[29] Dacharry, M., (1984). Spécificité de l'hydrologie urbaine. Bulletin de l'association de géographies français, 500-501:99-109.

[30] Jaglin, S. (2001). L'eau potable dans les villes en développement: les modèles marchands face à la pauvreté. Revue Tiers Monde, t. XLII, 166:275-303.

[31] Etienne, J. (2003). Eau et assainissement: Croyances, modes et modèles.... Afrique contemporaine, (1), 103-117.

[32] Théodat, J.-M., (2010). L'eau dans l'État, l'État nan dlo : dilution des responsabilités publiques et crise urbaine dans l'airemétropolitaine de Port-au-Prince. Bulletin de l'Association de géographes français, 87e année, 3:336-350.

[33] UNICEF Haïti (2013). Eau et assainissement : les défis. https://www.unicef.org/haiti/french/wes.html.

[34] Jérôme, Y., Emmanuel, E., Saffache, P. (2017). L'eau à canaan : quelles formes de participation à une gestion démocratique de ce bien commun ? In. : Bezunesh Tamru, Evens Emmanuel, Alphonse Yapi-Diahou, Anie Bras, Jean-Fritzner Etienne. Quel développement urbain pour la ville post-crise? Pétion-Ville : Editions Pédagogie Nouvelle S.A., pp 79-83.

[35] Prüss, A., David, K., Lorna F., Jamie, B. (2002). Estimating the burden of disease from water, sanitation, and hygiene at a global level. Environ Health Perspect 110(5);537-542. *http://ehpnet1.niehs.nih.gov/docs/2002/110p537542prüss/abstract.html*

[36] Guerrant, R. L., Kosek, M., Moore, S., Lorntz, B., Brantley, R., & Lima, A. A. (2002). Magnitude and impact of diarrheal diseases. Archives of medical research, 33(4), 351-355.

[37] Campbell, O. M., Benova, L., Gon, G., Afsana, K., & Cumming, O. (2015). Getting the basic rights–the role of water, sanitation and hygiene in maternal and reproductive health: a conceptual framework. Tropical medicine & international health, 20(3), 252-267.

[38] Fewtrell L, Fuge R & Kay D (2005) An estimation of the global burden of disease due to skin lesions caused by arsenic in drinking water. Journal of Water and Health 3, 101-107.

[39] IHE et ICF. (2018). Enquête Mortalité, Morbidité et Utilisation des Services (EMMUS-VI 2016-2017). Pétion-Ville:IHE (Institut Haïtien de l'Enfance), et Rockville:ICF.

[40] TRACTEBEL DEVELOPMENT (1998). Définition des périmètres de protection pour les sources exploitées par la CAMEP. Bruxelles.

[41] Emmanuel, E., Pierre, M.G., Perrodin, Y. (2009). Groundwater contamination by microbiological and chemical substances released from hospital wastewater: health risk assessment for drinking water consumers. Environment International, 35:718-726.

[42] Brasseur, P., Agnamey, P., Emmanuel, E., Pape, J. W., Vaillant, M., & Raccurt, C. P. (2011). Cryptosporidium contamination of surface and water supplies in Haiti. Archives of Environmental & Occupational Health, 66(1), 12-17.

[43] Damiani, C., Balthazard-Accou, K., Clervil, E., Diallo, A., Da Costa, C., Emmanuel, E., Totet, A., & Agnamey, P. (2013). Cryptosporidiosis in Haiti: surprisingly low level of species diversity revealed by molecular characterization of Cryptosporidium oocysts from surface water and groundwater. Parasite (Paris, France), 20, 45. https://doi.org/10.1051/parasite/2013045

[44] Pape J.W., Levine E., Beaulieu M.E., Marshall F., Verdier R. & Johnson W.D. (1987) Cryptosporidiosis In Haitian Children. The American Journal Of Tropical Medicine And Hygiene, 36, 333-337.

[45] Fayer R., Morgan U & Upton S.J. (1998) Epidemiology Of Cryptosporidium : Transmission Detection And Identification. International Journal For Parasitology, 30, 1305-1322.

[46] Balthazard-Accou, K., Emmanuel, E., Agnamey, P., Brasseur, P., Lilite, O., Totet, A., Raccurt, C., 2009. Presence of Cryptosporidium oocysts and Giardia cysts in the surface water and groundwater in the City of Cayes, Haiti. Aqua-LAC, 1:63-71.

[47] Butterlin J. Géologie générale de la République d'Haïti. Institut des Hautes Etudes de l'Amérique Latine, Paris, 1960.

[48] Emmanuel, E. et Lindskog P. (2002). Regards sur la situation actuelle des ressources en eau de la République d'Haïti. In Actes du Colloque International Gestion Intégrée de l'Eau en Haïti. Port-au-Prince: Laboratoire de Qualité de l'Eau et de l'Environnement: Université Quisqueya, pp. 30-52.

[49] Woodring, W.P., J.S. Brown, and W.S. Burbank. Geology of the Republic of Haiti. Department of Public Works, Baltimore, Maryland: Lord Baltimore Press, 1924.

[50] PNUD (Programme des Nations Unies), (1991a). République d'Haiti - Développement et gestion des ressources en eau. Disponibilité en eau et adéquate aux besoins. vol 4 Région Centre–Sud. New York, 80 p.

[51] Emmanuel E., Simon Y., Joseph O. (2014) Characterization of hardness in the groundwater of Port-au-Prince. An overview on the health significance of magnesium in the drinking water. Aqua-LAC, 5 (2):35-43.

[52] Rubenowitz – Lundin E., Hiscock M. K (2005). Water Hardness and Health Effects. In: Selinus O., Alloway J. B., Centeno A. J., Finkelman B. R., Fuge R., Lindh U., Smedley P. Essentials of Medical Geology. London: Elsevier Academic Press, pp. 331-345. ISBN: 0-12-636341-2.

[53] Berthollet A. (2003). Le magnésium: un nutriment important. Forum Med Suisse. 27: 638-640.

[54] Eisenberg M.J. (1992). Magnesium deficiency and sudden death. Am. Heart j., 124:544-549.

[55] France, G. (2012). Les maladies chroniques un fléau mondial et un problème majeur de santé publique. Bulletin Trimestriel d'Information Sanitaire, No. avril-juin 2012, p.5-8. https://www.mspp.gouv.ht/site/downloads/BulletinMSPP.pdf

[56] OMS (2018). Profils des pays pour les maladies non transmissibles (MNT), Haïti. https://www.who.int/nmh/countries/hti_fr.pdf?ua=1

[57] OMS (2020). Suivi des progrès dans la lutte contre les maladies non transmissibles 2020. https://apps.who.int/iris/bitstream/handle/10665/332337/9789240002593-fre.pdf

[58] Angerville R., Emmanuel E., Nelson J., Saint-Hilaire P. Evaluation of the fluorine concentration in the water resources of hydrographic area "Centre-Sud" of Haïti. Proceedings of 8th annual CWWA and 4th AIDIS region 1 conference. Kingston, Jamaica, October 4 to 8, 1999. CDROM.

[59] Gonfiantini, R., Simonot, M. (1989) Isotopic study of the groundwater of the flatland of Cul-de-Sac, Republic of Haiti (No. IAEA-TECDOC--502).

[60] Bois M., Emmanuel E., Prévilon E., Laraque E. (1999). Water salinity evaluation from the principal wells of Cul-de-Sac groundwater supplying tank trucks. Proceedings of 8th annual CWWA and 4th AIDIS region 1 conference. Kingston, Jamaica, October 4 to 8, 1999. CDROM.

[61] Isa NM, Aris AZ, Sulaiman WNAW (2012) Extent and severity of groundwater contamination based on hydrochemistry mechanism of sandy tropical coastal aquifer. Science of the Total Environment, 438:414-425.

[62] Fifi U. (2010). Impacts des eaux pluviales urbaines sur les eaux souterraines en zone tropicale : Mécanismes de transfert de métaux lourds à travers un sol modèle de Port-au-Prince (Haïti). *Cotutelle de thèse* École

Doctorale Chimie de Lyon (Chimie, Procédés et Environnement), Institut National des Sciences Appliquées de Lyon, et École Doctorale Société et Environnement, Université Quisqueya. https://uniq.edu.ht/upload/inside_articles_document/9534_these%20urbain%20fifi.pdf

[63] Emmanuel, E., Angerville, R., Joseph, O., Perrodin, Y. (2007). Human health risk assessment of lead in drinking water: A case study from Port-au-Prince Haiti. International Journal of Environment and Pollution, Vol. 31, Nos. 3/4, 280-291.

[64] Fifi, U., Winiarski, T., & Emmanuel, E. (2013). Assessing the mobility of lead, copper and cadmium in a calcareous soil of Port-au-Prince, Haiti. International journal of environmental research and public health, 10(11), 5830-5843.

[65] Emmanuel, E., de Tricornot, H., Theodat, J.-M., Lucien, G.E., Roy, P.-M., Bodson, P. (2012). L'habilitation urbaine post- séisme de Port-au-Prince : quel rôle pour les universités et la recherche?. Pré-actes du colloque international Réhabilitation urbaine de Port-au-Prince, 16-20 avril 2012. Port-au-Prince:Université Quisqueya,75p. https://www.researchgate.net/publication/324503451_Pre-actes_du_Colloque_international_habilitation_urbaine_post-seisme_de_Port-au-Prince_quel_role_pour_les_universites_et_la_recherche

[66] Ribordy, V., Yersin, B., & Vittoz, G. (2002). Catastrophe ou accident majeur: risques dans les pays industrialisés. Médecine et hygiène, 1424-1429.

[67] Desse, M., Clerveau, M., & Lucien, G. E. (2017). Crises et extension urbaine au cœur du pro-cessus de production des vulnérabilités pré et post catastrophes des années 2000 en Haïti. In. : Bezunesh Tamru, Evens Emmanuel, Alphonse Yapi-Diahou, Anie Bras, Jean-Fritzner Etienne. Quel développement urbain pour la ville post-crise? Pétion-Ville: Editions Pédagogie Nouvelle S.A., pp 93-96.

[68] Pigeon, P., (2012). Paradoxes de l'urbanisation. L'Harmattan, 280p.

[69] Gubry, P. (1996). L'environnement urbain. In. Population et environnement dans les pays du Sud. Paris : Karthala, pp.273-288.

[70] Holly, G. (1999). Les problèmes environnementaux de la région métropolitaine de Port-au-Prince. Port-au-Prince, ouvrage collectif, Commission pour la commémoration du 250è anniversaire de la fondation de la ville de Port-au-Prince.

[71] Corbet, A. (2014). Haïti : d'un camp à l'autre. Michel Agier. Un monde de camps, La Découverte, Hors collection Sciences humaines, pp.233-244, 9782707183224. ⟨halshs-01109909⟩

[72] Noël R. (2012). Reconstruction et environnement dans la région métropolitaine : Cas de Canaan ou la naissance d'un quartier ex-nihilo. Port-au-Prince: Group URD, [en ligne], http://www.urd.org/IMG/pdf/ReconstructionetEnvironnement_Rapport_Canaan_Nov2012.pdf.

[73] Corbet A (2012). Approche communautaire en Haïti: décryptage de la notion de communautés et recommandations. Rapport de recherche. Port-au-Prince : Groupe URD. https://hal.archives-ouvertes.fr/ha

[74] ONU-HABITAT (2015). Une vision stratégique et structure urbaine pour Canaan. Première Charrette de planification urbaine. Rapport. Port-au-Prince:ONU-HABITAT.

[75] Bodson, P., Emmanuel, E., Jérôme, Y., Thérasmé, K. (2018). Santé et conditions de vie à Canaan aux confins

de Port-au-Prince. In. : Perspectives de développement de l'Aire Métropolitaine de Port-au-Prince, Horizon 2030. Université du Québec à Montréal. Rapport de recherche, Programme de recherche dans le champ de l'urbain PRCU FED/2015/360-478. Port-au-Prince, pp 235-250. ⟨hal-01944107⟩

[76] Petter, A. M., Labbé, D., Lizarralde, G., & Goulet, J. (2020). City profile: Canaan, Haiti-A new post disaster city. Cities, 104, 102805.

[77] OXFAM GB (2014) Rapport final d'évaluation technique des menaces naturelles de la commune de Croix-des-Bouquets (Haïti) - Guide méthodologique. Londres: OXFAM GB. 77p. https://www.preventionweb.net/files/38544_38544rapportconsultationcartographi.pdf

[78] Herrera, J., Lamaute-Brisson, N., Milbin, D., Roubaud, F., Saint-Macary, C., Torelli, C., Zanuso, C. (2014). L'évolution des conditions de vie en Haïti entre 2007 et 2012 : la réplique sociale du séisme. Paris (FRA) ; Port-au-Prince : DIAL ; IHSI, 220 p. https://www.documentation.ird.fr/hor/fdi:010062827#

Chapter 6

Impact of Arsenic on Reproductive Health

Sweety Nath Barbhuiya, Dharmeswar Barhoi and Sarbani Giri

Abstract

Arsenic is ubiquitously present in the earth's crust. Population across the world gets exposed to arsenic mainly through drinking water, responsible for causing diseases like hypertension, skin pigmentation, skin lesion, cardiovascular diseases, and even cancer. However, arsenic also disturbs the male and female hormone balance in the body, thus, interfering with the process of spermatogenesis and oogenesis. This eventually leads to infertility in the reproductive system irrespective of gender. Cohort studies have revealed that when pregnant women get exposed to arsenic-contaminated water; it leads to abortion, preterm birth, and stillbirth. Thus, arsenic contamination from any source has a devastating effect on the life of organisms and also on the environment.

Keywords: arsenic, stillbirth, groundwater, testosterone, estrogen, endocrine disruptor

1. Introduction

Arsenic is one of the major environmental toxicant that is ubiquitously present all around the earth's crust. Arsenic holds the highest ranking concerning toxicity, frequency, and potential for human exposure since 1997 on the US Agency for Toxic Substances and Disease Registry (ATSDR) substance priority list [1]. Many countries are known to be highly contaminated with arsenic like Hungary, Argentina, Chile, Mexico, the United States of America, and also Asian countries *viz.* Bangladesh, China, Inner Mongolia, and Taiwan, including India [2]. According to World Health Organization (WHO) report, 140 million people from around 50 countries are exposed to arsenic through drinking arsenic-contaminated groundwater [3] at a concentration of 10 μg/L. Arsenic contamination in the groundwater occurs from natural geological sources and also anthropogenic activities [4]. Anthropogenic activities include combustion of fossil fuel, mining, utilization of arsenical pesticides, herbicides, and agricultural additives for livestock are responsible for enhancing arsenic in groundwater and soil [5]. There are two forms of inorganic arsenic: AsIII and AsV, and it is reported that AsIII is the most toxic species [6]. Intake of inorganic arsenic induces cancer of the skin, bladder, and lung [7]. Chronic arsenic exposure is reported to cause cardiovascular, respiratory, hepatic, hematological, neurological, diabetes, and reproductive effects in humans. Studies have reported that arsenic exposure for a longer period in animal models induces reproductive toxicity in both males and females; characterized by impaired ovarian and testicular steroidogenesis, alteration of tissue architecture, and cessation of spermatogenesis and folliculogenesis [8].

2. Chemistry of arsenic

In the natural environment, arsenic shows diverse chemical behavior. Arsenic has the potential to readily change oxidation state and bonding configuration, producing inorganic and organic forms [9]. In the periodic table, arsenic is in the 33rd position of the periodic table, secures a position in Group 15, being a member of the nitrogen family. The atomic number of arsenic is 33 and its atomic weight is 74.921, thus it is heavier than iron, nickel, and manganese but lighter than silver, lead or gold. The electronic configuration of the stable form of arsenic, As (0) is: $1s^2\ 2s^2\ 2p^6\ 3s^2\ 3p^6\ 3d^{10}\ 4s^2\ 4p^3$. There exist four oxidation states of arsenic *viz.* arsines and methyl arsines, elemental arsenic, arsenite, and arsenate, the inorganic form of arsenic is highly lethal and mobile in the atmosphere compared to the organic form. Arsenite is found to be 10 times more poisonous than arsenate [10].

3. Global scenario of arsenic contamination

Arsenic is a matter of global concern because of its adverse health effects. Arsenic is widespread at a high concentration in the groundwater throughout the world: Asia (Bangladesh, China, India, Inner Mongolia, and Taiwan), Europe (Hungary), and the Americas *viz.* Argentina, Chile, Mexico, and the northeast and western United States of America [2]. It was reported that about 150 million people across the world were affected by arsenic and the number is increasing as newly affected areas are discovered continuously [11]. In 2019, the number of affected people has increased to 500 million around the globe [12].

4. Sources of contamination

The establishment of a stable society largely depends upon the availability of safe and reliable water bodies. In the recent world, due to numerous anthropogenic actions, water bodies are contaminated with heavy metals like arsenic [13]. Millions of people across the globe are under the threat of arsenic-related diseases. There are various routes of arsenic exposure but the major one is through the drinking water available from the groundwater [14]. The main reason behind arsenic contamination in the groundwater may be attributed to both natural and anthropogenic activities, producing hazardous effects on health and the environment [11]. In developing countries, owing to a huge number of industries, unfortunately, pollute the air due to the generation of various chemicals, of which arsenic is one of the most toxic chemicals. The occurrence of arsenic in the air as particulate matter is considered to be associated with various diseases [14]. According to the World Health Organization guidelines, the recommended level of arsenic in the aquatic ecosystem, including drinking water is $<10\ \mu g/L$ and this threshold was chosen based on the limits of diagnostic and treatment techniques [15].

According to a recent study by Bundschuh et al. [16] in Latin America, seven possible sources of arsenic are being determined and they are as follows:

i. Volcanism and geothermalism

ii. Mining and related activities leads to deposition of natural lixiviation and accelerated mobilization from (mostly sulfidic) metal ore

iii. Deposition of coal and their exploitation

iv. Hydrocarbon reservoirs and water produced during exploitation

v. Transportation of solute and sediment via rivers to the sea

vi. Atmospheric Arsenic through dust and aerosol

vii. Exposure of arsenic through involuntary ingestion and geophagy.

Thus, there are several pathways through which people get exposed to arsenic in different regions but the outcome of the exposure is dangerous to both living organisms and the environment.

5. Reproductive health

5.1 Arsenic induced reproductive toxicity in human

A study was carried out among the population of Dhaka, Bangladesh; consisting of a total number of 192 participants (married women of reproductive age 15–49 years). From the study, it was observed that the women exposed

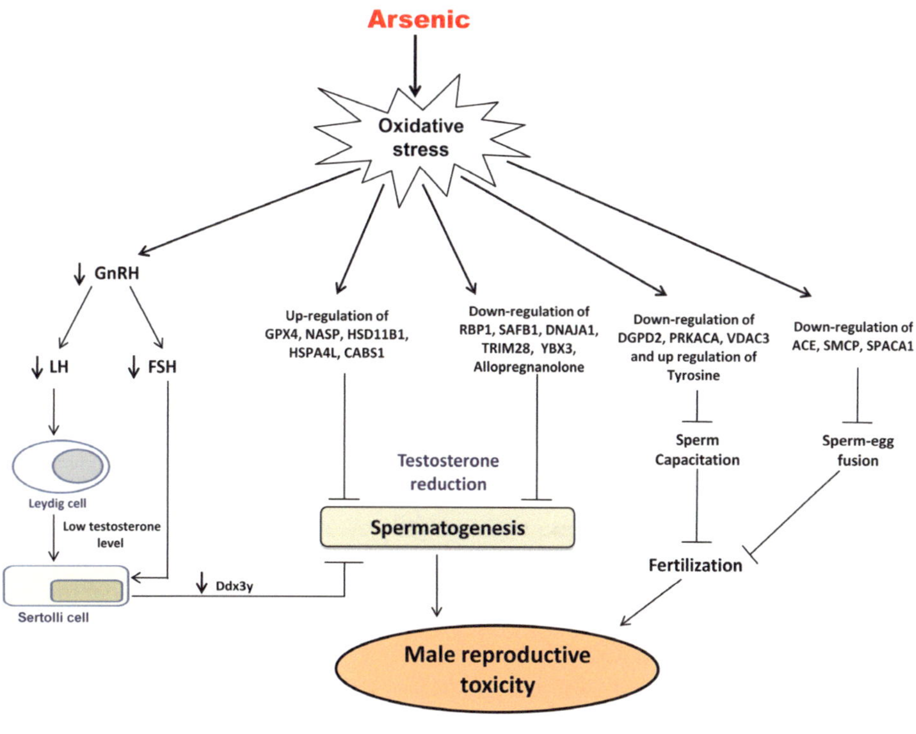

Figure 1.
Schematic representation of the pathways through which arsenic induces male reproductive toxicity. GPx4: glutathione peroxidase, NASP: nuclear autoantigenic sperm protein, HSD11B1: 11β-hydroxysteroid dehydrogenase, HSP4AL: heat shock 70 kDa protein 4-like, CABS1: calcium-binding and spermatid-specific protein 1, RBP1: retinol-binding protein 1, SAFB1: scaffold attachment factor B1, DNAJA1: DNAJ homolog subfamily a member 1, TRIM 28: transcription intermediary factor 1-beta, YBX3: Y-box binding protein 3, GPD2: glycerol-3-phosphate dehydrogenase, mitochondrial, PRKACA: cAMP-dependent protein kinase catalytic subunit alpha, VDAC3: voltage-dependent anion-selective channel protein 3, ACE: angiotensin-converting enzyme, SMCP: sperm mitochondrial-associated cysteine-rich protein and SPACA1: sperm acrosome membrane-associated protein 1.

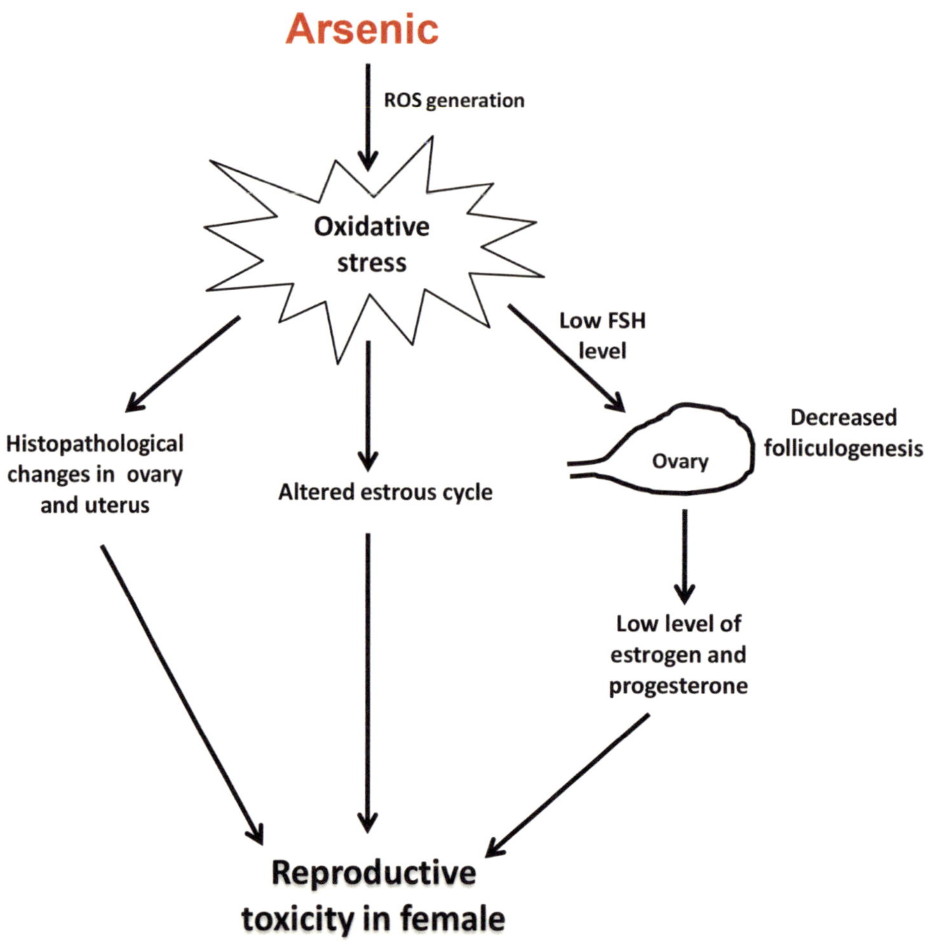

Figure 2.
Schematic overview of arsenic induced reproductive toxicity in female.

to arsenic-contaminated drinking water (>0.05 mg/L) had adverse pregnancy outcomes *viz.* abortion, stillbirth, and preterm birth at a much higher rate than the non-exposed (<0.02 mg/L) groups [17]. Another study conducted on 202 married women in West Bengal, India showed that pregnant women exposed to arsenic-contaminated drinking water had a six times higher rate of stillbirth than compared to non-exposed pregnant women [18]. According to a cohort study done in Bangladesh, comprising of 1458 women, it was observed that arsenic exposure is directly proportional to the adverse reproductive and maternal health of the exposed women [19]. In the year 2008, a group of researchers reported that drinking arsenic-contaminated water by the woman was associated with a higher risk of stillbirth. In this study, the total number of cases studied was n = 30,984 and it was conducted in the rural area of Bangladesh [20]. According to a report, there is an increase in the rate of arsenic methylation effectiveness and total arsenic content of urine in pregnant women (n = 1613) of Bangladesh. The samples (urine) were collected at two prenatal time periods: first at 4–16 weeks and the second at 21–37 weeks of pregnancy [21]. Arsenic is a well-known toxicant and a prospective study was taken up from two studies conducted in Matlab, Bangladesh. This study included 809 girls who participated at the age of their menarche and had a previous report of prenatal exposure to arsenic via the tube well water that was used by their mother during pregnancy. The outcome of the study is that girls prenatally exposed to arsenic have delayed menarche, indicating endocrine disruption that eventually may impair the total reproductive system [22]. Arsenic exerts its toxicity by following different pathways as detailed in **Figures 1** and **2**.

5.2 Arsenic mediated toxicity in animal models

5.2.1 Toxicological implications in the male reproductive system

Chemical	Animal model	Treatment	Observation	Reference
Arsenic	Swiss albino mice	Arsenic was administered at a concentration of 30 and 40 mg/L for a period of 30, 45, and 60 days via drinking water.	The results showed a relative decline in the testicular weight in experimental animals, with dose-dependent gradual diminution in seminiferous tubule diameter and gametogenic cell population. Leydig cell atrophy increased in the arsenic exposed groups, indicating the ill effects of arsenic on spermatogenesis.	[23]
Arsenic	Swiss albino mice	The experimental animals were exposed to arsenic at a level of 53.39, 133.47, 266.95, and 533.90 μmol/L for 35 days through drinking water.	The results revealed that at the lower doses (53.39, 133.47, and 266.95) μmol/L, the sperm count, motility, and morphological abnormalities are similar to the control group. However, at the highest dose, i.e., 533.90 μmol/L, a sharp decline in sperm count and motility, along with abnormal sperm cells was evident.	[24]
Arsenic	Swiss albino mice	Mice were treated with 53.39 μmol/L sodium arsenite (4 ppm As) via drinking water for 365 days.	A marked decrease in the absolute and relative testicular weight was observed. The sperm count, motility was decreased upon arsenic exposure while there is an increment in abnormal sperm. The long-term arsenic exposure decreased the activities of marker testicular enzymes such as sorbitol dehydrogenase, acid phosphatase, and 17β-hydroxysteroid dehydrogenase (17β-HSD), but those of lactate dehydrogenase and, y-glutamyl transpeptidase (y-GT) were significantly increased.	[25]
Arsenic	Rat	Arsenic (sodium arsenite) treatment of 5 mg/L through drinking water was given for 4 weeks	The results indicated decreased testicular weights, accessory sex organ weight, and low sperm count, as well as degeneration of a wide variety of germ cells at the 7th stage of the spermatogenic cycle.	[26]
Arsenic	Mice	Mice received arsenic (arsenic trioxide) through oral gavage daily at a level of 3 and 4 mg/kg BW for 56 days.	The study reveals that arsenic treatment causes damage to the spermatogonia and the testosterone level decreases with an increase in the extent of arsenic exposure.	[27]
Arsenic	Swiss albino mice	Mice were treated with arsenic at a level of 10, 25, 50, 100, and 200 ppm for 40 days.	Mice treated with arsenic showed a dose-dependent decline in testosterone level.	[28]

Chemical	Animal model	Treatment	Observation	Reference
Arsenic	Swiss albino mice	Arsenic trioxide at a dose of 3 and 4 mg/kg BW were administered orally to mice for 8 weeks.	Arsenic treatment causes decreased testosterone level and elevated luteinizing hormone. This indicated impairment of Leydig cells, leading to poor sperm production and eventually led to infertility in experimental animals.	[29]
Arsenic	Sprague-Dawley rat	Treatment of arsenic was given to rats (male) at a dose of 1, 5, and 25 mg/L for 6 months.	Arsenic concentration in serum was found to range from 0.18–0.67 μg/ml, while in testis it was recorded as 0.35–1.74 μg/ml. This suggests that arsenic can pass through the blood-testis barrier and accumulate in rat testis, causing adverse effects in the male reproductive system. In the present study, five proteins (GPX4, HSD11B1, NASP, HSP4AL and CABS1) were found to be upregulated while five other proteins (SAFB1, TRIM28, RBP1, DNAJA1, YBX3) were downregulated including one metabolite (Allopregnanolone) in response to arsenic exposure during spermatogenesis, causing impaired spermatogenesis and formation of low-quality sperm. Arsenic treatment represses three proteins (VDAC3, PRKACA and GPD2) as well as increases the L-tyrosine level, causing disruption of protein tyrosine phosphorylation, necessary for sperm capacitation, leading to inhibition of fertilization and male infertility. Arsenic exposure also affects fertilization by decreasing the expression levels of SPACA1, ACE and SMCP in rat testis, inhibiting the binding and fusion of sperm to egg. It was observed that the differential proteins and metabolites associated with male reproduction, was also found to be involved in ERK/AKT/NF-κ B pathway. The up-regulation of ERK1/2, PI3K, AKT, IKKγ and NFKB gene expression, alongwith enhanced phosphorylated ERK/AKT level in rat testis, it was reported that arsenic may induce male reproductive toxicity through activated ERK/AKT/NF-κ B pathway.	[30]
Arsenic	Wistar rats	Rats were treated with 0.1 and 10 mg/L of sodium arsenite and sodium arsenate daily for 56 days via drinking water.	Arsenic treatment showed a dose-dependent decrease in the sperm-count parameters and epididymal morphometry. This indicates arsenic exposure causes adverse effects to male reproductive functions in adult Wistar rats.	[31]
Arsenic	Mice	The experimental animals were treated with arsenic trioxide at a dosage of 1, 2 and 4 mg/L via drinking water for 60 days.	It was observed that subchronic arsenic exposure induces downregulation of Ddx3y expressions in the testis and epididymis, which may adversely affect spermatogenesis, leading to male reproductive toxicity.	[32]

5.2.2 Arsenic mediated toxicity in the female reproductive system

Chemical	Animal model	Treatment	Observation	Reference
Arsenic	Sprague-Dawley rats	50, 100, and 200 ppm of arsenic was administered to the animals through drinking water for 28 days.	Treatment of arsenic to immature rats showed decreased uterine diameter and epithelium height. The thickness of the endometrium and myometrium also got reduced.	[32]
Arsenic	Albino Wistar strain rats	10 mg/kg bodyweight of arsenic was administered orally to the experimental animals for 8 days.	The study showed reduced glutathione peroxidase, superoxide dismutase, and catalase activities. Treatment of arsenic also induced DNA break and necrosis in the uterine tissues. Arsenic exposure even leads to disruption in the steroidogenesis process.	[33]
Arsenic	Albino Wistar strain rats	The experimental animals were treated with an aqueous solution of arsenic trioxide at a dose level of 3 ppm/rat/day orally.	Serum estradiol level decreased due to arsenic exposure. Degeneration of Ovarian DNA was prominent in the treated groups.	[34]
Arsenic	Kunming mice	Arsenic is injected with distilled water as vehicle control to the experimental animals at a concentration of 8 mg/kg per day bodyweight on every alternate day for 16 days.	Treatment of arsenic increased reactive oxygen species (ROS) generation in the ovary of treated mice.	[35]
Arsenic	Wistar albino rats	Three doses 10, 30, and 50 μg/L of arsenic were administered to the mice via drinking water for 60 days.	Arsenic exposure disrupted the estrous cycle with a prolonged diestrous and metestrus phase. An increase in many follicular atresia was evident from the study.	[36]
Arsenic	Sprague-Dawley rats	The experimental animals were treated with a dose of 4 μg/ml per day for 28 days.	The results indicated that arsenic exposure disturbed the gonadotropins and estradiol levels, causing disintegration of the luminal epithelial, myometrial and stromal cells of the uterus. The study also showed that arsenic exposure leads to downregulation of the downstream components of the estrogen signaling pathway.	[37]
Arsenic	Albino rats	Albino rats were treated with arsenic (sodium arsenite) at a dose of 0.4 ppm for 28 days.	The arsenic-treated rats showed a prolonged diestrous phase. Treatment with arsenic also led to a significant diminution of the entire uterine diameter. It was also evident from the study that the endometrium is not well-defined and the lumen became narrow and unfolded, indicating damage in the reproductive system of the female upon exposure to arsenic.	[38]

Chemical	Animal model	Treatment	Observation	Reference
Arsenic	Wistar rats	Sodium arsenite was administered at a dose of 3 ppm during the pre-natal and post-natal development.	Arsenic exposure resulted in decreased folliculogenesis, the morphological characteristic of the ovaries were disturbed, and modified the adrenocortical cell number, causing the delayed onset of puberty.	[39]
Arsenic	Wistar rats	Rats were orally administered with sodium arsenite (0.4 ppm) for two time periods—16 and 28 days.	Arsenic treatment reduced ovarian steroidogenic dehydrogenase activity. The study also showed diminished levels of luteinizing hormone, follicle-stimulating hormone, and estrogen upon exposure to arsenic.	[40, 41]
Arsenic	Mice	Arsenic (arsenic trioxide) was administered at a dose of 0, 0.2, 2 and 20 ppm to the parents from 35 days before breeding and is continued until weaning. The female offspring received the same treatment until maturity.	Arsenic trioxide (As_2O_3) exposure at a higher dose in the prenatal or parental stage via drinking water induces autophagy in the ovaries of mature F1-female mice via activation of autophagic genes (PDK1, TSC2, P13K, P62, ATG13, AMPK, ULK1, ATG12, ATG5, LC3, Beclin1, ATG3, ATG7 and p62) and proteins (Beclin1, LC3-I, II and mTOR), resulting in decreased female gametes number as compared to the control.	[42]

6. Epigenetic effect of arsenic on reproductive system

Epigenetics is the study of how cells control gene activity without altering the DNA sequence. It was reported that arsenic causes hypermethylation of the of the p53 gene and thus, gained the attention of the researchers regarding the epigenetic effects of arsenic [43]. Exposure to inorganic arsenic is found to be associated with epigenetic modifications like gene specific DNA methylation, histone acetylation, phosphorylation, methylation and altered expression of miRNAs, which may induce carcinogenesis or other diseases [44]. According to a report, arsenic exposure during gestation increases the hypomethylation of active Long Interspersed Nuclear Element (LINE) and Long Terminal Repeat (LTR) subfamilies of the offspring sperm, causing transgenerational effects. The study indicates that retrotransposon methylomes in the sperm is one of the main targets of arsenic when exposed during gestation period [45]. Another study showed that arsenic (As_2O_3) exposure to parents at a dose of 1 mg/L has adverse transgenerational effects on the reproductive phenotype in both male and female offspring after attaining maturity, which may be due to an altered global DNA methylation pattern in gonadal tissue [46]. Thus the studies indicate that arsenic exposure at the gestation period is enough to induce toxicity in the reproductive system of the future generations.

7. Conclusion

Arsenic is a well-documented toxicant available all around the earth's crust. Arsenic has the potential to cause various diseases *viz.* cardiovascular diseases, hypertension, diabetes, skin lesion, and also cancer. So, its presence in the environment both in the groundwater or air is very harmful to the livelihood of organisms as well as for the atmosphere. Arsenic has the potential to decrease the male reproductive hormones like testosterone and may inhibit spermatogenesis. It can also adversely affect the folliculogenesis of females by disturbing the female monthly cycle. This is brought about by arsenic due to its massive capacity to reduce hormone synthesis (follicle stimulating hormone and estrogen). The exposure to arsenic in the case of a pregnant woman leads to severe implications like stillbirth, preterm birth, and abortion. Thus, sources of arsenic exposure may vary from region to region but the ill effects of it are very much prominent and thus, suitable techniques and methodologies are to be adopted to reduce the burden of diseases associated with arsenic exposure.

Author details

Sweety Nath Barbhuiya*, Dharmeswar Barhoi and Sarbani Giri
Laboratory of Cell and Molecular Biology, Department of Life Science and Bioinformatics, Assam University, Silchar, Assam, India

*Address all correspondence to: sweetynath91@gmail.com

References

[1] Shih YH, Islam T, Hore SK, Sarwar G, Shahriar MH, Yunus M, et al. Associations between prenatal arsenic exposure with adverse pregnancy outcome and child mortality. Environmental Research. 2017;**158**:456-461. DOI: 10.1016/j.envres.2017.07.004

[2] Wang A, Holladay SD, Wolf DC, Ahmed SA, Robertson JL. Reproductive and developmental toxicity of arsenic in rodents: A review. International Journal of Toxicology. 2006;**25**(5):319-331. DOI: 10.1080/10915810600840776

[3] World Health Organization (WHO). Fact sheets on Arsenic. Available from: http://www.who.int/news-room/fact-sheets/detail/arsenic. [Accessed: 25-08-2021]

[4] Ratnaike RN. Acute and chronic arsenic toxicity. Postgraduate Medical Journal. 2003;**79**(933):391-396

[5] Das N, Patel AK, Deka G, Das A, Sarma KP, Kumar M. Geochemical controls and future perspective of arsenic mobilization for sustainable groundwater management: A study from Northeast India. Groundwater for Sustainable Development. 2015;**1** (1-2):92-104. DOI: 10.1016/j.gsd.2015.12.002

[6] Ahmad SA, Khan MH, Haque M. Arsenic contamination in groundwater in Bangladesh: Implications and challenges for healthcare policy. Risk Management and Healthcare Policy. 2018;**11**:251. DOI: 10.2147/RMHP.S153188

[7] Mukherjee A, Sengupta MK, Hossain MA, Ahamed S, Das B, Nayak B, et al. Arsenic contamination in groundwater: A global perspective with emphasis on the Asian scenario. Journal of Health, Population, and Nutrition. 2006;**1**:142-163

[8] Khatun S, Maity M, Perveen H, Dash M, Chattopadhyay S. Spirulina platensis ameliorates arsenic-mediated uterine damage and ovarian steroidogenic disorder. FACETS Journal. 2018;**3**(1):736-753. DOI: 10.1139/facets-2017-0099

[9] O'Day PA. Chemistry and mineralogy of arsenic. Elements. 2006;**2**(2):77-83

[10] Jang YC, Somanna Y, Kim HJ. Source, distribution, toxicity and remediation of arsenic in the environment—A review. International Journal of Applied Environmental Sciences. 2016;**11**(2):559-581

[11] Shankar S, Shanker U. Arsenic contamination of groundwater: A review of sources, prevalence, health risks, and strategies for mitigation. The Scientific World Journal. 2014;**2014**: 1-18. DOI: 10.1155/2014/304524

[12] Shaji E, Santosh M, Sarath KV, Prakash P, Deepchand V, Divya BV. Arsenic contamination of groundwater: A global synopsis with focus on the Indian Peninsula. Geoscience Frontiers. 2020;**12**(2020):101079. DOI: 10.1016/j.gsf.2020.08.015

[13] Saikia KC, Gupta S. Assessment of surface water quality in an arsenic contaminated village. American Journal of Environmental Sciences. 2012;**8**(5): 523. DOI: 10.3844/ajessp.2012.523.527

[14] Chung JY, Yu SD, Hong YS. Environmental source of arsenic exposure. Journal of Preventive Medicine and Public Health. 2014;**47**(5): 253. DOI: 10.3961/jpmph.14.036

[15] Masuda H. Arsenic cycling in the Earth's crust and hydrosphere: Interaction between naturally occurring arsenic and human activities. Progress in Earth and Planetary Science. 2018;**5**(1):1-11. DOI: 10.1186/s40645-018-0224-3

[16] Bundschuh J, Schneider J, Alam MA, Niazi NK, Herath I, Parvez F, et al. Seven potential sources of arsenic pollution in Latin America and their environmental and health impacts. The Science of the Total Environment. 2021;**8**:146274. DOI: 10.1016/j.scitotenv.2021.146274

[17] Ahmad SA, Sayed MH, Barua S, Khan MH, Faruquee MH, Jalil A, et al. Arsenic in drinking water and pregnancy outcomes. Environmental Health Perspectives. 2001;**109**(6):629-631

[18] Von Ehrenstein OS, Guha Mazumder DN, Hira-Smith M, Ghosh N, Yuan Y, Windham G, et al. Pregnancy outcomes, infant mortality, and arsenic in drinking water in West Bengal, India. American Journal of Epidemiology. 2006;**163**(7):662-669. DOI: 10.1093/aje/kwj089

[19] Kile ML, Rodrigues EG, Mazumdar M, Dobson CB, Diao N, Golam M, et al. A prospective cohort study of the association between drinking water arsenic exposure and self-reported maternal health symptoms during pregnancy in Bangladesh. Environmental Health. 2014;**13**(1):1-3. DOI: 10.1186/1476-069X-13-29

[20] Cherry N, Shaikh K, McDonald C, Chowdhury Z. Stillbirth in rural Bangladesh: Arsenic exposure and other etiological factors: A report from Gonoshasthaya Kendra. Bulletin of the World Health Organization. 2008;**86**:172-177

[21] Gao S, Lin PI, Mostofa G, Quamruzzaman Q, Rahman M, Rahman ML, et al. Determinants of arsenic methylation efficiency and urinary arsenic level in pregnant women in Bangladesh. Environmental Health. 2019;**18**(1):1-4. DOI: 10.1186/s12940-019-0530-2

[22] Rahman A, Kippler M, Pervin J, Tarafder C, Lucy IJ, Svefors P, et al. A cohort study of the association between prenatal arsenic exposure and age at menarche in a rural area, Bangladesh. Environment International. 2021;**154**:106562. DOI: 10.1016/j.envint.2021.106562

[23] Sarkar S, Hazra J, Upadhyay SN, Singh RK, Chowdhury AR. Arsenic induced toxicity on testicular tissue of mice. Indian Journal of Physiology and Pharmacology. 2008;**52**(1):84-90

[24] Pant N, Kumar R, Murthy RC, Srivastava SP. Male reproductive effect of arsenic in mice. Biometals. 2001;**14**(2):113-117

[25] Pant N, Murthy RC, Srivastava SP. Male reproductive toxicity of sodium arsenite in mice. Human & Experimental Toxicology. 2004;**23**(8):399-403. DOI: 10.1191/0960327104ht467oa

[26] Jana K, Jana S, Samanta PK. Effects of chronic exposure to sodium arsenite on hypothalamo-pituitary-testicular activities in adult rats: Possible an estrogenic mode of action. Reproductive Biology and Endocrinology. 2006;**4**(1):1-3. DOI: 10.1186/1477-7827-4-9

[27] Kumar R, Khan SA, Dubey P, Nath A, Singh JK, Ali MD, et al. Effect of arsenic exposure on testosterone level and spermatogonia of mice. World Journal of Pharmaceutical Research. 2013;**2**:1524-1533

[28] Guvvala PR, Sellappan S, Parameswaraiah RJ. Impact of arsenic (V) on testicular oxidative stress and sperm functional attributes in Swiss albino mice. Environmental Science and Pollution Research. 2016;**23**(18):18200-18210. DOI: 10.1007/s11356-016-6870-3

[29] Ali M, Khan SA, Dubey P, Nath A, Singh JK, Kumar R, et al. Impact of arsenic on testosterone synthesis pathway and sperm production in mice.

Innovative Journal of Medical and Health Sciences. 2013;**4**:185-189

[30] Huang Q, Luo L, Alamdar A, Zhang J, Liu L, Tian M, et al. Integrated proteomics and metabolomics analysis of rat testis: Mechanism of arsenic-induced male reproductive toxicity. Scientific Reports. 2016;**6**(1):1-2. DOI: 10.1038/srep32518

[31] Souza AC, Marchesi SC, Ferraz RP, Lima GD, Oliveira JA, Machado-Neves M. Effects of sodium arsenate and arsenite on male reproductive functions in Wistar rats. Journal of Toxicology and Environmental Health, Part A. 2016;**79**(6):274-286. DOI: 10.1080/15287394.2016.1150926

[32] Li Y, Wang M, Piao F, Wang X. Subchronic exposure to arsenic inhibits spermatogenesis and downregulates the expression of ddx3y in testis and epididymis of mice. Toxicological Sciences. 2012;**128**(2):482-489. DOI: 10.1093/toxsci/kfs169

[33] Akram Z, Jalali S, Shami SA, Ahmad L, Batool S, Kalsoom O. Adverse effects of arsenic exposure on uterine function and structure in female rat. Experimental and Toxicologic Pathology. 2010;**62**(4):451-459. DOI: 10.1016/j.etp.2009.07.008

[34] Dash M, Maity M, Dey A, Perveen H, Khatun S, Jana L, et al. The consequence of NAC on sodium arsenite-induced uterine oxidative stress. Toxicology Reports. 2018;**5**:278-287. DOI: 10.1016/j.toxrep.2018.02.003

[35] Mondal S, Mukherjee S, Chaudhuri K, Kabir SN, Kumar MP. Prevention of arsenic-mediated reproductive toxicity in adult female rats by high protein diet. Pharmaceutical Biology. 2013;**51**(11):1363-1371. DOI: 10.1016/j.toxrep.2018.02.003

[36] Wang XN, Zhang CJ, Diao HL, Zhang Y. Protective effects of curcumin against sodium arsenite-induced ovarian oxidative injury in a mouse model. Chinese Medical Journal. 2017;**130**(9):1026. DOI: 10.4103/0366-6999.204927

[37] Mehta M, Hundal SS. Effect of sodium arsenite on reproductive organs of female Wistar rats. Archives of Environmental & Occupational Health. 2016;**71**(1):16-25. DOI: 10.1080/10915810600840776

[38] Chatterjee A, Chatterji U. Arsenic abrogates the estrogen-signaling pathway in the rat uterus. Reproductive Biology and Endocrinology. 2010;**8**(1):1-1

[39] Elshawarby AM, Saleh HA, Attia AA, Negm EA. Arsenic-induced toxicity in the endometrium of adult albino rat and the possible role of human chorionic gonadotropin hormone: A histological study. Egyptian Journal of Histology. 2014;**37**(2):327-338. DOI: 10.1097/01.EHX.0000446582.73701.1b

[40] Dávila-Esqueda ME, Jiménez-Capdeville ME, Delgado JM, De la Cruz E, Aradillas-García C, Jiménez-Suárez V, et al. Effects of arsenic exposure during the pre-and postnatal development on the puberty of female offspring. Experimental and Toxicologic Pathology. 2012;**64**(1-2):25-30. DOI: 10.1016/j.etp.2010.06.001

[41] Chattopadhyay S, Pal SG, Chaki S, Debnath J, Ghosh D. Effect of sodium arsenite on plasma levels of gonadotrophins and ovarian steroidogenesis in mature albino rats: Duration-dependent response. The Journal of Toxicological Sciences. 1999;**24**(5):425-431

[42] Ommati MM, Shi X, Li H, Zamiri MJ, Farshad O, Jamshidzadeh A, et al. The mechanisms of arsenic-induced ovotoxicity, ultrastructural alterations, and autophagic related

paths: An enduring developmental study in folliculogenesis of mice. Ecotoxicology and Environmental Safety. 2020;**204**:110973. DOI: 10.1016/j.ecoenv.2020.110973

[43] Mass MJ, Wang L. Arsenic alters cytosine methylation patterns of the promoter of the tumor suppressor gene p53 in human lung cells: A model for a mechanism of carcinogenesis. Mutation Research, Reviews in Mutation Research. 1997;**386**(3):263-277. DOI: 10.1016/S1383-5742(97)00008-2

[44] Ray PD, Yosim A, Fry RC. Incorporating epigenetic data into the risk assessment process for the toxic metals arsenic, cadmium, chromium, lead, and mercury: Strategies and challenges. Frontiers in Genetics. 2014;**5**:201. DOI: 10.3389/fgene.2014.00201

[45] Nohara K, Nakabayashi K, Okamura K, Suzuki T, Suzuki S, Hata K. Gestational arsenic exposure induces site-specific DNA hypomethylation in active retrotransposon subfamilies in offspring sperm in mice. Epigenetics & Chromatin. 2020;**13**(1):1-4

[46] Nava-Rivera LE, Betancourt-Martínez ND, Lozoya-Martínez R, Carranza-Rosales P, Guzmán-Delgado NE, Carranza-Torres IE, et al. Transgenerational effects in DNA methylation, genotoxicity and reproductive phenotype by chronic arsenic exposure. Scientific Reports. 2021;**11**(1):1-6. DOI: 10.1038/s41598-021-87677-y

Chapter 7

Fluoride Content in Drinking Water and the Health Implications of Fluoride-Rich Water Consumption: An Overview of the Situation in Canada and Nigeria

Ochuko Orakpoghenor, Talatu Patience Markus, Meshack Inotu Osagie and Paul Terkende Hambesha

Abstract

Fluoride is an inorganic monatomic anion of fluorine and forms part of essential reagents used by the chemical industry. It occurs naturally in several minerals and in trace quantities in water. Fluoride has been used to prevent tooth decay and in the treatment of osteoporosis. Extensive research has consistently demonstrated the safety and effectiveness of fluorides in the prevention of dental caries following the practice of water fluoridation. Despite these benefits, fluorides pose danger as an endocrine disruptor thus, affecting bones, brain, thyroid gland, pineal gland and blood sugar levels. In Canada, water fluoridation remains a contentious issue although dental decay constitutes the most common chronic disease. However, several Canadians are receiving the benefits of water fluoridation and about 1% have access to naturally fluoridated water. In Nigeria, the prevalence of dental caries has been documented to be greatly reduced following fluoridation of public water supplies in areas where the condition was endemic. Fluoride is therefore the only medicine added to public water, and at the recommended level, fluoride is safe and effective in the reduction of dental decay and poses no risk for health problems. Hence, this article highlighted fluoride content in drinking water and the health implications of consuming fluoride-rich water with a focus on the situation in Canada and Nigeria.

Keywords: fluoride, water, dental decay, health

1. Introduction

Fluoride, an inorganic monatomic anion, is the simplest anion of fluorine and represented by the chemical formula F^-. Fluoride salts and minerals are essential chemical reagents and industrial chemicals used in the production of hydrogen fluoride for fluorocarbons. Fluoride ions occur on earth in several minerals, particularly fluorite, but are only present in trace quantities in water and contribute a distinctive bitter taste [1, 2]. Fluoride is added to public drinking water, toothpaste and mouthwashes to prevent tooth decay by protecting teeth from bacteria in plaque [3–5]. Also, fluoride is taken orally for the treatment of osteoporosis as well as for the prevention of bone loss in people with rheumatoid arthritis by promoting new bone formation [6]. Since the inception of water fluoridation, extensive research has consistently demonstrated the safety and effectiveness of fluorides in the prevention of dental caries [7–9]. Furthermore, there has been continual monitoring of this scientific literature by the world's major National and International Health Organizations, committees of experts and special councils of governments [8].

2. Effects of fluoride in the body (fluorosis)

Many assumption states that consuming fluoride only pose risk on dental health [10]. However, fluoride affects many tissues in the body besides the teeth [3]. Fluoride has been reported to be an endocrine disruptor that can affect the bones, brain, thyroid gland, pineal gland and blood sugar levels. The ability of fluoride to cause brain damage constitutes one of the most active areas of fluoride research and many studies have demonstrated that fluoride is a neurotoxin (a chemical that can damage the brain) [11]. Studies have demonstrated association of fluoride toxicity with varieties of health problems including increased lead absorption, disruption of collagen synthesis and muscle disorders, hyperactivity and/or lethargy, thyroid disease and lowered thyroid function, arthritis, bone fractures and bone cancer (osteosarcoma), dementia, genetic damage and cell death, increased cancer rate, disruption of the immune system and inhibition of antibodies formation and damage of sperms and increased infertility [3, 11–13].

Most developed countries do not fluoridate their water and countries that fluoridated their water do not have less tooth decay than countries that do not fluoridate their water [3]. Based on the few data available on fluoride in drinking water, there is an established relationship between dental caries and environmental fluoride in drinking water [14]. Although with decline in the water supply systems in most parts of Nigeria due to increasing human population demand, about 90% of people use groundwater (well and borehole) for drinking and other domestic purposes [15]. About 40% of American teenagers show visible signs of fluoride overexposure. In infants, fluoridated water provides no benefits but only risks. However, swallowing fluoride tablets provides little benefit to the teeth [14].

3. Water fluoridation in Canada

In North America, dental decay constitutes the most common chronic disease with over 96% of Canadians being affected [11]. The use of water fluoridation for the prevention of tooth decay has been used for over 60 years and is endorsed by various organizations, including Health Canada, the Canadian Public Health Association, the Canadian Dental Association, the Canadian Medical Association and the World Health Organization [3]. Approximately, 42.6% of public water supplies in Canada receive water fluoridation [16]. Over 13 million Canadian's are receiving the benefits of water fluoridation, while another 1% (270,000 people) has access to naturally fluoridated water [14]. As of 2011, the large Canadian cities without water fluoridation were Vancouver, Regina, Montreal and Calgary [4].

DOI: http://dx.doi.org/10.5772/intechopen.97209

The recommended optimal level of fluoride (0.7 mg/L) [8] is set to promote public health benefits of fluoride for preventing tooth decay while minimizing the chance for dental fluorosis. The Guidelines for Canadian Drinking Water Quality states that the maximum acceptable concentration of fluoride in public water supplies is 1.5 mg/L to protect against health risks from exposure to too much fluoride [11]. However, with fluoride levels above 1.5 mg/L over a period of time, the effects of fluorosis are observed [8].

Water fluoridation remains a contentious issue in Canada and many communities chose to fluoridate their water supply [3]. As of 2007, 45.1% of the Canadian population had access to fluoridated water supplies [9, 11]. The main argument for and against fluoridation have changed very little over the years, with supporters (including the World Health Organization and Health Canada) citing evidence that shows fluoridation as a safe and effective method of caries prevention, while detractors cite high costs and potential health risks [17].

4. Water fuoridation in Nigeria

The mottling and staining of teeth (dental caries) previously believed to be an identity of certain ethnic groups or communities in Nigeria has been described to be associated with fluorosis [18]. Hence dental caries has extended beyond tribal or communal barriers as foreigners that came from far away Asia also showed evidence of this disease condition [15]. From records, the prevalence of dental caries was greatly reduced in areas where dental caries was endemic following fluoridation of public water supplies [3]. However in Nigeria, dental caries is endemic and epidemic mainly in the North Eastern half of Nigeria both in the crystalline basement and sedimentary areas. Also, fluoride values (0.2–8 mg/L) above the 1.5 mg/L WHO recommended level have been recorded in groundwater in Nigeria (**Figure 1**) [15, 20].

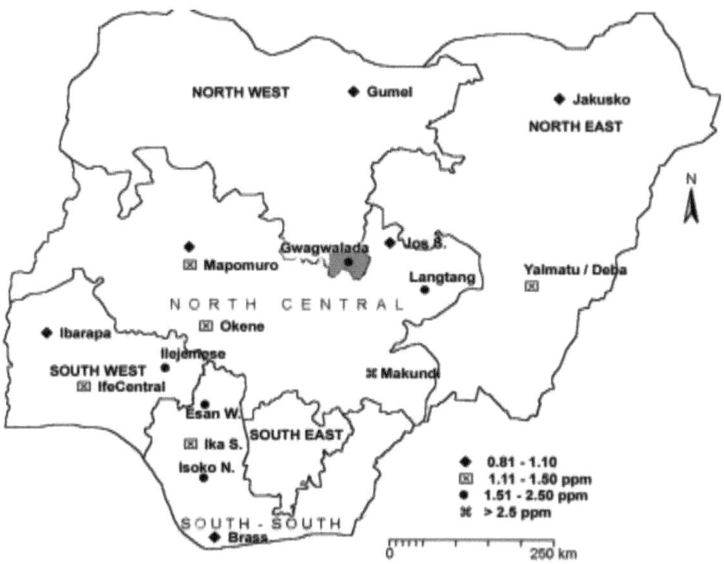

Figure 1.
Areas with drinking water containing fluoride levels higher than 0.8 ppm in the six geopolitical zones of Nigeria [19].

5. Conclusion

Fluoride is the only medicine added to public water, and water fluoridation at the recommended level is safe and effective in the reduction of dental decay and poses no risk for health problems. Hence, it will be of public health benefit to ascertain that the well-being of the populace is safe guarded by knowing the level of fluoride is within the acceptable limit. Also, there should be recommendation for compliance with the WHO guidelines to the permissible limit by the policy makers.

Conflict of interest

The authors declare no potential conflict of interest.

Author details

Ochuko Orakpoghenor[1*], Talatu Patience Markus[2], Meshack Inotu Osagie[3] and Paul Terkende Hambesha[4]

1 Department of Veterinary Pathology, Ahmadu Bello University, Zaria, Nigeria

2 Department of Veterinary Microbiology, Ahmadu Bello University, Zaria, Nigeria

3 Department of Veterinary Public Health and Preventive Medicine, Ahmadu Bello University, Zaria, Nigeria

4 Veterinary Teaching Hospital, Federal University of Agriculture, Makurdi, Nigeria

*Address all correspondence to: ochuko.orakpoghenor@gmail.com

References

[1] Aigueperse J, Mollard P, Devilliers D, Chemla M, Faron R, Romano R, Cuer JP. Ullmann's Encyclopedia of Industrial Chemistry. 2000

[2] Liteplo DR, Gomes R, Howe P, Malcolm H. Fluorides - Environmental Health Criteria 227: 1st draft. Geneva: World Health Organization. 2002

[3] World Health Organization (WHO). Fluoride in drinking-water. 2004

[4] Tiemann M. Fluoride in Drinking Water: A Review of Fluoridation and Regulation Issues. Congressional Research Service. 2013. p. 3. Retrieved 6 May 2016.

[5] Griffin SO, Regnier E, Griffin PM, Huntley V. Effectiveness of fluoride in preventing caries in adults. Journal of Dental Research. 2007;86 (5): 410-415.

[6] Haguenauer D, Welch V, Shea B, Tugwell P, Adachi JD, Wells G. Fluoride for the treatment of postmenopausal osteoporotic fractures: a meta-analysis. Osteoporosis International. 2000;11(9): 727-738.

[7] Singh KA, Spencer AJ, Armfield JM. Relative effects of pre- and post-eruption water fluoride on caries experience of permanent first molars. Journal of Public Health and Dentistry. 2003;63(1):11-9.

[8] National Toxicology Program. Toxicology and carcinogenesis studies of sodium fluoride (CAS No. 7681-49-4) in F344/N rats and B6C3F mice (drinking water studies). ResearchTriangle Park, NC: National Institute of Health, Public Health Services, 1990.

[9] Centers for Disease Control and Prevention (CDC). Using Fluoride to Prevent and Control Tooth Decay in the United States. Community Water Fluoridation. [Online] January 7, 2011. [Cited: July 25, 2011.] http://www.cdc.gov/fluoridation/fact_sheets/fl_caries.htm

[10] Malinowska E, Inkielewicz I, Czarnowski W, Szefer P. (2008). Assessment of fluoride concentration and daily intake by human from tea and herbal infusions. Food Chemistry and Toxicology. 2008; 46(3): 1055-1061.

[11] JCDA. www.cda-adc.ca/jcda. July/August 2009, Vol. 75, No. 6

[12] McDonagh MS, Whiting PF, Wilson PM, Sutton AJ, Chestnutt I, Cooper J, Misso K, Bradley M, Treasure E, Kleijnen J. Systematic review of water fluoridation. British Medical Journal. 2000;321(7265): 855-859.

[13] Levy M, Leclerc BS. Fluoride in drinking water and osteosarcoma incidence rates in the continental United States among children and adolescents. Cancer Epidemiology. 2012;36 (2): 83-88.

[14] Health Canada. Report on the Findings of the Oral Health Component of the Canadian Health Measures Survey 2007-2009. Ottawa : 2010.

[15] Lar AU, Dibal H, Schoeneich K. Fluoride in Groundwater in Nigeria: Origin and Human Health Impact. American Journal of Environmental Protection. 2014;3(6-2): 66-69.

[16] Health Canada. Fluoride and Human Health. Healthy Living: It's Your Health. 2011. http://www.hc-sc.gc.ca/hl-vs/iyh-vsv/environ/fluor-eng.php#prov.

[17] Yeung CA. A systematic review of the efficacy and safety of fluoridation. Evid. Based Dent. 2008;9 (2): 39-43.

[18] Wongdem JG, Aderinokun GA, Sridhar MR, Selkur, S. Prevalence and distribution pattern of enamel fluorosis in Langtang Town. African Journal of Medical Science. 2003;35: 120-135.

[19] Akpata ES, Danfillo IS, Otoh EC, Mafeni JO. Geographical mapping of fluoride levels in drinking water sources in Nigeria. African Health Science. 2009;9(4): 227-233.

[20] Dibal HU, Lar UA. Preliminary survey of fluoride concentrations in the groundwater of Kaltungo area, Gombe State, northeastern Nigeria. Journal of Environmental Sciences. 2005; 9(2): 41-52.

Section 3

Air, Water and the Earth

Chapter 8

Sustainable Use of Biochar in Environmental Management

*Ammal Abukari, Ziblim Abukari Imoro,
Abubakari Zarouk Imoro and Abudu Ballu Duwiejuah*

Abstract

Conversion of agricultural wastes into eco-friendly and low cost biochar is not only a smart recycling strategy but a panacea to environmental pollution management. Agricultural wastes biochar can be an effective alternative technique for controlling contaminants due to its low cost, high-efficiency, simple to use, ecological sustainability and reliability in terms of public safety. Biochars have made substantial breakthroughs in reducing greenhouse gases emissions, reducing soil nutrient leaching, sequester atmospheric carbon into the soil, increasing agricultural productivity, and reducing bioavailability of environmental contaminants. Recent advances in the understanding of biochars warrant a proper scientific evaluation of the relationship between its properties and impact on soil properties, environmental pollutant remediation, plant growth, yield, and resistance to biotic and abiotic stresses. The main factors controlling biochar properties include the nature of feedstock, heat transfer rate, residence time and pyrolysis temperature. Biochar efficacy in pollutants management largely depends on its elemental composition, ion-exchange capacity, pore size distribution and surface area, which vary with the nature of feedstock, preparation conditions and procedures. The chapter explored the possibility of using biochar from agricultural wastes as a suitable alternative for the remediation of environmental pollutants, soil conditioning and the long-term biochar application in the environment.

Keywords: agricultural waste, biochar, elemental composition, carbon sequestration, environmental pollution

1. Introduction

Agricultural waste has been widely studied for at least 6 decades now [1]. This waste stream continues to increase in line with agricultural production [2]. This has negative impacts on the environment (soil, water and air) and human health [1]. Though agriculture accounts for 21% of global greenhouse emissions [1], it is its solid waste that is most obvious and an immediate environmental problem. Meanwhile, the world is fighting for zero solid waste [3]. Some uses of agriculture waste include; the fertilisation of farms through animal manure, the use of agriculture solid waste as adsorbents (ie, for heavy metal remediation), production of biochar from agricultural waste, use of agricultural waste as animal feed and as heating (energy) sources. Renewable energy (biofuels) can also be produced from agriculture waste [4]. The reduction in the quantity or total elimination of agricultural solid waste is an important consideration in the promotion of environmental health. One viable method to safely reduce agricultural solid waste is to convert them into biochar.

Biochar is a carbon-rich by-product produced from the thermochemical conversion of biomass feedstock under partial or total absence of oxygen (pyrolysis) [5]. Principally, biochar is produced through various thermochemical conversion methods such as low pyrolysis, fast pyrolysis, and gasification, under different process parameters [6]. Biochar production and application has increased significantly recently. Significant attention has been given to biochar in relation to agriculture, climate, energy and environment [7]. The adsorption capability of biochar can largely be accrued to its surface chemistry, specific area, and pore structure [8]. Humans over the years have used biochar for various activities due to its naturally occurring characteristics like surface functional groups, thermal recalcitrance, cation exchange capacity, calorific value, specific surface area, porosity, electrical conductivity, volatile contents, fixed carbon and pH [8]. These properties have been traversed for numerous beneficial application such as the amendment of soil [8]. Due to the continuous increase in food insecurity, greenhouse gases emissions and environmental safety demands, biochar in recent years have been linked to the development of sustainable agriculture and soil management as well as carbon sequestration [9].

Biochar application has proven to be a very favourable method for simultaneously solving the numerous multipronged issues. The bioavailability of toxic metals in water and soil can be reduced using biochar, hence, biochar aids in subsiding toxic metal pollution as well as enhancing the quality of contaminated water and soil [9]. Biochar is capable of removing inorganic and organic contaminants due to its intrinsic properties and characteristics such as high cation exchange capacity, non-carbonised fraction, coupled with high surface area and oxygen-rich functional groups on surface [10].

The emission of greenhouse gases poses a great challenge to the industrial world we have today [11]. This has greenhouse gas emissions have a significant adverse impact on the environment including air pollution and inducing climate change [12]. Industrialisation is required for human perpetuity and development hence pollutants generated through the processes cannot stopped, however, it can be reduced by replacing toxic substances and polluting compounds with less toxic substances that has both political and economic feasibilities [13]. There is the need to manage and protect soil, water and air sustainably during large scale agricultural practices and massive industrial activities. This can be done through the use of biochar which is carbonaceous product of biomass pyrolysis.

Biochar has been widely known for its ability to serve as remediator of contaminant, plays a vital role climate change mitigation and bioenergy production. Biochar could have an important effect on soil biological and nutritional properties as well as greenhouse emissions. It is evident that most of the Sustainable Development Goals (SDGs) can be achieved through biochar application and production. It has been proven that biochar could be a sustainable solution for numerous problems that is putting the earth at risk, hence, much research needs to be carried out on the production and application of biochar as one of the most important and beneficial steps to take.

1.1 Conversion of agricultural waste into biochar

Most agricultural solid waste can be converted into biochar [14, 15] and there are different methods for the production of biochar from this waste stream. These include hydrothermal carbonisation [16], gasification and pyrolysis [15]. However, pyrolysis is the most used method for the production of biochar [14]. This involves the irreversible thermal decomposition of organic substances at higher temperatures under anoxic conditions. Biochar from pyrolysis can be used as an energy source [17] and for soil quality improvements. With the production and use of biochar from agricultural waste, a circular economy within the agricultural industry can be realised. Besides biochar, pyrolysis also produces volatile liquids and could either be slow, fast, flash and intermediate pyrolysis [18]. Slow pyrolysis is usually carried out below the temperature of 450 °C [18], at atmospheric pressure [15] and takes several hours to complete. A heating rate of 17 °C min^{-1} may be used [19]. The main product of slow pyrolysis is char [18]. Traditional Kilns and special reactors (ie, Elsa barrel pyrolyser) are used for slow pyrolysis. The source of feedstock for biochar production can influence its quality in terms of environmental safety and sustainable use. Thus feedstocks (wastewater sludge, municipal and industrial solid wastes, etc) which are potential sources of pollutants (heavy metals, PAHs, PCBs, etc) should be avoided. Biochar from these feedstocks can therefore serve as secondary pollutants [20] and require further treatment before use.

1.2 Biochar elemental composition

The characteristics and application of a substance is determined by the composition and structure of that substance. According to literature the composition of biochar is made up of elements such as carbon (C), hydrogen (H), oxygen (O), nitrogen (N), sulphur (S), phosphorus (P), potassium (K), calcium (Ca), magnesium (Mg), sodium (Na), and silicon (Si). Carbon takes up more 60% of the biochar contents followed by H and O. The ash contains mainly the mineral elements [21]. The C found in biochar is aromatic carbon which are in irregular piles or stack of stable aromatic rings [22]. Different variants of carbon compounds most likely consists of alcohols, fatty acids, phenols, esters, humic acid and fulvic acid. Relatively, humic acid and fulvic acids are found in fresh biochar, livestock manure biochar and low temperature pyrolytic biochar [23]. Biochars within a C-N heterocyclic structure have nitrogen to be largely present on the surface and the available N is very low in biochar [9]. Phosphorus is relatively low in biochar. The availability of P greatly varies, and has a negative correlation with carbonisation temperature. This differences may be as a result of high pH value and phosphates containing Ca and Mg formed during carbonisation processes [24, 25]. The contents of K, Ca, Mg, and Na is largely dependent on the type of biochar. Low-valence metal ions such as K and Na are more available than the high-valence metal ions such as Al, Ca, and Mg in biochar. In general, the elemental composition and activity of biochar are related to raw materials, conditions of carbonisation process and pH [24].

Biochar's mineral component has been given less attention as compared to carbon. Current studies suggested that minerals biochar can significantly impact biochar attributes, hence affecting its use either directly or indirectly. According to literature Mg, Ca, K, and P in biochar can become a direct source of mineral nutrients thus promoting plant growth attributes and anions including CO_3^{2-}, OH^-, SO_4^{2-} and PO_4^{3-} leached from biochar are largely significant in eliminating toxic metals through the formation of metal precipitates [26]. Mineral components and carbon of biochar contribute significantly to the removal of toxic metals from solutions [26]. Biochar contain sulphur are much more efficient in making complex surfaces and could be useful in heavy metal removal from contaminated water. The porosity and surface area of biochars are important physical features which affects the adsorption of heavy metals capability from water. In terms of environmental application, molar ratios (i.e. O/C and H/C) are important factors that plays significant roles in determining interface interactions between the surface of the biochar and target matrices [27]. The meso-porous and macro structure of biochars derived from plants are known to be reliant on the intrinsic makeup of the feedstock, which is very vital for determining pollutant adsorptive and water-holding capacity in soil and solution systems [28]. A well-developed pore structure of biochars that consist of stable aliphatic chain structure, and high mineral content [29], have the potential to control water pollution, mitigate greenhouse gas emissions, and remediate soils [30]. The potential to utilise biochar for various applications is related to its properties.

Biochar with high porosity and plenty of liming and fertiliser-related elements (such as N, P and K) is preferred for improving soil properties [31]. A study conducted by [32] also indicated that the innate minerals of biomass could affect biochar properties significantly through interaction with its organic contents during pyrolysis process. However, removal of these intrinsic minerals before the pyrolysis process could significantly increase the optimum pyrolysis temperature (370 vs. 350 °C) required for the conversion of the biomass into biochar, as compared to untouched biomass. Interestingly, about 30.1% of C content of biomass could be secluded into biochar when there are no inherent biomass materials, simultaneously, lower amounts of low-molecular-weight organic compounds would be emitted during pyrolysis [32]. Therefore, the type and amount of minerals in biomass must be optimised according to the intended environmental application of biochar.

1.3 Role of biochar in pollution management

The continuous increase in the world population has cause an accompanying increase in anthropogenic polluting activities. This situation has caused several problems including global increments in atmospheric temperatures, droughts, floods, acid rains and increments in the spread of diseases. Effective and affordable solutions to these problems are yet to be arrived at. Biochar has been found to possess the potential to directly and indirectly alleviate the occurrences and effects of these problems. It uses are broad and includes the removal of pollutants (organic and inorganic) from wastewater [33]. Biochar have used been to remove antibiotics from wastewaters. Heavy metals (Cu, Pb, Ni, Cd) [34] and nutrients (nitrogen and phosphorus) [35] in wastewater have also been removed with biochar. Biochar can be used to either replace or augment sand filters in wastewater treatment because of its ability to remove particulate matter and pollutants such as pathogens [16]. It has also been used for chemical oxygen demand (COD) removal efficiency of 74 ± 18% was recorded in a treatment process [36].

The environment or surrounding systems are often degraded by contaminants discharged from residential, commercial and industrial sources. Literature reveals that soil and water media are more affected by both organic and inorganic contaminants in an ecosystem which is largely the cause of anthropogenic activities. Over the years, there is a rapid increase in technological advancement in soil and water remediation. One of the most paramount technologies is the reduction of bioavailable contaminants which would in turn lead to a significant decrease in the accumulation of toxic substance in plants and animals.

Materials that are carbonaceous have been adopted as sorbents for organic and inorganic contaminants in soil and water for a very long time now [37]. The multifunctional properties of biochar showed the potential as a sorbent for organic and inorganic contaminants in soil and water. The greatest concern of organic contaminants such as pesticides, herbicides, polycyclic aromatic hydrocarbons, dyes, and antibiotics have been a concern due to its toxicity and accumulative properties [38]. In the soil medium, biochar has been used for heavy metal sequestration [39, 40]. In this process, heavy metals are immobilised not removed and maybe converted into hydroxide, carbonate, and phosphate precipitates [40]. Sequestration of pesticides from polluted soils [15] and carbon sequestration (climate change mitigation measure) have also been achieved in soils amended with biochar [15]. In recent years biochar has become a focus for most researchers in the field of soil environment due its increasing potential to serve as carbon sinks, reducing greenhouse gas emissions, reducing the pressure on the burning of stray and finally remediating contaminated soil.

Properties of biochar such carbonaceous materials, degree of aromatization, elemental composition, pH, pore structure, surface chemistry, etc., plays vital roles in its ability to adsorb organic pollutants [41]. Biochar therefore reduces CO_2 emissions into the atmosphere [39]. The indiscriminate exploitation of natural resources and the rapid growth of environmental destruction resulting from anthropogenic activities have already posed a burden on efforts to sustain natural environment. Biochar's uses also includes the neutralisation of acidic soils and this is because of its calcium and magnesium carbonate contents [39] and ability to elevate pH [40]. Reducing acidity may however negatively affect acid loving worms and fungi in the soil environment [42]. Moreover, biochar can be used to enhance the biodegradation of organic pollutants because of the availability of suitable surfaces for microbial attachments [40] and the introduction of nutrients such as N, P and K [20]. In anaerobic digesters, biochar has been used to limit the effect of NH_4^+ [43] and may as well be used as buffering agents in these digesters [44].

Biochar has also been found to have many uses in air quality improvements. It has been used to control the release of air pollutants like NO_2 and NO which respectively presents greenhouse effects and localised ozone formations [45]. For instance, biochar has been used to achieve a 67% NO removal from soils [46]. This is achieved through biochar's ability to reduce the bioavailability of nitrogen to soil microorganisms for their metabolic activities [47]. The removal of gaseous mercury has also been achieved using biochar [48]. Several research reports show that, biochar surfaces are usually negatively charge thus have high affinity for positively charged metal ions [48] including Hg^{2+}. Removal efficiency usually depend on biochar properties (surface and elemental properties), feedstock and pyrolysis conditions under which biochar was prepared [48]. Though biochar can be used to reduce CO_2 emissions, it has low affinity for CO_2 and thus requires modifications for effective CO_2 capture [48]. One modification method is impregnating biochar with nitrogen and this improves biochar removal of CO_2 of up to 55% [49]. For H_2S gas, biochar has been used to achieve as high as 95% removal efficiency from a biogas production process [50]. It was shown that H_2S removal is better in the presence of hydroxide and carboxylic functional groups [51]. Other gases that have been removed with biochar include; ammonia and toluene [52], ozone [53], benzene [54], methyl tert- butyl ether and [55]. Though agriculture wastes are abundant for the production of biochar, it is however necessary to practice the sustainable utilisation of biochar (**Figure 1**). This is particularly necessary because biochar production consume energy and may release pollutants (gaseous and particulate matter). Sustainable utilisation of biochar includes the reuse of biochar, production biochar from feedstock which are less likely to contain pollutants and the use of calculated/optimised quantities in field applications.

It is having been demonstrated in numerous studies, the excellent performance of biochar in the removal of organic contaminants as well as inorganic contaminants. Generally, the adsorption of inorganic contaminants by biochar depends on biochar surface properties, contaminant type and pH. Phosphate adsorption in biochar is decreased by high aqueous pH values. The effect of P on the remediation of Cd by biochar was studied by [56]. The adsorbed P remains bioavailable, allowing the formulation of slow release of P fertilisers. Leaching of P in agricultural soil could be minimised by 89.25% by introducing biochars imbued with Mg whilst the

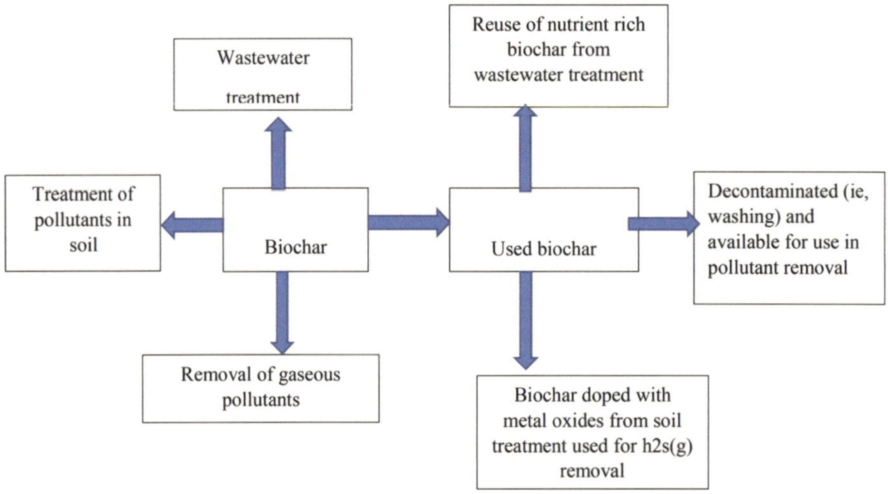

Figure 1.
An illustration showing a pathway for the sustainable utilisation of biochar.

availability of P of the surface at the same time is increased by 3.5 folds as compared to the soil without biochar [57].

Recent studies have been demonstrated the use of biochar for water treatment and purification have gained a lot of attention. Xiao et al. [58] indicated that micro-nano-engineered nitrogenous cow bone biochar (pyrolysed at 600 °C) was created which was able to adsorb 165.7, 287.6 and 558.9 mg/g of Cd(II), Cu(II), and Pb from water, respectively. Also a different study demonstrated the adsorption of ammonium from water using ball mining bamboo biochar where the adsorption was even more than three folds as compared to pristine biochar (7.0 vs. 22.9 mg/g) [59]. Toxic metals in soil medium can be remediated just like how toxic metal remediation in water medium is being remediated using biochar. For instance, calcium-based magnetic biochar minimised the bioavailability of Cd and As in soil through the transformation of thew metals into fractions that are stable [60]. The pH and cation exchange capacity of the soil increases due to the addition of porous biochar which lead to Cd remediation. The remediation of Pb and Cd polluted soil was also performed using thoil-modified biochar and the maximum adsorption capacities recorded were 61.4 mg/g and 45.1 mg/g, respectively [61]. Addition of biochar into soil may indirectly remediate toxic metals via the enrichment of microorganisms that are capable of remediating toxic metals [62].

Besides the removal of inorganic contaminant by biochar, it has the potential to remove hazardous organic compounds such as dyes, antibiotics, pesticides, oils, phenolics, polynuclear aromatics and persistent organic pollutants. The type of contaminant and biochar surface properties dictates how organic compounds are adsorbed. The mechanism for adsorbing organic compounds can be classified as pore-filling, p–p interaction, electrostatic attraction, cation exchange, hydrophobic interactions, complexes adsorption, and partition uncarbonised fraction [63]. Biochars engineered have been greatly used to remove organic contaminants. A typical example is the improvement of levofloxacin removal by cerium trichloride-treated biochar [64]. The treatment of cerium could be correlated with increasing the O-containing functional groups on the surface of biochar. Also, the structure of CeO_2 mesoporous, hence, its adsorption capacity as biochar can be improved [64]. In order to improve the surface area and the sizes of each pores, the surface polarity was also increased due to higher presence of O-functional groups [65]. The availability of these functional groups enhances the sorption organic contaminants via the bind of H_2 and complexation between biochar and organic compounds [66].

Biochars that are engineered are also good at adsorbing biological contaminants from water. For instance, developing wood biochar through H_2SO_4 oxidation and the resulting increase in surface area of the biochar and also resulting in an improved retention of *Escherichia coli* from stormwater [67]. Recently, the characteristics as well as the properties of pristine biochar developed from pyrolysed banana pseudostem biomass at 600 °C was improved significantly by Fe_3O_4 coating [68]. This engineered biochar demonstrated superparamagnetic properties and a significantly high surface area and was used for removal of the antibiotic furazolidone from wastewater efficiently. Adsorption of antibiotics from wastewaters/ agricultural drainage is crucial in order to halt the prevalence of drug-resistant pathogens [69] and to avoid new threats to human and animal health [70]. Also, the breakdown or depletion of these compounds does not actually make them less lethal or harmless. For example, degradation of furazolidone biologically may lead to the formation and development of carcinogenic metabolites [71]. This further depicts the relevance of biochar application in removing them via the adsorption mechanism.

Biochar engineering increases its efficiency in pesticides removal. In a successful field experiment, steam activated (800 °C for 45 min) almond shell biochar that was slowly pyrolyzed at 650 °C for 1 h under N_2 was used for the removal of dibromo chloropropane from well waters [72]. Biochar can also be used for the adsorption of solvents from water. Trichloroethylene, for example, has been eliminated from water using biochars developed from soybean stover [73]. The pyrolysis temperature is the major determinant of biochar adsorption capacity. Specifically, the highest adsorption capacity for trichloroethylene (32.02 mg/g) by the biochar was produced at the highest temperature (700 °C) depicted [73]. Biochar can be employed in water purification processes via the development of hybrid techniques such as permeable reactive barriers, biochar-augmented biofilters and biochar-based membrane filtration [74]. In general, the removal capacity of biochars can be greatly enhance or improved through bioengineering can be achieved via hybridisation techniques.

1.4 Role of biochar in environmental safety and sustainable agriculture

Agricultural lands are now degrading due to continuous farming leading to nutrient mining and decreased soil organic matter levels. Reduced levels of soil fertility in agricultural fields are nowadays becoming the prime concern for cultivating crops. The waning of soil on agricultural fields remains until improved management practices improve them. Soil health is the basis of the vital and supportable food system. Nutrient cycling and release and nutrient uptake are usually disturbed as the agricultural land is continuously cultivated, which affects the natural supplies of vital nutrients for plant development to decline and inhibits the growth rate of crops of farm soils. Biochar improves soil health, improves soil fertility, improves crop yields, and sequester carbon depending on the application rates, type of feedstocks, and temperature.

The incorporation of biochar into the soil improves plant health and crop productivity which been linked to four main mechanisms. The first mechanism is in connection with the capability of the biochar to stimulate beneficial microbes in the rhizosphere [75]. As a source of reduced carbon compounds and by increasing the availability of micronutrients, biochar provide beneficial sites to microbial populations [76] and other plant-growth-promoting microbes [77]. However, increase in microbial biomass resulting from microbial growth following biochar application has been reported to be as a result of the; effect of nutrient and water retention, creation of active surfaces that provided optimal habitat for microorganisms, weak alkalinity and partial inhibition of destructive and simultaneous support for beneficial microorganisms [78].

Secondly, the high water retention capacity of biochar leads to enhancement of water regime of the soil, and this is of special advantage to sandy soil area where the biochar will lessen the leaching away of moisture, thereby reducing water loss, whilst it reduces the risk of water-logging in clay soil by promoting water drainage [79]. The third mechanism is related to the capability of biochar to adsorb and neutralise phytotoxic organic molecules such as anthropogenic, xenobiotics and natural allelopathic compounds. This detoxifying ability is directly associated with the increases of specific surface area that occur during pyrolysis [10]. Increase in soil pH is the fourth mechanism, which is significantly beneficial to acidic soils [80].

1.4.1 Biochar effect on soil properties

Applying biochar to infertile soil reduces the bulk density and enhances the soil's total pore volume and water holding capacity to retain and mobilise nutrients to the soil-root system [81]. Primarily, biochar has a marginal effect on compaction. Still, on a long-term scale, with the ageing of biochar, modification is projected [82]. The application of biochar significantly influences several chemical properties such as pH, electrical conductivity (EC), cation exchange capacity (CEC), organic carbon, availability of nutrients. The use of biochar in the soil decreases soil acidity by enhancing soil pH as it is alkaline [9]. It also helps increase CEC, organic C, and exchangeable cations (such as Ca, K, Mg) [83]. By enhancing soil pH and CEC, it increases the availability of nutrients to plants. Soil fertility is improved by biochar treatment, primarily through two mechanisms: nutrients (like K, P, many micronutrients) and the soil or nutrient retention from other sources, including nutrients from the soil itself. Biochar shows a net positive effect on crop growth by increasing nutrient elements' availability (C, N, P, Ca and Mg) as it absorbs and slowly releases fertilisers [84]. Higher CEC of biochar treated soil binds cations to retain nutrients on biochar surface, humus, and clay rather than leached, making them further accessible for plants' uptake. Naturally, aged biochar generally shows a higher negative charge that promotes more soil aggregation and nutrient availability than fresh biochar or artificially old biochar [82]. The rise in plant-available water by biochar proposes that biochar could reduce irrigation frequency in croplands, mainly in low water areas. Biochar's positive effect on upsurging water holding capacity can be more extensive in sandy soils with lower micro-porosity and a smaller specific surface area than clayey soil.

Various life forms, including fungi, bacteria, nematodes, protozoa, earthworms, arthropods, indicate good healthy soil. Biochar addition has different influences on abundance, activity, and soil biological communities' multiplicity than fresh organic matter [76]. Research shows that biochar treatment results in higher microbial respiration by enhancing soil biodiversity and creating pores for soil microbes due to the complex aromatic structure, absence of carbon in biochar, and higher biochar stability than other fresh organic matters. Biochar can act as a habitat for microorganisms as it has a highly porous nature, and it can alter enzyme activity on or around biochar particles. Besides, by providing a more favourable habitat to microorganisms, it can modify soil's physical and chemical environment [76]. Moreover, microbial biomass and composition can also be affected by biochar addition. The pores of biochar can physically protect soil microorganisms. The buffering capacity of biochar that can resist changes in pH helps maintain favourable pH and abate pH instabilities in biochar particles supporting increasing microbial growth in micro-habitats [85].

The addition of biochar to soil sequester carbon and retain nutrients, thus promoting soil health and fertility and agronomic benefits. Moreover, nutrient availability also varies with the physico-chemical properties of biochar and the type of feedstock materials. Generally, biochar produced from feedstocks like manures and animal products is considered rich in nutrients related to those made from plant materials, mostly from hardwoods [86]. Biochar and other aromatic black carbons persist in soil for a more extended period and retain cations than any other organic carbon form. The ageing of biochar retains more cations than fresh biochar. Continuous fertilisers in the soil cause nutrient leaching from the soil that can deplete soil fertility, increase soil acidity, reduce crop yield and most notably deprive soil and environmental health. Higher absorption of cations and anions (like phosphate) due to biochar to soil restrict excess nutrients' leaching. Besides, biochar decreases the leaching of nutrients like N, P, Mg, Ca, nitrate and ammonium from soil [87].

1.4.2 Interaction of biochar with soil, plant and microorganisms

Biochar provides sites that can hold nutrients and other organic compounds as it exhibits natural oxidation through the formation of functional groups [82]. Biochar particles are highly associated with clay and silt-sized minerals, and oxidised biochar particles may be bound to soil minerals, in so doing decreasing the potential of its decomposition [88]. This association enhances the ability of soil-biochar-complex to adsorb organic compounds available in the soil whereas the biochar also interrelate directly with organic matter of soil by sorption [89]. Largely, amending soils with biochar helps to restore the health of the soils by increasing organic matter content and water holding capacity, balancing its pH, and re-establishing microbial populations. It also results in easing compaction, allowing the establishment of vegetation, recreation of ecological function of soils, decreasing bioavailability of toxic pollutants, leachability and mobility of contaminants, as well as improve soil drainage compared to the traditional remediation techniques [90]. The positively charged particles in biochar after pyrolysis are usually transmuted into oxides, hydroxides, and carbonates (ash) which behave as liming agents when incorporated into soil. Biochar is composed of low density material that The incorporation of biochar enhances reduction in soil bulk density as result of the composed low density material, thereby increasing root penetration, water infiltration, soil aeration and aggregate stability [87].

1.4.3 Impact of biochar application on nitrogen fixation and plant productivity

Amending soils with biochar enhances biological nitrogen fixation. The nitrogen available in the biochar is usually higher than that of the soil due to the high carbon/nitrogen (C/N) ratio of the biochar, and the resulting N immobilisation [76]. The incorporation of biochar in the soil results in the combination of factors related to soil nutrient availability and simulation of plant microbe interaction, along with increases in nitrogen/nutrient levels. Rondon et al. [91] reported an enhanced biological N-fixation in leguminous crops in soils amended with biochar. The increase in the availability of major plant nutrients due to biochar application is as a result of the release of some small amounts of nutrients that would be available to soil biota [92].

Biochar promotes plant productivity and yield through a number of mechanisms. It changes the physical conditions of plants. The dark colour of biochar alters the thermal dynamics and facilitates rapid germination of plants, allowing more time for growth compared with soils that are not amended with biochar [93]. Amendment of soils with biochar must be done based on extensive field testing since there are no specific recommended application rates. Chan et al. [94] opined that incorporation of 5–50 tonnes of biochar per hectare, with proper nutrient management gave positive effects on crop yields. Poultry litter biochar has been reported to improve the yield of corn, cowpea and radishes by 140, 100 and 96% respectively [94]. Field incorporation of biochar below 30 tonnes/ha has been reported to increase crop productivity for legume crops (30%), vegetables (29%) and grasses (14%) compared to corn (8%), wheat (11%) and rice (7%) [95]. Additionally, incorporation of biochar produced from wastewater sludge resulted in 64% increased production of cherry tomatoes above the control soil conditions at the rate of 10 tons/ha [96]. According to [97] sawdust and rice husk biochar significantly improved uptake of N, P and K by maize plants, and also significantly enhanced plant height, number of leaves, fresh and dry weight of cobs of maize.

1.4.4 Role of biochar in sustainable plant disease management

The ever increasing desire to increase agricultural efficiency in terms of producing maximum crop yields and produce is only achievable if pest and disease agents affecting crop productions are effectively monitored. Interventions such as cultural, biological, chemical and regulatory measures are the main approaches to plant disease management. The chemical method, since its adoption over a century ago, had assumed a position of significance and preferred over the existing cultural method as a result of its effectiveness in the management of diseases and pests. The availability, stability and quick-action, relatively low cost of the chemicals and ease with which they can be used, limits the harm done to crops. With the apprehension of the havoc, however, caused by continuous and persistent use of chemicals either by misuse or abuse, with the consequent degradation of ecological community of most of the farm sites based on their effects on both the target and non-target organisms, has led to the destruction of beneficial organisms and the natural predator in the eco-system. The normal functioning of the ecosystem is obstructed if the organisms develop resistance to the chemicals used, thus resulting in pests evolution. Consequently, agricultural workers suffer occupational exposure to pesticides whilst the general population is exposed to pesticides pollution principally through the food chain and drinking water contaminated with pesticide residues which are carcinogenic [98].

1.5 The role of biochar in mitigating climate change

Biochar can satisfy the following targets: achieving food security by enhancing crop productivity, promoting soil health and quality by improving soil properties, avoiding land degradation, reduction of greenhouse gas emissions minimises climate change, and adsorbing hazardous elements onto its surface. The conversion of *terra preta* soil into highly fertile soil due to biochar application is excellent evidence of biochar's role in soil sustainability and the environment. Many greenhouse gases are from the agricultural sector primarily due to many crop residues burning. A considerable amount of CO_2 is released from the fields, hampering the quality of the environment. The use of biochar has been well-thought-out, a novel technique to make a slow continuing elimination of CO_2 from the terrestrial atmosphere due to its complex aromatic structure and recalcitrant nature. The conversion of residue into biochar is considered a better alternative against burning. About 50% C retains in the soil in converting biomass C to biochar C than traditional conservation agriculture and microbial degradation, providing a more stable soil C sink than burning or direct biomass application [9]. Thus, applying biochar to soils can play an essential role in C sequestration to mitigate climate change as its residence time is up to millennial time scales [99]. On a global ranking of removing C from the atmosphere, biochar-bioenergy can play a significant role in inhibiting erratic climate change. It helps to capture and store C from the atmosphere at lower prices, where biochar addition significantly enhances the crop yield. About 62–66% of CO_2 emissions could sequester within biochar [100]. Thus, biochar can be an advantageous element to sequester more CO_2 from the soil's atmosphere to mitigate climate change. Besides CO_2, the emission of other greenhouse gases such as methane (CH_4), nitrous oxide (N_2O) has become a significant threat to the environment. Biochar application to the soil decreases the emission of CH_4 by suppressing the oxidation of ambient CH_4 depending upon soil type, the properties of biochar, and environmental conditions. On the other hand, the impact of biochar on the nitrogen transformation process is still unknown. Compared with other fresh organic materials, biochar application helps reduce N_2O emission and NH_4^+ leaching from the soil. Biochar reduces N_2O emission at reduced paddy fields due to the oxidative reactions on the biochar surfaces with ageing [86]. The biochar addition at the rate 20 and 40 Mg ha^{-1} reduced the total release of N_2O by 10.7% to 41.8%, respectively [101]. Furthermore, soil N_2O fluxes have also decreased to 79% in biochar treated soil [102].

1.6 How safe is the use of biochar on the environment?

The process of biochar production transforms the easily oxidised carbon fractions present in organic residues into more stable forms [5] that can persist in soils for years [103]. The incorporation of biochar reduces the emissions of greenhouses gases [104] and can be considered as a climate change mitigation strategy [105]. On the other side of the coin, required quantities of this conditioner to improve soil productivity might be less comparable with compost or other organic amendments on the long run. Consequently, biochar also known as "the black diamond" is offered as a promising soil amendment of high economic and environmental value [106]. However, several environmental traits should be taken into consideration whilst using this amendment. The primary one to consider is the production process. During the pyrolysis process of biochar, significant emissions of CO_2 occur and this probably may raise the levels of greenhouse gases in atmosphere [107]. The second important issue has to do with the degradation of biochar in the soil. Under warm climatic conditions, biochar degradation is reported to be relatively high [6] and therefore, further emissions of greenhouse gases might take place from biochar-amended soils. The third relates to ethylene production, which is a by-product of the pyrolysis process of biochar [108]. Ethylene is increased considerably in biochar-amended soils to subdue several soil microbial processes [82]. Soil biota not only affects the physical and chemical properties of soil but also improves plant health [80]. Several researches have established the positive influences of amending soils with biochar on increasing crop productivity. Soils Amended with biochar have been proven to significantly improve macro- and micro-nutrients availability [6], even though many biochar additives have an alkaline nature [76]. Furthermore, amending soils with biochar reduces nitrate (NO_3) loss through leaching as well as the gaseous loss through release of nitrous oxide [92], which can positively boost plant growth [93].

However, the effects of amending soils with biochar are not always the similar and depend mainly on the features of the biochar used such as grain size and pyrolysis temperature. Fine biochar decreases soil hydraulic conductivity (EC), whilst the coarse biochar (particles were coarser than sand) did not affect the hydraulic conductivity of soils [95]. In addition, the pyrolysis temperature for the production of the biochar has a significant effect on ash content, pH, EC, and basic functional groups as well as carbon stability, which increases in biochar with increasing pyrolysis temperature [109]. Another positive influence of biochar as a soil conditioner is related to its ability to mitigate salinisation of arable lands [110]. It is noted that biochar plays positive significant influence on regulating the contaminants present in water and soils [111]. Conversely, many contaminants such as atrazine and acetochlor that are sorbed on biochar [107] may also originate from biochar [112] and this may reduce its efficacy [98]. Although biochar plays important positive roles on environmental sustainability, there is a stream of knowledge regarding the recommended application rates to soils to evade its negative potential effects on the environment.

2. Conclusion

The chapter explored the possibility of using biochar from agricultural wastes as a suitable alternative for the remediation of environmental pollutants, soil conditioning and the long-term biochar application in the environment. Agricultural wastes biochar can ensure environmental safety and sustainability. Minerals biochar can significantly impact biochar attributes therefore, the type and amount of minerals in biomass must be optimised for the intended environmental application. Biochars have made substantial breakthroughs in reducing greenhouse gases emissions, reducing soil nutrient leaching, sequester atmospheric carbon into the soil, increasing agricultural productivity, and reducing bioavailability of environmental contaminants. Biochar has been widely known for its ability to serve as remediator of contaminant, plays a vital role climate change mitigation and bioenergy production. The incorporation of biochar into the soil improves plant health and crop productivity.

Acknowledgements

The authors are very grateful to the editors and anonymous reviewers for their suggestions and comments for improving the book chapter quality.

Conflict of interest

The authors declare no conflict of interest.

Author details

Ammal Abukari[1*], Ziblim Abukari Imoro[2], Abubakari Zarouk Imoro[3] and Abudu Ballu Duwiejuah[4]

1 Department of Forestry and Forest Resources Management, Faculty of Natural Resources and Environment, University for Development Studies, Tamale, Ghana

2 Department of Biodiversity Conservation and Management, Faculty of Natural Resources and Environment, University for Development Studies, Tamale, Ghana

3 Department of Environment, Water and Waste Engineering, School of Engineering, University for Development Studies, Tamale, Ghana

4 Department of Biotechnology, Faculty of Biosciences, University for Development Studies, Tamale, Ghana

*Address all correspondence to: aammal@uds.edu.gh

References

[1] Duque-Acevedo M, Belmonte-Ureña LJ, Cortés-García FJ, Camacho-Ferre F, Agricultural waste: Review of the evolution, approaches and perspectives on alternative uses. Global Ecology and Conservation. 2020;22:1-23, e00902. DOI:10.1016/j.gecco.2020.e00902.

[2] Obi FO, Ugwuishiwu BO, Nwakaire JN. Agricultural waste concept, generation, utilization and management. Nigerian Journal of Technology. 2016;35(4):957-964. DOI: 10.4314/njt.v35i4.34.

[3] United Nations. Programme Performance Report 2018. UN Environment Programme. 2019. https://wedocs.unep.org/bitstream/handle/20.500.11822.

[4] Food and Agriculture Organization of the United Nations (FAO) & United Nations Environment Programme (UNEP). A decision support tool for sustainable bioenergy. 2010. www.fao.org/docrep/013/am237e/am237e00.pdf. (Accessed 3 January 2021).

[5] Atkinson NJ, Urwin PE. The interaction of plant biotic and abiotic stresses: From genes to the field. Journal of Experimental Botany. 2012;63(10):3523-3543.

[6] Bonanomi G, Ippolito F, Scala F. A "black" future for plant pathology? Biochar as a new soil amendment for controlling plant diseases. Journal of Plant Pathology. 2015; 97(2):223-234.

[7] Sanchez-Monedero MA, Cayuela M, Roig A, Jindo K, Mondini C, Bolan N. Role of biochar as an additive in organic waste composting. Bioresour. Technol. 2018; 247:1155-1164, 10.1016/j.biortech.2017.09.193.

[8] Oginni O, Singh K. Influence of high carbonization temperatures on microstructural and physicochemical characteristics of herbaceous biomass derived biochars. Journal of Environmental Chemical Engineering. 2020;8: 104169.

[9] Lehmann J, Gaunt J, Rondon M. Bio-char sequestration in terrestrial ecosystems - a review. Mitig Adapt Strat Glob Change. 2006;11:403-427.

[10] Ahmad M, Rajapaksha AU, Lim JE, Zhang M, Bolan N, Mohan D, Vithanage M, Lee SS, Ok YSik. Biochar as a sorbent for contaminant management in soil and water: A review. Chemosphere. 2014; 99:19-33.

[11] Aghbashlo M, Hosseinpour S, Tabatabaei M, Soufiyan MM. Multiobjective exergetic and technical optimization of a piezoelectric ultrasonic reactor applied to synthesize biodiesel from waste cooking oil (WCO) using soft computing techniques. Fuel. 2019; 235:100-112.

[12] Panahi KSH, Dehhaghi M, Aghbashlo M, Karimi K, Tabatabaei M. Shifting fuel feedstock from oil wells to sea: Iran outlook and potential for biofuel production from brown macroalgae (ochrophyta; phaeophyceae). Renew. Sustain. Energy Rev. 2019;112:626-642.

[13] Soltanian S, Aghbashlo M, Almasi F, Hosseinzadeh-Bandbafha H, Nizami AS, Ok YS, Lam SS, Tabatabaei M. A critical review of the effects of pretreatment methods on the exergetic aspects of lignocellulosic biofuels. Energy Convers. Manag. 2020;212:112792.

[14] Suman S, Gautam S. In: Energy systems and environment. Biochar derived from agricultural waste biomass act as a clean and alternative energy source of fossil fuel inputs. IntechOpen. 2018; 207-220. DOI: 10.5772/intechopen.73833.

[15] Zabaniotou A, Stamou K. Balancing waste and nutrient flows between urban agglomerations and rural ecosystems: biochar for improving crop growth and urban air quality in the Mediterranean region. Atmosphere. 2020; 11:539. DOI:10.3390/atmos11050539.

[16] Enaime G, Baçaoui A, Yaacoubi A, Lübken M. Biochar for wastewater treatment conversion technologies and applications. 2020;10:3492. DOI:10.3390/app10103492

[17] Lee M, Lin YL, Chiueh PT, Den W. Environmental and energy assessment of biomass residues to biochar as fuel: A brief review with recommendations for future bioenergy systems. Journal of Cleaner Production. 2020;251: 119714.

[18] Eliasson J, Carlsson V. Agricultural waste and wood waste for pyrolysis and biochar - an assessment for Rwanda. Examensarbete Inom Teknik, Grundnivå, 15 Hp Stockholm, Sverige. 2020.

[19] Ronsse F, Van Hecke S, Dickinson D, Prins W. Production and characterization of slow pyrolysis biochar: influence of feedstock type and pyrolysis conditions. GCB Bioenergy. 2013;5:104-115. DOI: 10.1111/gcbb.12018.

[20] Cheng S, Chen T, Xu W, Huang J, Jiang S, Yan B. Application research of biochar for the remediation of soil heavy metals contamination: a review. Molecules. 2020;25:3167. DOI:10.3390/molecules25143167.

[21] Yuan JH, Xu RK, Zhang H. The forms of alkalis in the biochar produced from crop residues at different temperature. Bioresource Technology. 2011;102:3488-3497.

[22] Lehmann J, Joseph S. Biochar. Environ Manag Sci Technol Implement, 2nd edn. Routledge, London. 2015.

[23] Bruun EW, Ambus P, Egsgaard H, Hauggaardnielsen H. Effects of slow and fast pyrolysis biochar on soil C and N turnover dynamics. Soil Biol Biochem. 2012; 46:73-79.

[24] Chan KY, Zwieten LV, Meszaros I, Downie A, Joseph S. Agronomic values of greenwaste biochar as a soil amendment. Aust J Soil Res. 2007;45:629-634.

[25] Cao XD, Harris W. Properties of dairy-manure-derived biochar pertinent to its potential use in remediation. Biores Technol. 2010; 101:5222-5228.

[26] Inyang MI, Gao B, Yao Y, Xue YW, Zimmerman A, Mosa A, Pullammanappallil P, Ok YS, Cao XD. A review of biochar as a low-cost adsorbent for aqueous heavy metal removal. Critical Reviews in Environmental Science and Technology. 2016; 46(4):406-433.

[27] Elnour AY, Alghyamah AA, Shaikh HM, Poulose AM, Al-Zahrani SM, Anis A, Al Wabel MI. Effect of pyrolysis temperature on biochar microstructural evolution, physicochemical characteristics, and its influence on biochar/ polypropylene composites. Appl. Sci. 2019;9:1149.

[28] Ok YS, Uchimiya SM, Chang SX, Bolan N. Biochar: production, characterization, and applications. CRC Press. 2015.

[29] Cha JS, Park SH, Jung S, Ryu C, Jeon J, Shin M, Park Y. Production and utilization of biochar: A review. J. Ind. Eng. Chem. 2016;40:1-15.

[30] Pukalchik M, Mercl F, Terekhova V, Tlustoš P. Biochar, wood ash and humic substances mitigating trace elements stress in contaminated sandy loam soil: Evidence from an integrative approach. Chemosphere. 2018;203:228-238.

[31] Ding Y, Liu Y, Liu S, Li Z, Tan X, Huang X, Zeng G, Zhou L, Zheng B.

Biochar to improve soil fertility. A review. Agron. Sustain. Dev. 2016;36:36.

[32] Nan H, Yang F, Zhao L, Masek O, Cao X, Xiao Z. Interaction of inherent minerals with carbon during biomass pyrolysis weakens biochar carbon sequestration potential. ACS Sustain. Chem. Eng. 2018;7:1591-1599.

[33] Deng Y, Zhang T, Wang Q. In: Engineering application of biochar. Biochar adsorption treatment for typical pollutants removal in livestock wastewater: a review. IntechOpen. 2017; 71-82. DOI: 10.5772/intechopen.68253.

[34] Inyang M, Gao B, Yao Y, Xue Y, Zimmerman AR, Pullammanappallil P, Cao X. Removal of heavy metals from aqueous solution by biochars derived from anaerobically digested biomass. Bioresource Technology. 2012;110:50-56.

[35] Cheng W, Li H, Yang Y, et al. Study on preparation of biochar and its adsorption of nitrogen and phosphorus by pyrolysis of anaerobic fermentation residue from municipal sludge. Acta Chimica Sinica. 2016;4:1541-1548.

[36] Kaetzl K, Lübken M, Nettmann E, Krimmler S, Wichern M. Slow sand filtration of raw wastewater using biochar as an alternative filtration media. Sci. Rep. 2020; 10: 1229.

[37] Ahmad M, Hashimoto Y, Moon DH, Lee SS, Ok YS. Immobilization of lead in a Korean military shooting range soil using eggshell waste: an integrated mechanistic approach. J. Hazard Mater. 2012;209:392-401.

[38] Xu G, Lv Y, Sun J, Shao H, Wei L. Recent advances in biochar applications in agricultural soils: benefits and environmental implications. Clean. 2012;40:1093-1098.

[39] Antonangelo JA, Zhang H. In: Applications of biochar for environmental safety. The use of biochar as a soil amendment to reduce potentially toxic metals (ptms) phytoavailability. IntechOpen. 2020:1-15. DOI: http://dx.doi.org/10.5772/intechopen.92611.

[40] Guo M, Song W, Tian J. Biochar-facilitated soil remediation: Mechanisms and efficacy variations. Frontiers. Frontiers Environmental Science. 2020; 8:521512. DOI: 10.3389/fenvs.2020.521512.

[41] Chen Y, Jiang Z, Wu D, Wang H, Li J, Bi M, Zhang Y. Development of a novel bio-organic fertilizer for the removal of atrazine in soil. J Environ Manag. 2019; 233:553-560.

[42] Anyanwu IN, Alo MN, Onyekwere AM, Crosse JD, Nworie O, Chamba EB. Influence of biochar aged in acidic soil on ecosystem engineers and two tropical agricultural plants. Ecotoxicol. Environ. Saf. 2018;153: 116-126.

[43] Lü F, Luo C, Shao L, He P. Biochar alleviates combined stress of ammonium and acids by firstly enriching methanosaeta and then methanosarcina. Water Research. 2016;90:34-43.

[44] Cao GL, Guo WQ, Wang AJ, Zhao L, Xu CJ, Zhao QL, Ren NQ. Enhanced cellulosic hydrogen production from lime-treated cornstalk wastes using thermophilic anaerobic microflora. International Journal of Hydrogen Energy. 2012;37:13161-13166.

[45] Pourhashem G, Rasool QZ, Zhang R, Medlock KB, Cohan DS, Masiello CA. Valuing the air quality effects of biochar reductions on soil NO emissions. Environmental Science and Technology. 2017;51(17):9856-9863. DOI: 10.1021/acs.est.7b00748.

[46] Nelissen V, Saha BK, Ruysschaert G, Boeckx P. Effect of different biochar and fertilizer types on N_2O and

NO emissions. Soil Biology and Biochemistry. 2014;70:244-255.

[47] Mørkved PT, Dörsch P, Bakken LR. The N_2O product ratio of nitrification and its dependence on long-term changes in soil pH. Soil Biology and Biochemistry. 2007;39(8):2048-2057.

[48] Gwenzi W, Chaukura N, Wenga T, Mtisi M. Biochars as media for air pollution control systems: Contaminant removal, applications and future research directions. Science of the Total Environment. 2021;753:142249. DOI:10.1016/j.scitotenv.2020.142249 .

[49] Xu Y, Luo G, He S, Deng F, Pang Q, Xu Y, Yao H. Efficient removal of elemental mercury by magnetic chlorinated biochars derived from co-pyrolysis of Fe (NO_3) 3-laden wood and polyvinyl chloride waste. Fuel. 2019;239:982-990.

[50] Oliveira FR, Patel AK, Jaisi DP, Adhikari S, Lu H, Khanal SK. Environmental application of biochar: Current status and perspectives. Bioresource Technology. 2017;246:110-122.

[51] Shang G, Shen G, Wang T, Chen Q. Effectiveness and mechanisms of hydrogen sulfide adsorption by camphor-derived biochar. Journal of the Air and Waste Management Association. 2012;62(8):873-879.

[52] Bhandari PN, Kumar A, Huhnke RL. Simultaneous removal of toluene (Model Tar), NH_3, and H_2S, from biomass-generated producer gas using biochar-based and mixed-metal oxide catalysts. Energy Fuels. 2014;28(3):1918-1925. DOI:10.1021/EF401687.

[53] Zhou L, Richard C, Ferronato C, Chovelon JM, Sleiman M. Investigating the performance of biomass-derived biochars for the removal of gaseous ozone, adsorbed nitrate and aqueous bisphenol A. Chemical Engineering Journal. 2018; 334:2098-2104.

[54] Khan A, Szulejko JE, Samaddar P, Kim K, Liu B, Maitlo HA, Yang X, Ok YS. The potential of biochar as sorptive media for removal of hazardous benzene in air. Chemical Engineering Journal. 2018;361:1576-1585. DOI: 10.1016/j.cej.2018.10.193.

[55] Pongkua W, Dolphen R, Thiravetyan P. Effect of functional groups of biochars and their ash 1456 content on gaseous methyl tert-butyl ether removal. Colloids and Surfaces A. 2018;558:531-537.

[56] Han B, Song L, Li H, Song H. Immobilization of Cd and phosphorus utilization in eutrophic river sediments by biochar-supported nanoscale zerovalent iron. Environ. Technol. 2020; pp 1-18.

[57] Chen Q, Qin J, Cheng Z, Huang L, Sun P, Chen L, Shen G. Synthesis of a stable magnesium-impregnated biochar and its reduction of phosphorus leaching from soil. Chemosphere. 2018;199:402-408.

[58] Xiao J, Hu R, Chen G. Micro-nano-engineered nitrogenous bone biochar developed with a ball-milling technique for high-efficiency removal of aquatic Cd (II), Cu (II) and Pb (II). J. Hazard Mater. 2020;387:121980.

[59] Qin Y, Zhu X, Su Q, Anumah A, Gao B, Lyu W, Zhou X, Xing Y, Wang B. Enhanced removal of ammonium from water by ball-milled biochar. Environ. Geochem. Health. 2019; pp 1-9.

[60] Wu J, Li Z, Huang D, Liu X, Tang C, Parikh SJ, Xu J. A novel calcium based magnetic biochar is effective in stabilization of arsenic and cadmium co-contamination in aerobic soils. J. Hazard Mater. 2020; 122010.

[61] Fan J, Cai C, Chi H, Reid BJ, Coulon F, Zhang Y, Hou Y. Remediation of cadmium and lead polluted soil using thiol-modified biochar. J. Hazard Mater. 2020;122037.

[62] Hamedi J, Dehhaghi M, Mohammdipanah F. Isolation of extremely heavy metal resistant strains of rare actinomycetes from high metal content soils in Iran. Int. J. Environ. Res. 2015; p 9.

[63] Dai Y, Zhang N, Xing C, Cui Q, Sun Q. The adsorption, regeneration and engineering applications of biochar for removal organic pollutants: a review. Chemosphere. 2019;223:12-27.

[64] Yi S, Sun Y, Hu X, Xu H, Gao B, Wu J. Porous nano-cerium oxide wood chip biochar composites for aqueous levofloxacin removal and sorption mechanism insights. Environ. Sci. Pollut. Res. 2018;25:25629-25637.

[65] Alghazwi M, Smid S, Musgrave I, Zhang W. In vitro studies of the neuroprotective activities of astaxanthin and fucoxanthin against amyloid beta (Ab1-42) toxicity and aggregation. Neurochem. Int. 2019; 124:215-224.

[66] Liu W, Zhang J, Zhang C, Ren L. Sorption of norfloxacin by lotus stalk based activated carbon and iron-doped activated alumina: mechanisms, isotherms and kinetics. Chem. Eng. J. 2011;171:431-438.

[67] Lau AY, Tsang DC, Graham NJ, Ok YS, Yang X, Li XD. Surface-modified biochar in a bioretention system for *Escherichia coli* removal from stormwater. Chemosphere. 2017;169: 89-98.

[68] Gurav R, Bhatia SK, Choi TR, Park YL, Park JY, Han YH, Vyavahare G, Jadhav J, Song HS, Yang P. Treatment of furazolidone contaminated water using banana pseudostem biochar engineered with facile synthesized magnetic nanocomposites. Bioresour. Technol. 2020;297:122472.

[69] Mohammadipanah F, Panahi HKS, Imanparast F, Hamedi J. Development of a reversed-phase liquid chromatographic assay for the quantification of total persipeptides in fermentation broth. Chromatographia. 2016;79:1325-1332.

[70] Panahi HKS, Mohammadipanah F, Dehhaghi M. Optimization of extraction conditions for liquid-liquid extraction of persipeptides from *Streptomyces zagrosensis* fermentation broth. Eur. Chem. Bull. 2016;5:408-415.

[71] Lewkowski J, Rogacz D, Rychter P. Hazardous ecotoxicological impact of two commonly used nitrofuran-derived antibacterial drugs: furazolidone and nitrofurantoin. Chemosphere. 2019;222:381-390.

[72] Klasson KT, Ledbetter CA, Uchimiya M, Lima IM. Activated biochar removes 100% dibromochloropropane from field well water. Environ. Chem. Lett. 2013;11:271-275.

[73] Mohan D, Sarswat A, Ok YS, Pittman CU Jr. Organic and inorganic contaminants removal from water with biochar, a renewable, low cost and sustainable adsorbent - A critical review. Bioresource Technology. 2014;160:191-202.

[74] Palansooriya KN, Yang Y, Tsang YF, Sarkar B, Hou D, Cao X, Meers E, Rinklebe J, Kim KH, Ok YS. Occurrence of contaminants in drinking water sources and the potential of biochar for water quality improvement: a review. Crit. Rev. Environ. Sci. Technol. 2020;50:549-611.

[75] Thies J, Rilling M, Graber ER. Biochar effects on the abundance, activity and diversity of the soil biota.

In: Lehmann J, Joseph S, editors. Biochar for Environmental Management: Science and Technology. 2nd ed. London, UK: Earthscan. 2015.

[76] Lehmann J, Rillig MC, Thies J, Masiello CA, Hockaday WC, Crowley D. Biochar effects on soil biota–a review. Soil biology and biochemistry. 2011;43(9):1812-1836.

[77] Kolton M, Harel YM, Pasternak Z, Graber ER, Elad Y, Cytryn E. Impact of biochar application to soil on the root-associated bacterial community structure of fully developed greenhouse pepper plants. Applied and Environmental Microbiology. 2011;14:4924-4930.

[78] Schulz H, Dunst G, Glaser B. Positive effects of composted biochar on plant growth and soil fertility. Agronomy for Sustainable Development. 2013;33(4):817-827.

[79] Barnes RT, Gallagher ME, Masiello CA, Liu Z, Dugan B. Biochar-induced changes in soil hydraulic conductivity and dissolved nutrient fluxes constrained by laboratory experiments. PLoS One. 2014;9(9):108-340.

[80] Jeffery S, Verheijen FGA, Van Der Velde M, Bastos AC. A quantitative review of the effects of biochar application to soils on crop productivity using meta-analysis. Agriculture, Ecosystems and Environment. 2011;144:175-187.

[81] Case SD, McNamara NP, Reay DS, Stott AW, Grant HK, Whitaker J. Biochar suppresses N_2O emissions whilst maintaining N availability in a sandy loam soil. Soil Biology and Biochemistry. 2015;81:178-185.

[82] Cheng CH, Lehmann J, Engelhard MH. Natural oxidation of black carbon in soils: changes in molecular form and surface charge along a climosequence. Geochimica et Cosmochimica Acta. 2008;72(6):1598-1610.

[83] Van Zwieten L, Kimber S, Morris S, Chan KY, Downie A, Rust J, Joseph S, Cowie A. Effects of biochar from slow pyrolysis of papermill waste on agronomic performance and soil fertility. Plant and soil. 2010;327(1-2):235-246.

[84] DeLuca TH, Gundale MJ, MacKenzie MD, Jones DL. Biochar effects on soil nutrient transformations. Biochar for environmental management: science, technology and implementation. 2015;2:421-454.

[85] Rousk J, Bååth E, Brookes PC, Lauber CL, Lozupone C, Caporaso JG, Knight R, Fierer N. Soil bacterial and fungal communities across a pH gradient in an arable soil. The ISME journal. 2010;4(10):1340-1351.

[86] Singh B, Singh BP, Cowie AL. Characterisation and evaluation of biochars for their application as a soil amendment. Soil Research. 2010;48(7):516-525.

[87] Laird D, Fleming P, Wang B, Horton R, Karlen D. Biochar impact on nutrient leaching from a Midwestern agricultural soil. Geoderma. 2010;158(3-4):436-442.

[88] Brodowski S, John B, Flessa H, Amelung W. Aggregate-occluded black carbon in soil. European Journal of Soil Science. 2006;57:539-546.

[89] Hammes K, Schmidt WI. Changes of biochar in soil. In: Lehmann J, Joseph S, editors. Biochar for Environmental Management: Science and Technology. London: Earthscan. 2009; pp 169-182.

[90] U.S. EPA. The use of soil amendments for remediation, revitalization and reuse. Hazardous Waste Clean-up Information System

(Clu-In). Available from: www. Clu-in. org/pub1.cfm. 2007.

[91] Rondon M, Lehmann J, Ramirez J, Hurtado M. Biological nitrogen fixation by common beans (*Phaseolus vulgaris* L.) increases with bio-char additions. Biology and Fertility of Soils. 2007; 43:699-708

[92] Yamato M, Okimori Y, Wibowo IF, Anshiori S, Ogawa M. Effects of the application of charred bark of *Acacia mangium* on the yield of maize, cowpea and peanut, and soil chemical properties in South Sumatra, Indonesia. Soil Science and Plant Nutrition. 2006;52:489-458.

[93] Genesio L, Miglietta F, Baronti S, Vaccari FP. Biochar increases vine-yard productivity without affecting grape quality: Results from a four years field experiment in Tuscany. Agriculture, Ecosystems and Environment. 2015;201:20-25.

[94] Chan KY, van Zwieten L, Meszaros I, Downie A, Joseph S. Using poultry litter biochars as soil amendments. Australian Journal of Soil Research. 2008;46:437-444.

[95] Liu X, Zhang A, Ji C, Joseph S, Bian R, Li L, Pan G, Paz-Ferreiro J. Biochar's effect on crop productivity and the dependence on experimental conditions: A meta-analysis of literature data. Plant and Soil. 2013;373:583-594.

[96] Brantley KE, Savin MC, Brye KR, Longer DE. Pine woodchip biochar impact on soil nutrient concentrations and corn yield in a silt loam in the mid-southern U.S. Agriculture. 2015;5(1):30-47.

[97] Ndor E, Ogara JI, Bako DA, Osuagbalande JA. Effect of biochar on macronutrients release and plant growth on degraded soil of Lafia, Nasarawa State, Nigeria. Asian Research Journal of Agriculture. 2016;2(3):1-8.

[98] Tariq MI, Afzal S, Hussain I, Sultana N. Pesticides exposure in Pakistan: A review. Environment International. 2007;33:1107-1122

[99] Woolf D, Amonette JE, Street-Perrott FA, Lehmann J, Joseph S. Sustainable biochar to mitigate global climate change. Nature communications. 2010;1(1):1-9.

[100] Roberts KG, Gloy BA, Joseph S, Scott NR, Lehmann J. Life cycle assessment of biochar systems: estimating the energetic, economic, and climate change potential. Environmental science & technology, 2010;44(2):827-833.

[101] Zhang A, Liu Y, Pan G, Hussain Q, Li L, Zheng J, Zhang X. Effect of biochar amendment on maize yield and greenhouse gas emissions from a soil organic carbon poor calcareous loamy soil from Central China plain. Plant and Soil.2012;351:263-275.

[102] Castaldi S, Riondino M, Baronti S, Esposito FR, Marzaioli R, Rutigliano FA, Vaccari FP, Miglietta F. Impact of biochar application to a Mediterranean wheat crop on soil microbial activity and greenhouse gas fluxes. Chemosphere. 2011;85:1464-1471.

[103] International Biochar Initiative. Standardized product definition and product testing guidelines for biochar that is used in soil. IBI biochar standards. 2015. Available from: https://www.biochar-international. org/wp content/uploads/2018/04/ IBI_Biochar_Standards_V2.1_Final.pdf [Last accessed: 21-05-2019]

[104] Conversa G, Bonasia A, Lazzizera C, Elia A. Influence of biochar, mycorrhizal inoculation, and fertilizer rate on growth and flowering of Pelargonium (*Pelargonium zonale* L.) plants. Frontiers in Plant Science. 2015;6:429.

[105] Harder B. Smoldered-earth policy: Created by ancient Amazonian natives, fertile, dark soils retain abundant carbon. Science News. 2006;169:133

[106] Elad Y, Cytryn E, Harel YM, Lew B, Graber ER. The biochar effect: Plant resistance to biotic stresses. Phytopathologia Mediterranea. 2011;50:335-349.

[107] Sohi SP, Krull E, Lopez-Capel E, Bol RA. Review of biochar and its use and function in soil. Advances in Agronomy. 2010;105:47-82.

[108] Kumar S, Nakajima T, Mbonimpa EG, Gautam S, Somireddy UR, Kadono A, Lal R, Chintala R, Rafique R, Fausey N. Long-term tillage and drainage influences on soil organic carbon dynamics, aggregate stability, and carbon yield. Soil Science & Plant Nutrition. 2014;60: 108-118.

[109] Hossain MK, Strezov V, Chan KY, Nelson PF. Agronomic properties of wastewater sludge biochar and bioavailability of metals in production of cherry tomato (*Lycopersicon esculentum*). Chemosphere. 2010;78:1167-1171.

[110] Kammann C, Ratering S, Eckchard C, Muller C. Biochar and hydrochar effects on greenhouse gas fluxes from soils. Journal of Environmental Quality. 2015;41:1052-1066.

[111] Subedi R, Kammann C, Pelissetti S, Taupe N, Bertora C, Monaco S, et al. Does soil amended with biochar and hydrochar reduce ammonia emissions following the application of pig slurry? European Journal of Soil Science. 2015;66:1044-1053.

[112] Raghunath S, Chiara B, Laura Z, Carlo G. Crop response to soils amended with biochar: Expected benefits and unintended risks. Italian Journal of Agronomy. 2017;12:161-173.

Chapter 9

Reproductive Toxicity of Arsenic: What We Know and What We Need to Know?

Hafiz Ishfaq Ahmad, Muhammad Bilal Bin Majeed, Abdul Jabbar, Ruqia Arif and Gulnaz Afzal

Abstract

In the most recent the environmental provident and threatening conduct of arsenic has increased the consideration of the world due to its pollution and hazardous effects throughout the world. Arsenic contamination is serious issue throughout the world and is substantial risk factor in most of countries including China, U.S.A, India, Bangladesh, Mexico and Argentina. Several experimental models have been established to understand the diseases caused by arsenic exposure. However reproductive and developmental toxicity have been poorly understood. The objectives of this study are to discuss current landscapes and future horizons of arsenic toxicity in human and animals in relation to various toxicity routes including oral route involving food and water or through inhalation of agricultural pesticides. Addition of current evidence on the development of destiny and actions of arsenic toxicity in human and animal population and other species will lessen the uncertainties in the hazard assessment for arsenic. This effort would help to protect the public health against the toxic and carcinogenic effects associated with arsenic exposure.

Keywords: arsenic, reproduction, toxicity, endocrine, spermatogenesis

1. Introduction

In the most recent the environmental provident and threatening conduct of arsenic has increased the consideration of the world due to its pollution and hazardous effects throughout the world [1, 2]. Arsenic contamination is serious issue throughout the world and is substantial risk factor in most of countries including China, U.S.A, India, Pakistan, Bangladesh, Mexico and Argentina. Human revelation to arsenic is through oral route involving food and water or through inhalation of agricultural pesticides [3–5]. According to World Health Organization fact sheet, arsenic contamination is major public issue requires emergency amendments [6]. As the arsenic contamination of ground water is most serious issue for human health in China, India, Pakistan, inner-Mongolia and Bangladesh [7]. Arsenic is present round the earth in environment and is extremely toxic for life. It is metalloid occurring 20th in earth crust, 14th in sea water and 12th in human body [8]. Toxic effects of arsenic on health is wide spread in both humans and animals [9], as epidemiological substantiation proved that chronic arsenic exposure is associated with increased risk of liver, bladder and skin cancer, cardiovascular diseases, diabetes mellitus neuropathies, and ocular diseases [10–12]. Arsenic ingestion leads to accumulation in liver, kidney and lungs and small amount in gastrointestinal tract, muscle nervous system and spleen because these organs are rich in oxidative enzymes [13]. The toxic effects of arsenic mostly occur from chronic exposure to humans and animals. Epidemiological studies have revealed that chronic arsenic exposure is associated with elevated risk of liver, lung, kidney, and skin cancer in addition to other ailments such as vascular, diabetic, reproductive and neurologic [14, 15]. On the contrary arsenic has been considered as an effective chemotherapeutic agent in the treatment of human cancer [16]. Various experimental models have been developed to understand the diseases caused by arsenic exposure. However reproductive and developmental toxicity have been poorly understood. Numerous studies documented elevated spontaneous abortion and stillbirth and decreased birth weight by utero arsenic exposure [17]. Arsenic as a risk factor for developing fetus has primarily been studied through murine studies, signifying the reproductive toxicity of arsenic. In animal's studies on arsenic toxicities revealed that arsenic is associated with spermatotoxicity [18] inhibition of testicular steroidogenesis and reduction of weight of testes and accessory organs [19]. In the current review, we try to summarize the existing information on arsenic toxicity from the available literature. We initiate by describing how and when the arsenic contamination took place by considering the course through current literature lens. We present an overview of how human and animals have been affected in the light of colors of various exposure sources by considering the relationship between arsenic toxicity and environment influenced by human activities. Furthermore, we conclude with a preview of future directions and challenges for this field.

Endocrine Disruption.

The gene regulation of mineralocorticoid, glucocorticoids, and androgen and progesterone receptors is disrupted by arsenic [20]. The mechanistic effect of arsenic on these four steroid hormones is studies on glucocorticoids receptors. Arsenic altered receptor of transcription regulation of DNA dependent glucocorticoids, signifying that transcriptional machinery is required for glucocorticoids regulation [21]. Comprehensive mutational investigation of glucocorticoids revealed that only receptor is not the causal target for arsenic effect, as studies that entire C-terminal and N-terminal domains can be removed from glucocorticoids receptors without altered arsenic effects, which indicate the primary mediator of the response of central DNA binding domain. However mutation of almost all the predicted sites of DNA binding domains did not eliminate function and also did not ablate the arsenic effects [21] Abnormalities of male reproductive system such as hypospadias, prostate, testicular cancer and cryptorchidism, may instigate through endocrine disruption [19].

2. Male reproductive effects

Male reproductive system is directly affected by arsenic exposure, as it targets particular reproductive organs and neuroendocrine system and it also disrupt sertoli cells during fetal development. Sertoli cells propagate during prepubertal, fetal, neonatal period and these stages are chiefly susceptible to adverse effects of arsenic (**Figure 1**) [22]. The interruption of spermatogenesis at cell differentiation stage can decline the overall sperm count, and cause sperm DNA damage [23]. Arsenic accumulation in seminal vesicles, prostate and epididymis reduces the progressive sperm motility [24]. Beyond this arsenic also cause hormonal disturbance through affecting endocrine system, disturbing the secretion of androgen from leyding cells, it has significant association between arsenic exposure and

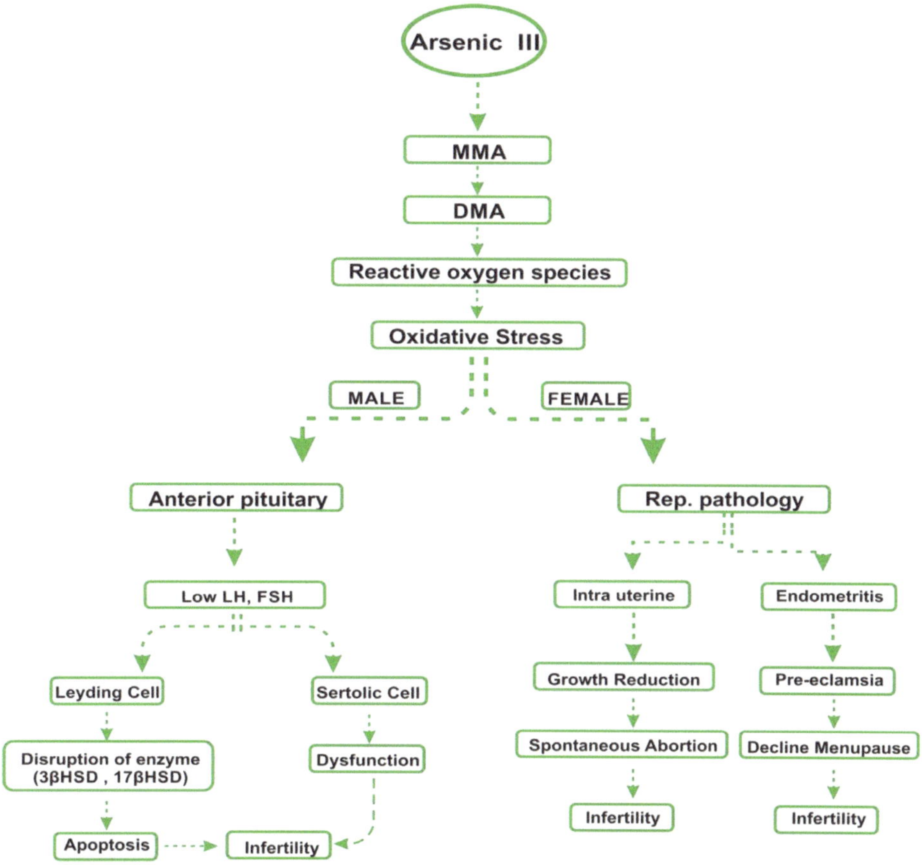

Figure 1.
Reproductive toxicity of arsenic.

sperm motility in arsenic exposed patients [24]. Environmental epidemiological evidences show that in general environmental conditions there is association between arsenic exposure and sperm quality in male [25]. The total arsenic concentration and sperm concentration are strongly correlated in the in the seminal plasma of heavily exposed human population [26]. The quality of semen of arsenic exposed population is decreased and there was a strong association between sperm percentage of the group exposed by arsenic, as the sperm concentration was lower in arsenic exposed group than non-exposed group [27].

3. Effects on spermatogenesis

The interference in spermatogenesis at cell differentiation stage can reduce the overall sperm count, increased anomalous sperms, and impaired constancy of sperm [28]. As accumulation of arsenic in seminal vesicles, seminal fluid, prostate, and epididymis may impair the sperm progressive motility [29]. In addition arsenic causes hormonal disproportion affecting neuroendocrine system and androgens, as there is strong evidence that oxidative stress vulnerably affect the spermatozoa due to extreme production of reactive oxygen species resulting in the peroxidation of poly unsaturated fatty acids in the plasma membrane [30]. Arsenic increase the reactive oxygen species production and decrease the glutathione, and other antioxidant level which lead to lipid per oxidation of cell membrane causing apoptosis leads to oxidative DNA damage [31, 32]. Damage of sperm membrane reduces sperm motility and ability to fuse with oocyte, whereas the sperm DNA damage compromise parental genomic involvement to the embryo [33] and increase the risk of infertility, and serious disease in offspring [34].

4. Effects on male fertility

In addition to affecting sperm quality, some epidemiological studies documented that arsenic exposure in the environment is increasing the sterility risks in populations which result in decrease androgen hormones level in body, sexual dysfunction and chromosomal aberration (**Figure 2**) [36]. As level of hormones and arsenic concentration is measured in the blood of infertile males which indicated that the concentration of arsenic and blood luteinizing hormones are strongly negatively correlated. LH can stimulate testosterone production in interstitial cell, the dysfunction or absence of testosterone lead to male infertility [37]. Epidemiological studies revealed that in Taiwan due to drinking of arsenic contaminated water the risk of prostate cancer is 6 times more than other population [38]. In many studies it is documented that risk of arsenic exposure affect genetic integrity in chromosome repeat region and it has certain effect on Y chromosome [38]. A group reported that arsenic exposure may increase erectile dysfunction; the experimental showed that the risk of erectile dysfunction was 3.4 fold higher in arsenic exposed population [39].

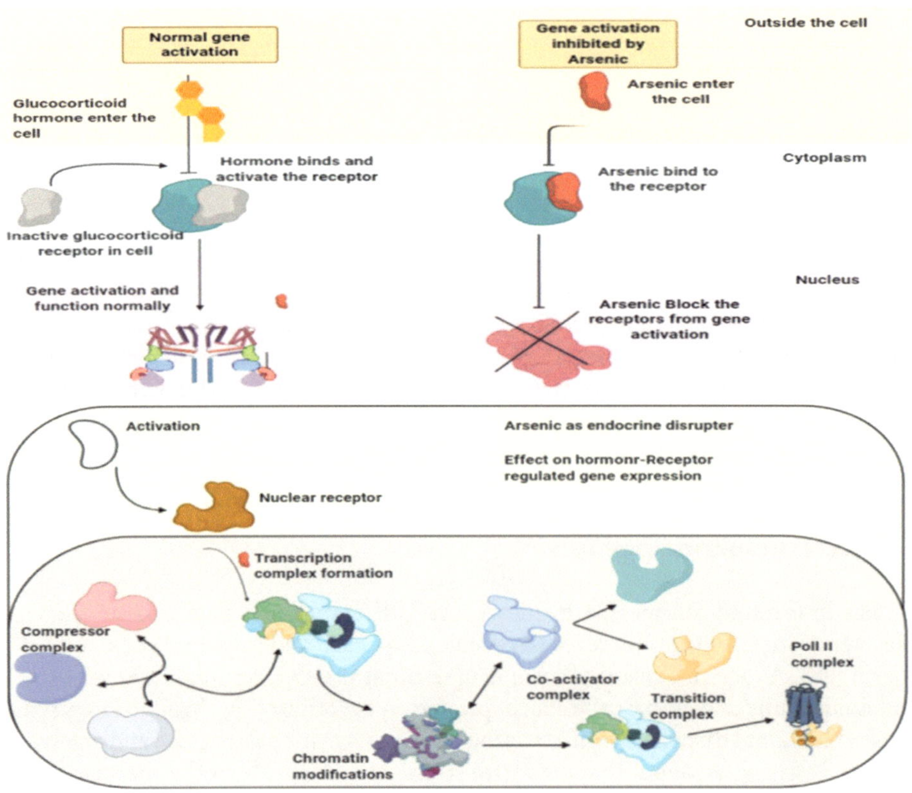

Figure 2.
Genotoxicity of arsenic adapted from [35].

5. Female reproductive toxicity

Recent data has summarized toxicological effects on female reproductive system in humans and animals implicating impaired fertility effects [40]. Infertility has been predicted as substantial public health hazard and becoming medical challenge round the globe [41], as it ahead of any uncertainty that lifestyle and quality of ambient environment can play fundamental role in reproductive success in both human and animal population [42]. It is demonstrated that exposure to toxic metals such as arsenic, lead and cadmium may be extremely involved in impaired fertility [43]. Arsenic is highly toxic and hazardous for pregnant humans and animals because it can disrupt the neuroendocrine system as it may inhibit estrogen binding receptors and un-regulate the progesterone receptors and it is potential source of estrogen dependent diseases such as breast cancer, endometritis and spontaneous abortions in human population [44]. Elevated endometrial cancer risk is associated with intake of arsenic [45]. Arsenic exposure may also affect angiogenesis in endometrium during pregnancy which is the most important for embryogenesis. These ailments lead to endometrial dysfunction, premature birth, subfertility, sterility and spontaneous abortions [17].

6. Female endocrine disruption

Arsenic is well recognized for its reproductive toxicity, as in case of male reproductive system it is accounted that to hinder activities of spermatogenetic enzymes and impede spermatogenesis [28]. Arsenic may act on brain or pituitary or and on germ line cells and affect the female reproductive system such as it reduce ovarian steroidogenesis, prolong diestrus, degenerate ovarian follicles and decrease the plasma level of estradiol and progesterone [46]. Furthermore reduced plasma gonadotrophin level may decline activities of ovarian 3β- HSD (Hydroxysteroid dehydrogenase) and 17β- HSD (Hydroxysteroid dehydrogenase), which are essential regulatory enzymes for steroidogenesis [47]. As it is observed that low plasma level of estradiol may be the cause of diestrus. Furthermore, arsenic exposure in human causes reproductive toxicity, including elevated incidence of miscarriages, still birth and low birth weight in offspring [17]. Similarly, it also effect on viability in the conceptus, dam mortality and weight gain of fetus [48]. Arsenic plays a potential role in disruption of female hormonal function, such as interfering hormone synthesis and hormone normal function. All hormones are differing in their structure and function and have various routes of synthesis with numerous steps. Arsenic exposure through pesticides and other products may disrupt the chain of hormone synthesis such as inhibition of estrogen biosynthesis [49], by preventing the conversion of androgen into estrogen [50]. Methylated arsenic may interfere in dopamine beta hydroxylase activity resulting in reduced conversion of dopamine into nor-epinephrine [19] which may lead to hindrance of hypothalamic catecholamine activity involved in generation of pro-estrus surge in LH, which stimulates ovulation [51]. It also inhibits various other enzymes which are involved in progesterone synthesis [52]. Disruption in LH timing surge could alter the viability and quality of oocytes [51] and inhibition of progesterone secretion may lead to poor conception (**Figure 1**) [48]. The distorted estrogen signaling may cause over expression of estrogen receptors through promoter region hypo-methylation and cause epigenetic change to produce estrogen like effect by direct or indirect stimulation of estrogen receptors.

7. Developmental toxicity

Inorganic arsenic affect the nervous system causing behavioral changes and peripheral neuropathies [53], as chronic exposure of arsenic during pregnancy may affect fetal brain development as a result mutilation of behavioral skills, including cognitive abilities and social competency. It is further conformed that exposure of chronic arsenic increase the risk of spontaneous abortions and stillbirths [54]. Significant association of arsenic exposure was found during pregnancy causing spontaneous abortions and stillbirth [3, 55]. It was reported that the elevated the risk of still birth and neonatal mortality amongst 200 married women in Bengal [55, 56]. All pregnant women were provided proper care in arsenic exposed area, showed significant association between arsenic concentration and birth defects. In the recent study spontaneous abortions and still births were observed between exposed and unexposed women, which included 240, women living in arsenic exposed area in West Bengal of India with high concentrated arsenic drinking water [55, 57] as well as [58] documented the most common arsenic exposed regions in West Bengal, and miscarriage was observed due to arsenic contaminated water. However spontaneous abortions and still births were observed in almost all the arsenic exposed areas throughout the world [55]. Furthermore, a hospital based study was conducted in Texas community with low level of arsenic exposure through inhalation primarily arsenic based agricultural products reported spontaneous abortions and stillbirths [59].

8. Effect on female fertility

According to WHO documentation more than 10% of women are at the risk of infertility through the exposure of heavy metals such as arsenic which are the major environmental contaminant which may cause reproductive disorders [60]. WHO surveyed that the problem of infertility was pre dominantly greater in female than in males. Ovulation disturbances account for common cause of sub fertility in women [61, 62], as ovulation disturbances are present in uneven or lacking menstrual periods and can overcome through reproductive hormones. The risk of infertility increased in women due to hormonal disturbance, delay ovulation, chromosomal aberration in oocytes by higher exposure level of toxicity. Hormonal imbalance is an important cause of infertility in females due to endocrine disruption by arsenic toxicity which is the major cause of infertility in females (**Figure 2**) [40]. It may also cause cycle abnormality, such as decline in estrus cycle number and elevated duration of diestrus [63]. Ovulation issues, endocrine interference with estrogenic properties may inhibit ovulation and the mid cycle LH surge from pituitary gland in females which may lead to female fertility problems [40, 64]. However, most studies revealed that the arsenic exposure through pesticides and insecticides is the major cause of infertility in females, as these decrease the number of mature follicles and elevate the number of atretic follicles and this indicates potential reduction in fertility [65]. Increased exposure to methylated arsenic may lead to decrease in uterus weight which may affect implantation and increase pre-implantation embryonic loss which leads to infertility in females [66]. A recent study revealed that the women exposed to pesticides have longer menstrual cycle and increased probability of missed periods, as studied in USA; infertile women were observed have three times more exposure to pesticides, in which whole chain of gametogenesis is affected [67].

9. Genotoxicity of arsenic

Several studies have documented the elevated inter individual variability in receptiveness of arsenic toxicity underlying genetic factor as a cause of variability. The genotoxicity of arsenic cause deoxyribonucleic acid modification such as chromosomal aberrations, mutation, micronuclei formation, deletion, sister chromatid exchange [68]. Numerous studies have been done to explain the genotoxic effect of arsenic, over and above stimulation of oxidative stress and distorted DNA repair [69]. For the purpose of understanding several studies confirmed the manipulation of genetic polymorphism in gene coding enzymes involved in mechanism of arsenic metabolism and detoxification [70]. It has been demonstrated that arsenic does not affect DNA directly and is considered a poor mutagen, as regardless of its low mutagenicity it affects the mutagenicity of other carcinogens. For illustration, an elevated increase in mutagenicity of arsenic with ultraviolet light has been observed in mammalian cells [71]. Progression of experimentation proposed that arsenic genotoxicity is associated with the generation of reactive oxygen species during its biotransformation [68]. The generation of reactive oxygen species is able to break DNA strands, cross links and chromosomal aberration [72]. One of the mechanisms of arsenic destroys to DNA is base adjustment in particular 8-oxoguanine is one of the most frequently formed DNA nuclease modifications which are a mutagenic miscoding lesion that lead to G: C to T: A transverse [73].

Moreover arsenic can induce DNA strand breaks even at low concentration [70], as single strand breaks are caused by reactive oxygen species on DNA base directly or indirectly during base excision repair mechanism [74]. As it was observed that human fibroblast cells demonstrate single strand break and chromatid substitute interfering with polyadenosinediphosphate ribose polymerase activity which is a protein important for single strand DNA break and double strand DNA break repair process (**Figure 2**) [75]. Recent studies revealed that chronic arsenic exposure induces oxidative DNA damage, reduced thymic functions and subsequent immunosuppression in childhood [76]. Arsenic is well known inducer of chromosomal aberration which involves both clastogenic and a euploidogenic [77]. Recent studies documented cytogenetic monitoring by using chromosomal aberration and micronuclei assay in order to observe genotoxic effects of arsenic in human and animal population [78]. Inhibition of DNA repair is considered one of the most important effects of genotoxicity of arsenic. Nucleotide excision repair and base excision repair are the two process of DNA repair which are inhibited by reactive oxygen species of arsenic [79]. Earlier studies revealed that arsenic exposure may hinder the nucleotide excision repair mechanism of DNA repair but in recent studies it is observed that it also inhibit the base excision repair mechanism (**Figure 2**) [80]. Changes in DNA repair mechanisms have been confirmed in human exposed population, as arsenic exposure was linked with reduced expression of excision repair to at low dose. They have found that arsenic metabolites can affect several processes in the cell [81–83]. Particularly cellular activity of human 8-oxoguanine DNA glycosylase was the most sensitively affected by dimethylmonoarsenic acid [80]. Recently, epidemiological studies revealed that arsenic may affect single nucleotide polymorphism in genes of DNA repair pathways [84]. Arsenic causes DNA damage and changes cellular capacity for DNA repair. Consequently alterations in DNA repair capacity is associated to the presence of polymorphisms in DNA repair genes which are related to risk of developing disturbance induced by arsenic [85].

10. Conclusions

One of the most important revelations is the effect of toxic metals on reproductive system in mammals. In the preceding section we attempted to provide a recent and clear glimpse in all aspects regarding arsenic toxicity on reproduction in mammals. It is the most important concern that should be explored for better understanding and seeking preventive measures to get rid of this striking issue. Arsenic is an important environmental toxicant that affects the reproductive system of mammals. These toxic effects are influenced by variant sources and routes as well as doses and periods of exposure. Integration of novel information on the formation of fate and actions of arsenic toxicity in human and animal population and other species will reduce the uncertainties in the risk assessment for arsenic. This effort would help to protect the public health against the toxic and carcinogenic effects associated with arsenic exposure.

Acknowledgements

Authors are thankful to anonymous reviewers for their valuable comments in critical review of the manuscript.

Author details

Hafiz Ishfaq Ahmad[1]*, Muhammad Bilal Bin Majeed[1], Abdul Jabbar[2], Ruqia Arif[3] and Gulnaz Afzal[4]

1 Department of Animal Breeding and Genetics, University of Veterinary and Animal Sciences, Lahore, Punjab, Pakistan

2 Department of Clinical Medicine, University of Veterinary and Animal Sciences, Lahore, Punjab, Pakistan

3 Institute of Biochemistry and Biotechnology, University of Veterinary and Animal Sciences Lahore, Punjab, Pakistan

4 Department of Zoology, The Islamia University, Bahawalpur, Pakistan

*Address all correspondence to: ishfaq.ahmad@uvas.edu.pk

References

[1] Rahman M, Sohel N, Yunus FM, Alam N, Nahar Q, Streatfield PK, et al. Arsenic exposure and young adult's mortality risk: A 13 year follow-up study in Matlab, Bangladesh. Environment international. 2019;123:358-67.

[2] Liao N, Seto E, Eskenazi B, Wang M, Li Y, Hua J. A comprehensive review of arsenic exposure and risk from rice and a risk assessment among a cohort of adolescents in Kunming, China. International journal of environmental research and public health. 2018;15(10):2191.

[3] Rahman MM, Bodrud-Doza M, Muhib MI, Hossain KFB, Hossain MS, Akter S, et al. Human Health Risk Assessment of Nitrate and Trace Metals Via Groundwater in Central Bangladesh. 2019.

[4] Landrigan PJ, Fuller R, Acosta NJ, Adeyi O, Arnold R, Baldé AB, et al. The Lancet Commission on pollution and health. The Lancet. 2018;391(10119):462-512.

[5] Shahid M, Niazi NK, Dumat C, Naidu R, Khalid S, Rahman MM, et al. A meta-analysis of the distribution, sources and health risks of arsenic-contaminated groundwater in Pakistan. Environmental pollution. 2018;242:307-19.

[6] Ahmad SA, Khan MH, Haque M. Arsenic contamination in groundwater in Bangladesh: implications and challenges for healthcare policy. Risk Management and Healthcare Policy. 2018;11:251.

[7] Bhowmick S, Pramanik S, Singh P, Mondal P, Chatterjee D, Nriagu J. Arsenic in groundwater of West Bengal, India: A review of human health risks and assessment of possible intervention options. Science of the Total Environment. 2018;612:148-69.

[8] Khalid S, Shahid M, Bibi I, Sarwar T, Shah A, Niazi N. A review of environmental contamination and health risk assessment of wastewater use for crop irrigation with a focus on low and high-income countries. International journal of environmental research and public health. 2018;15(5):895.

[9] Zubair M, Martyniuk CJ. A review on hemato-biochemical, accumulation and patho-morphological responses of arsenic toxicity in ruminants. Toxin Reviews. 2018:1-11.

[10] Keshavarzi B, Seradj A, Akbari Z, Moore F, Shahraki AR, Pourjafar M. Chronic arsenic toxicity in sheep of Kurdistan province, Western Iran. Archives of environmental contamination and toxicology. 2015;69(1):44-53.

[11] Rana T, Bera AK, Bhattacharya D, Das S, Pan D, Das SK. Chronic arsenicosis in goats with special reference to its exposure, excretion and deposition in an arsenic contaminated zone. Environmental toxicology and pharmacology. 2012;33(2):372-6.

[12] Thakur BK, Gupta V. Arsenic-Contaminated Drinking Water and the Associated Health Effects in the Shahpur Block of Bihar: A Case Study From Five Villages. Arsenic Water Resources Contamination: Springer; 2020. p. 257-71.

[13] Sarma SD, Hussain A, Sarma JD. Advances made in understanding the effects of arsenic exposure on humans. Current science. 2017;112(10):2008.

[14] Sinha D, Prasad P. Health effects inflicted by chronic low-level arsenic contamination in groundwater: A global

public health challenge. Journal of Applied Toxicology. 2020;40(1):87-131.

[15] Chen C-J. Health hazards and mitigation of chronic poisoning from arsenic in drinking water: Taiwan experiences. Reviews on environmental health. 2014;29(1-2):13-9.

[16] Khairul I, Wang QQ, Jiang YH, Wang C, Naranmandura H. Metabolism, toxicity and anticancer activities of arsenic compounds. Oncotarget. 2017;8(14):23905.

[17] Milton AH, Hussain S, Akter S, Rahman M, Mouly TA, Mitchell K. A review of the effects of chronic arsenic exposure on adverse pregnancy outcomes. International journal of environmental research and public health. 2017;14(6):556.

[18] Waalkes MP, Ward JM, Liu J, DiwanBA.Transplacentalcarcinogenicity of inorganic arsenic in the drinking water: induction of hepatic, ovarian, pulmonary, and adrenal tumors in mice. Toxicol Appl Pharmacol. 2003;186(1):7-17.

[19] Kim M, Seo S, Sung K, Kim K. Arsenic exposure in drinking water alters the dopamine system in the brains of C57BL/6 mice. Biological trace element research. 2014;162(1-3):175-80.

[20] Davey JC, Nomikos AP, WungjiranirunM, ShermanJR, IngramL, Batki C, et al. Arsenic as an endocrine disruptor: arsenic disrupts retinoic acid receptor–and thyroid hormone receptor–mediated gene regulation and thyroid hormone–mediated amphibian tail metamorphosis. Environmental health perspectives. 2008;116(2):165-72.

[21] Meakin CJ, Szilagyi JT, Avula V, Fry RC. Inorganic arsenic and its methylated metabolites as endocrine disruptors in the placenta: Mechanisms underpinning glucocorticoid receptor (GR) pathway perturbations. Toxicology and Applied Pharmacology. 2020:115305.

[22] Amann RP. The cycle of the seminiferous epithelium in humans: a need to revisit? J Androl. 2008;29(5):469-87.

[23] Hess RA. Effects of environmental toxicants on the efferent ducts, epididymis and fertility. JOURNAL OF REPRODUCTION AND FERTILITY-SUPPLEMENT-. 1998:247-59.

[24] Renu K, Madhyastha H, MadhyasthaR,MaruyamaM,VinayagamS, Gopalakrishnan AV. Review on molecular and biochemical insights of arsenic-mediated male reproductive toxicity. Life sciences. 2018;212:37-58.

[25] Li P, Zhong Y, Jiang X, Wang C, Zuo Z, Sha A. Seminal plasma metals concentration with respect to semen quality. Biol Trace Elem Res. 2012;148(1):1-6.

[26] Xu W, Bao H, Liu F, Liu L, Zhu Y-G, She J, et al. Environmental exposure to arsenic may reduce human semen quality: associations derived from a Chinese cross-sectional study. Environmental Health. 2012;11(1):46.

[27] Sanocka D, Miesel R, Jedrzejczak P, Kurpisz MK. Oxidative stress and male infertility. J Androl. 1996;17(4):449-54.

[28] Zeng Q, Yi H, Huang L, An Q, Wang H. Reduced testosterone and Ddx3y expression caused by long-term exposure to arsenic and its effect on spermatogenesis in mice. Environmental toxicology and pharmacology. 2018;63:84-91.

[29] Bashandy SA, El Awdan SA, Ebaid H, Alhazza IM. Antioxidant potential of Spirulina platensis mitigates oxidative stress and reprotoxicity induced by sodium arsenite in male rats. Oxidative medicine and cellular longevity. 2016;2016.

[30] Koppers AJ, De Iuliis GN, Finnie JM, McLaughlin EA, Aitken RJ. Significance of mitochondrial reactive oxygen species in the generation of oxidative stress in spermatozoa. The Journal of Clinical Endocrinology & Metabolism. 2008;93(8):3199-207.

[31] Jones R, Mann T, Sherins R. Peroxidative breakdown of phospholipids in human spermatozoa, spermicidal properties of fatty acid peroxides, and protective action of seminal plasma. Fertil Steril. 1979;31(5):531-7.

[32] Wellejus A, Poulsen HE, Loft S. Iron-induced oxidative DNA damage in rat sperm cells in vivo and in vitro. Free Radical Res. 2000;32(1):75-83.

[33] Aitken RJ, Koppers AJ. Apoptosis and DNA damage in human spermatozoa. Asian journal of andrology. 2011;13(1):36.

[34] Meeker JD, Rossano MG, Protas B, Padmanahban V, Diamond MP, Puscheck E, et al. Environmental exposure to metals and male reproductive hormones: circulating testosterone is inversely associated with blood molybdenum. Fertil Steril. 2010;93(1):130-40.

[35] Bustaffa E, Stoccoro A, Bianchi F, Migliore L. Genotoxic and epigenetic mechanisms in arsenic carcinogenicity. Arch Toxicol. 2014;88(5):1043-67.

[36] Ahangarpour A, Oroojan AA, Alboghobeish S, Khorsandi L, Moradi M. Toxic Effects of Chronic Exposure to High-Fat Diet and Arsenic on the Reproductive System of the Male Mouse. Journal of Family & Reproductive Health. 2019;13(4):181.

[37] Zubair M, Ahmad M, Saleemi MK, Gul ST, Ahmad M, Martyniuk CJ, et al. Sodium arsenite toxicity on hematology indices and reproductive parameters in Teddy goat bucks and their amelioration with vitamin C. Environmental Science and Pollution Research. 2020:1-10.

[38] Ali S, Ali S. Genetic integrity of the human Y chromosome exposed to groundwater arsenic. BMC medical genomics. 2010;3(1):35.

[39] Jang DH, Hoffman RS. Heavy metal chelation in neurotoxic exposures. Neurol Clin. 2011;29(3):607-22.

[40] Rattan S, Zhou C, Chiang C, Mahalingam S, Brehm E, Flaws JA. Exposure to endocrine disruptors during adulthood: consequences for female fertility. Journal of Endocrinology. 2017;233(3):R109-R29.

[41] Shahab A, Qi S, Zaheer M. Arsenic contamination, subsequent water toxicity, and associated public health risks in the lower Indus plain, Sindh province, Pakistan. Environmental Science and Pollution Research. 2019;26(30):30642-62.

[42] Sharpe RM, Franks S. Environment, lifestyle and infertility--an inter-generational issue. Nat Cell Biol. 2002;4.

[43] Rzymski P, Rzymski P, Tomczyk K, Niedzielski P, Jakubowski K, Poniedziałek B, et al. Metal status in human endometrium: relation to cigarette smoking and histological lesions. Environ Res. 2014;132:328-33.

[44] Borja-Aburto VH, Hertz-Picciotto I, Lopez MR, Farias P, Rios C, Blanco J. Blood lead levels measured prospectively and risk of spontaneous abortion. Am J Epidemiol. 1999;150(6):590-7.

[45] Salnikow K, Zhitkovich A. Genetic and epigenetic mechanisms in metal carcinogenesis and cocarcinogenesis: nickel, arsenic, and chromium. Chem Res Toxicol. 2007;21(1):28-44.

[46] Ghersevich S, Nokelainen P, Poutanen M, Orava M, Autio-Harmainen H, Rajaniemi H, et al.

Rat17beta-hydroxysteroiddehydrogenase type 1: primary structure and regulation of enzyme expression in rat ovary by diethylstilbestrol and gonadotropins in vivo. Endocrinology. 1994;135(4):1477-87.

[47] Schroeder HA, Mitchener M. Toxic effects of trace elements on the reproduction of mice and rats. Archives of Environmental Health: An International Journal. 1971;23(2): 102-6.

[48] Calderon J, Navarro M, Jimenez-Capdeville M, Santos-Diaz M, Golden A, Rodriguez-Leyva I, et al. Exposure to arsenic and lead and neuropsychological development in Mexican children. Environ Res. 2001;85(2):69-76.

[49] Chatterjee A, Chatterji U. Arsenic abrogates the estrogen-signaling pathway in the rat uterus. Reprod Biol Endocrinol. 2010;8(1):80.

[50] Mason JI, Carr BR, Murry BA. Imidazole antimycotics: selective inhibitors of steroid aromatization and progesterone hydroxylation. Steroids. 1987;50(1):179-89.

[51] Chattopadhyay S, Ghosh D. The involvement of hypophyseal-gonadal and hypophyseal-adrenal axes in arsenic-mediated ovarian and uterine toxicity: Modulation by hCG. Journal of Biochemical and Molecular Toxicology. 2010;24(1):29-41.

[52] Fugo N, Butcher RL. Overripeness and the mammalian ova: I. Overripeness and early embryonic development. Fertil Steril. 1966;17(6):804-14.

[53] Sárközi K, Horváth E, Vezér T, Papp A, Paulik E. Behavioral and general effects of subacute oral arsenic exposure in rats with and without fluoride. International journal of environmental health research. 2015;25(4):418-31.

[54] Rahman A, Kumarathasan P, Gomes J. Infant and mother related outcomes from exposure to metals with endocrine disrupting properties during pregnancy. Science of the Total Environment. 2016;569:1022-31.

[55] Von Ehrenstein O, Guha Mazumder D, Hira-Smith M, Ghosh N, Yuan Y, Windham G, et al. Pregnancy outcomes, infant mortality, and arsenic in drinking water in West Bengal, India. American journal of epidemiology. 2006;163(7):662-9.

[56] Sen J, Chaudhuri A. Arsenic exposure through drinking water and its effect on pregnancy outcome in Bengali women. Archives of Industrial Hygiene and Toxicology. 2008;59(4):271-5.

[57] Mukherjee SC, Rahman MM, Chowdhury UK, Sengupta MK, Lodh D, Chanda CR, et al. Neuropathy in arsenic toxicity from groundwater arsenic contamination in West Bengal, India. Journal of Environmental Science and Health, Part A. 2003;38(1):165-83.

[58] Barchowsky A, Roussel RR, Klei LR, James PE, Ganju N, Smith KR, et al. Low levels of arsenic trioxide stimulate proliferative signals in primary vascular cells without activating stress effector pathways. Toxicol Appl Pharmacol. 1999;159(1):65-75.

[59] Lei H-L, Wei H-J, Ho H-Y, Liao K-W, Chien L-C. Relationship between risk factors for infertility in women and lead, cadmium, and arsenic blood levels: a cross-sectional study from Taiwan. BMC Public Health. 2015;15(1):1220.

[60] Apostoli P, Catalani S. Metal ions affecting reproduction and development. Met Ions Life Sci. 2011;8(5):263-303.

[61] Upadhyay Y, Chhabra A, Nagar JC. A Women Infertility: An Overview. Asian Journal of Pharmaceutical Research and Development. 2020;8(2):99-106.

[62] Naz B, Batool SS. Infertility related issues and challenges: perspectives of patients, spouses, and infertility experts. Pakistan Journal of Social and Clinical Psychology. 2017;15(2):3-11.

[63] Biswas P, Mukhopadhyay A, Kabir SN, Mukhopadhyay PK. High-protein diet ameliorates arsenic-induced oxidative stress and antagonizes uterine apoptosis in rats. Biological trace element research. 2019;192(2):222-33.

[64] Ashby J, Tinwell H, Stevens J, Pastoor T, Breckenridge C. The effects of atrazine on the sexual maturation of female rats. Regul Toxicol Pharmacol. 2002;35(3):468-73.

[65] Stoker TE, Goldman JM, Cooper RL. The dithiocarbamate fungicide thiram disrupts the hormonal control of ovulation in the female rat. Reprod Toxicol. 1993;7(3):211-8.

[66] Ma W-g, Song H, Das SK, Paria BC, Dey SK. Estrogen is a critical determinant that specifies the duration of the window of uterine receptivity for implantation. Proceedings of the National Academy of Sciences. 2003;100(5):2963-8.

[67] Nurminen T. Maternal pesticide exposure and pregnancy outcome. J Occup Environ Med. 1995;37(8):935-40.

[68] Liu S-X, Davidson MM, Tang X, Walker WF, Athar M, Ivanov V, et al. Mitochondrial damage mediates genotoxicity of arsenic in mammalian cells. Cancer research. 2005;65(8):3236-42.

[69] Pierce BL, Kibriya MG, Tong L, Jasmine F, Argos M, Roy S, et al. Genome-wide association study identifies chromosome 10q24. 32 variants associated with arsenic metabolism and toxicity phenotypes in Bangladesh. PLoS Genet. 2012;8(2):e1002522.

[70] Martinez VD, Vucic EA, Adonis M, Gil L, Lam WL. Arsenic biotransformation as a cancer promoting factor by inducing DNA damage and disruption of repair mechanisms. Mol Biol Int. 2011;2011.

[71] Yin Y, Meng F, Sui C, Jiang Y, Zhang L. Arsenic enhances cell death and DNA damage induced by ultraviolet B exposure in mouse epidermal cells through the production of reactive oxygen species. Clinical and experimental dermatology. 2019;44(5):512-9.

[72] Jomova K, Jenisova Z, Feszterova M, Baros S, Liska J, Hudecova D, et al. Arsenic: toxicity, oxidative stress and human disease. Journal of Applied Toxicology. 2011;31(2):95-107.

[73] Grollman AP, Moriya M. Mutagenesis by 8-oxoguanine: an enemy within. Trends Genet. 1993;9(7):246-9.

[74] Kligerman AD, Malik SI, Campbell JA. Cytogenetic insights into DNA damage and repair of lesions induced by a monomethylated trivalent arsenical. Mutation Research/Genetic Toxicology and Environmental Mutagenesis. 2010;695(1):2-8.

[75] Qin X-J, Hudson LG, Liu W, Timmins GS, Liu KJ. Low concentration of arsenite exacerbates UVR-induced DNA strand breaks by inhibiting PARP-1 activity. Toxicol Appl Pharmacol. 2008;232(1):41-50.

[76] Ahmed S, Ahsan KB, Kippler M, Mily A, Wagatsuma Y, Hoque AW, et al. In utero arsenic exposure is associated with impaired thymic function in newborns possibly via oxidative stress and apoptosis. Toxicol Sci. 2012;129(2):305-14.

[77] Huang H-W, Lee C-H, Yu H-S. Arsenic-Induced Carcinogenesis and Immune Dysregulation. International journal of environmental research and public health. 2019;16(15):2746.

[78] Ghosh P, Basu A, Mahata J, Basu S, Sengupta M, Das JK, et al. Cytogenetic

damage and genetic variants in the individuals susceptible to arsenic-induced cancer through drinking water. Int J Cancer. 2006;118(10):2470-8.

[79] Lai Y, Zhao W, Chen C, Wu M, Zhang Z. Role of DNA polymerase beta in the genotoxicity of arsenic. Environ Mol Mutag. 2011;52(6):460-8.

[80] Ebert F, Weiss A, Bültemeyer M, Hamann I, Hartwig A, Schwerdtle T. Arsenicals affect base excision repair by several mechanisms. Mutation Research/ Fundamental and Molecular Mechanisms of Mutagenesis. 2011;715(1-2):32-41.

[81] Andrew AS, Karagas MR, Hamilton JW. Decreased DNA repair gene expression among individuals exposed to arsenic in United States drinking water. Int J Cancer. 2003;104(3):263-8.

[82] Andrew AS, Burgess JL, Meza MM, Demidenko E, Waugh MG, Hamilton JW, et al. Arsenic exposure is associated with decreased DNA repair in vitro and in individuals exposed to drinking water arsenic. Environ Health Perspect. 2006;114(8):1193.

[83] Mauro M, Caradonna F, Klein CB. Dysregulation of DNA methylation induced by past arsenic treatment causes persistent genomic instability in mammalian cells. Environmental and molecular mutagenesis. 2016;57(2):137-50.

[84] Fujihara J, Soejima M, Yasuda T, Koda Y, Kunito T, Iwata H, et al. Polymorphic trial in oxidative damage of arsenic exposed Vietnamese. Toxicol Appl Pharmacol. 2011;256(2):174-8.

[85] Kundu M, Ghosh P, Mitra S, Das J, Sau T, Banerjee S, et al. Precancerous and non-cancer disease endpoints of chronic arsenic exposure: the level of chromosomal damage and XRCC3 T241M polymorphism. Mutation Research/Fundamental and Molecular Mechanisms of Mutagenesis. 2011;706(1):7-12.

Chapter 10

Chemical Pollution of Drinking Water in Haiti: An Important Threat to Public Health

Alexandra Emmanuel and Evens Emmanuel

Abstract

The geophysical environment of the Republic of Haiti is characterized by hydrological and biogeographical climatic phenomena, and a relief marked by its rugged appearance. Most of the territory is occupied by mountains formed of limestone. The differences in level are very marked. Fragmentation is another feature of the relief. These environmental imperfections juxtaposed with difficult socioeconomic conditions and anthropogenic actions raise questions about possible chemical metal pollution of the country's water resources. Indeed, the predominance of limestone in the Haitian geology generate water hardness, and in the case where the magnesium concentration is less than 7 mg/l, this water may be the source of cardiovascular diseases. Studies carried out on several water points show a total hardness greater than 200 mg/l. In Port-au-Prince, concentrations of lead ranging from 40 μg/L to 90 μg/L and high Cr (III) risks were measured and estimated in groundwater and drinking water. Concentration of fluorine ranging from 0 to 2 mg/l were obtained from water resources. Concentration above 1.5 mg/l have been found from alluvial aquifers. Chronic public health risks, such as cardiovascular diseases, deterioration of the psychological development of children, irreversible functional and morphological renal changes, and dental fluorosis, strain Haiti's water resources. Chemicals' exposures seem to pose a threat to public health in Haiti, which need to be studied. The aim of this study is: (i) to analyze the contribution of geology and anthropogenic actions in the alteration of water quality, (ii) to review the toxicology of chemicals detected in water distributed in Port-au-Prince.

Keywords: chemical pollutions, drinking water, environmental health, medical geology, One Health, Haiti

1. Introduction

Water is essential for sustaining life, yet it is also the source of many diseases for living things [1]. With the increase in population and the development of industrial activities, surface water resources and groundwater have become increasingly polluted. Thus, humans are exposed to many chemicals found in drinking water.

Several chemicals (organic and inorganic) have been identified in drinking water, and the sources of pollution of the drinking water system are multiple [2]. Among these pollutants, the literature reports particularly chlorine disinfection by-

IntechOpen

products [3–5], fluorine [6–8], lead [9, 10] chromium [11–13], cadmium [14, 15], nitrates [16, 17], pesticides [18, 19], hardness [20, 21], arsenic [22, 23], etc. The presence of chemical substances in the municipal drinking water is a major health concern. Indeed, some substances detected in drinking water have been the subject of epidemiological studies [1]. The health effects reported in the literature are different cases of cancer, reproductive problems (malformations) cardiovascular and neurological diseases. Drinking water is therefore an important route of exposure to chemicals.

Pollutants, particularly heavy metals are released into the environment from a wide spectrum of natural and anthropogenic sources [24]. Heavy metals are omnipresent in the environment, occurring in varying concentrations in air, bedrock, soil, water, and all biological matter [25, 26]. The principal anthropogenic sources are industrial and urban effluents, runoff water, drinking water production and distribution equipment and drinking water treatment processes [1]. The presence of heavy metals in the environment constitutes a potential source of both soil and groundwater pollution.

In Haiti, the work carried out in the field of the physicochemical quality of water intended for pollutants such as: lead, chromium [27], fluorine [28]. Excessive concentrations of hardness have also been observed in water resources [29]. These concentrations of natural origin are added to those generated by anthropogenic actions, such as poor management of solid waste, the absence of urban sanitation networks and water treatment plants only increase the rate of human exposures to these pollutants. These exposures to chemical substances continue to put Haitians at risk, and several examples shed light on the realities of risk management with respect to toxic chemicals in developing Countries [30]. The fact that the hydrographic basin of Port-au-Prince consists mainly of karst aquifers [31], rainwater, polluted by atmospheric particles of substances originating from industrial activities, and urban wastewater feeds, through the dominant geology, groundwater, thus leading to suppose that the water resources of this region are subject to significant chemical pollution.

The impact on human health of natural materials such as water, rocks and minerals has been known for thousands of years, but there have been few systematic and multidisciplinary studies on the relationship between geologic materials and processes and human health (the field of study commonly referred to as medical geology) [32]. In order to achieve a better understanding in urban and rural areas of Haiti of the different routes of exposure and the causes of a number of environmental health problems generated by exposure to high concentrations of essential and non-essential chemicals for the organism that are detected in drinking water, it seems relevant that geoscientists, environmental and health science researchers; as well as public health specialists combine their skills to approach the problem of pollution of water intended for human consumption by taking into account the two main sources of the qualitative degradation of water: "geological contributions and anthropogenic actions". The aim of this study is: (i) to analyze the contribution of geology and anthropogenic actions in the alteration of water quality, (ii) to review the toxicology of chemicals detected in water distributed in Port-au-Prince.

2. Medical geology and environmental health in the geographical context of Port-au-Prince

2.1 Environmental health and assessment of health risks associated with chemical mixtures in drinking water

During the 1950s, forms of anxiety gradually manifested themselves regarding the state of environmental degradation and its harmful consequences for the survival of ecosystems and for development [33]. Indeed, since the said decade, the environment-human health relationship has become a major concern in the field of public health. The questions of contaminated soil, emanations from landfills, destruction of the ozone layer, global warming, food contamination, radiation emitted by household appliances, new biological hazards … are among the subjects of intervention by government authorities [34].

Abenhaim [35] argues "Environmental health issues are among the most complex for scientists to study and the most difficult for policy makers to resolve. First, because it is rare that the exhibitions are pure, thus leaving room for many confounding factors. Then, because the contaminations are generally in relatively small quantity, at the limits of the observable effects. Finally, because the consequences of exposure often occur over the long term" [35]. Exposure to chemical mixtures is a reality that would seem to dictate the need to pay much attention to hazard identification, exposure assessment and risk characterization [36], of mixtures in water intended for human consumption. Contrary to this environmental reality, the toxicological reality is that until recently most of the research carried out in this field has been devoted to studies on the effects of substances acting independently, without considering the interactions or combined effects between pollutants at the inside the human organism [37].

In Haiti, all the work carried out on the health risk linked to the pollution of drinking water by chemical substances, the risk characterization was made based on the independent effects of the pollutants studied. This approach provides information on the level of exposure of the population to a substance but does not make it possible to assess the interactions of the various pollutants detected in the distributed water. It is now widely recognized that studying the combined effects of chemical mixtures in drinking water is an integral part of public health [37]. Characterizing the combined actions of chemical mixtures involves the challenge of how to define the antagonistic, additive, or synergistic effect. It is therefore important to understand the terminology that describes the combined effect of the agents in terms of the mechanism of action. Seventy years ago, three basic concepts of common action or the interaction of the combination of chemicals were defined by biomathematicians [38–40] and they are still valid today.

Indeed, Bliss [38] identified three modes of action of constituents within a mixture vis-à-vis living organisms:

1. "*Independent joint action*": in this type of action, the constituents act on different sites of action and the biological response of one constituent is not influenced by another.

2. "*Similar joint action*": the constituents act on the same sites of action and the biological response of one constituent is not influenced by another. This is the approach most used for the study of mixtures.

3. "*Synergistic action*": where the response of a mixture cannot be known by the isolated responses of the constituents. The response of a mixture depends on the combined effects of its constituents.

All three basic principles of common action of pollutants are theoretical. However, these concepts will most likely need to be addressed at the same time, especially when the mixtures consist of more than two compounds and when the targets (individuals rather than cells) are more complex.

Fox et al. [41] considers the risk assessment of chemical mixtures or the cumulative risk assessment (CRA) as the most recent step in the evolution of assessment.

USEPA [42, 43] defines this approach as an analysis, characterization, and possible quantification of the combined risks to human health or the environment due to multiple substances or stressors. This definition suggests that additivity is the initially accepted mode of action for the implementation of ERC.

U.S. EPA [44] developed for the implementation of cumulative risk assessment, the Hazard Index (HI) method. This approach first assesses the effects of a substance acting independently of the others. HI is calculated by dividing the measured or estimated exposure concentration by the reference concentration (RfC):

$$HI = \text{Measured or estimated exposure concentration}/RfC$$

For $HI < 1$, the exposure concentration is below the cutoff value, so no health effect can be expected. On the other hand, for $HI \geq 1$, the exposure concentration exceeds the threshold value, further research on the health effects of the pollutant is recommended, by calculating the Hazard metric HM.

$$HM = \text{Measured or estimated exposure concentration}/\text{NOAEL or adjusted LOAEL}$$

Based on the additive action of pollutants, the application of the HI or HM model to assess the concentration of exposure due to chemical mixtures can be also expressed:

$$LCE = \frac{C_1}{M_1} + \frac{C_2}{M_2} + \frac{C_n}{M_n} \leq 1 \quad (1)$$

LCE: Limit of exposure concentration

C1, C2 and Cn: observed concentrations.

M: Maximum acceptable concentration (threshold value)

In the distribution units where chlorination is applied to raw water rich in organic matter, a quite common situation or process in Haiti, the populations served are exposed to a certain number of chemical substances (by example Disinfection by-products (DBPs)), very known for their adverse effects on human health, especially the occurrence of cancers [45, 46]. In the absence of national standards for the quality of drinking water, Haiti applies the guidelines of the World Health Organization. The application of the HI or HM model in the evaluation of the combined effects of by-products could be, in a simplified manner, carried out from:

$$THMs = \frac{EcCHBr_3}{TS_{WHO}CHBr_3} + \frac{EcCHBr_2Cl}{TS_{WHO}CHBr_2Cl} + \frac{EcCHBrCl_2}{TS_{WHO}CHBrCl_2} + \frac{EcCHCl_3}{TS_{WHO}CHCl_3} < 1 \quad (2)$$

THMs: Trihalomethanes

EC: Exposure concentration

CHBr3: Bromoform

CHBr2Cl: Chlodibromomethane

CHBrCl2: Bromodichlomethane

CHCl3: Chloroform

TSWHO: WHO threshold value Different types of complex mixtures require different approaches, and the usefulness of a certain approach depends on the context in which one is confronted with a mixture, and on the amount, type and quality of the available data on the chemistry and the toxicity of the mixture [47]. Scientific literature reports the occurrence of several detected in drinking water in Haiti [26–29]. Moreover, MSPP and WHO [48] note "the quality of water intended for human consumption is not subject to any control. In such a context, the study of the combined effects of several chemical substances in drinking water and the assessment of the risks generated for human health constitute an important topic of transdisciplinary public health research.

2.2 Medical geology and ONE HEALTH approach in health risks assessment of drinking water in Haiti

Located between 18° and 20°6' Northern latitude and between 71°20′ and 74°30' Western longitude, Haiti divides with Dominican Republic "the island of Hispaniola" which is the second biggest island of the Caribbean. Its capital, Port-au-Prince, is settled at the bottom of the Gulf of "La Gonâve", in the south border of Plain of Cul-de-sac and in the north catchment area of the "Massif de la Selle" piedmont (**Figure 1**). The main municipalities which constitute urban community of Port-au-Prince are Port-au-Prince, Delmas, Pétion-ville, Croix-des-bouquets, Gressier and Carrefour.

Haiti is exposed to a considerable ecological imbalance, characterized by catastrophic flooding associated to torrential rains and hurricanes, devastating earthquakes, and deforestation [50]. Other problems, resulting from this imbalance include land use forming the immediate perimeter of headwaters and wells, wetlands draining, arable soils erosion, the decrease of the headwaters flow and groundwater, seawater intrusion, sewers obstruction and fecal pollution [51]. In addition, Haiti is one of the most vulnerable countries to climate change [52]. In general, Haiti's geophysical environment is characterized by rugged relief. Most of the territory is occupied by mountains formed of limestone and karst aquifers [31, 53–55]. The existence of karst aquifers conditions in rainy weather the contamination of groundwater by surface pollution. Indeed, the main characteristics of

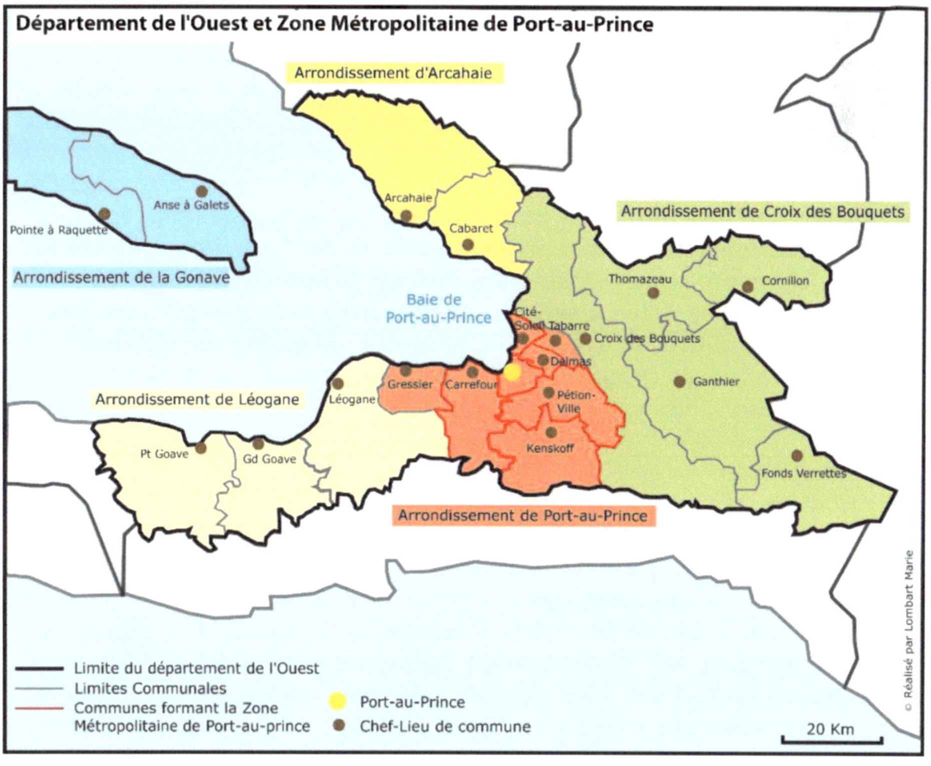

Figure 1.
Map of the west department of Haiti and metropolitan area of Port-au-Prince [49].

karst aquifers are the existence of irregular networks of pores, cracks, fractures and pipes of various shapes and sizes. Such a structure, of significant physical and geometric heterogeneity, causes complex hydraulic conditions and the spatial and temporal variability of hydraulic parameters. After a downpour, rapid and turbulent groundwater recharge occurs through drainage in large conduits with high volume of unfiltered water [56].

Groundwater resources at Port-au-Prince are vulnerable to contamination related to polluted water infiltration such as leachates, cesspools and septic tanks, stormwater runoff, waste oil discharging, over-irrigation and industrial discharging [50]. These sources of groundwater recharge may contain organic and inorganic compounds which can be in dissolved and colloidal forms or associated to particles. Microbiological and physicochemical characterization of groundwater resources in the metropolitan area of Port-au-Prince, among other things, highlight the presence of heavy metals [57], fecal coliforms [27] and Cryptosporidium oocysts [58]. In addition to bacterial and metal contaminations, it was found that aquifers in Haiti are also exposed to seawater pollution [50]. According to Gonfiantini and Simonot [59], the salt water is slightly enriched with heavy isotopes with respect to fresh groundwater, not showing any deviation from the straight line of meteoric waters. In the area of Port-au-Prince, the salinity of the groundwater is the result of seawater intrusion because of intensive exploitation [59].

The geophysical environment of Port-au-Prince, the inefficiency of the sanitation system (collection and treatment of solid waste, drainage, and treatment of wastewater, etc.), which contribute to the microbiological and physicochemical quality of the water distributed by public networks to the population gives rise to a particular epidemiological environment where the water generates several dangers for the health of consumers. In such a context, the assessment and management of health risks associated with water intended for human consumption require a multidisciplinary approach and call on researchers, technicians, and specialists in several fields of life and earth sciences as well as the humanities and social sciences.

The 2030 Agenda for Sustainable Development of the United Nations (UN) establishes goals and targets in areas of critical importance for humanity [60, 61], Ramirez-Mendoza et al., 2020 [62]. Indeed, the SDGs are linked to one another, the success of one often depending on the resolution of problems generally associated with another objective [60]. They thus constitute a universal and transversal approach concerning all countries, in the North as in the South. Regarding the issue of water, objective 6 - access to safe water and sanitation - aims to meet the challenges of drinking water, sanitation, and hygiene for populations, as well as issues concerning aquatic ecosystems. In the absence of quality and sustainable water resources and sanitation, progress in several other areas of the Sustainable Development Goals, including health, education and reduce of poverty, will also be delayed [60]. This objective, taken in the prism of the situation of the urban and hydrological context, as well as the geophysical environment of Haiti, raises concerns. However, the launching by public authorities and funding agencies of large research programs with the objective of generating and applying knowledge, promoting innovations in the life and earth sciences, as well as in human and social sciences, in a context of transdisciplinary would be of great use, even essential for the development to achieve the various objectives [63]. Indeed, Medical geology, the science that deals with the relationship between natural geological factors and human and animal health problems [32], and the One Health approach, an approach that attempts to bringing together medical/public health researchers, veterinary researchers, and environmental scientists to tackle health problems, provides an adequate theoretical framework to address environmental health problems resulting from the degradation of natural environment in Port-au- Prince.

The interconnectedness of human, animal, and environmental health is at the heart of One Health, an increasingly important prism through which governments, NGOs (nongovernmental organizations), and practitioners view human health) [64]. Mazet et al., [65] note "An important implication of the One Health approach is that integrated policy interventions that simultaneously and holistically address multiple and interacting causes of poor human health—unsafe and scarce water, lack of sanitation, food insecurity, and proximity between animals and humans—will yield significantly larger health benefits than policies that target each of these factors individually and in isolation. By its very nature, the One Health approach is transdisciplinary, since it is predicated on agricultural scientists, anthropologists, economists, educators, engineers, entomologists, epidemiologists, hydrologists, microbiologists, nutritionists, physicians, public health professionals, sociologists, and veterinarians working collaboratively to improve and promote both human and animal health" [65].

3. Chemistry and toxicology of selected pollutants detected in water distributed in Port-au-Prince

3.1 Presence of fluoride in drinking water and risk for human health

Fluoride, the 13th most abundant element in the earth's crust, is essential to human life [66]. Elemental fluorine almost never occurs in nature, but fluoride is widely distributed in the Earth's crust, mainly as the mineral's fluorspar, cryolite, apatite, mica, hornblende, and fluorite [67, 68]. **Table 1** shows certain physical and chemical properties of fluoride.

Fluoride participates in the formation of bones and teeth and contributes to their solidification. It enters the body in the form of fluorides through drinking water, food, air, drugs, and cosmetics. It is known to have beneficial and harmful effects on humans [69]. Indeed, its deficiency has long been linked to the incidence of dental caries [70], while prolonged excessive intake has been associated with fluorosis [71]. Large populations throughout parts of the developing world suffer the effects of chronic endemic fluorosis [70].

The most important source of fluoride intake in the human body is drinking water [72]. According to WHO [73], the guideline value for fluoride in drinking-water is 1.5 mg/L, based on increasing risk of dental fluorosis at higher

	Fluoride
Molecular formula	F_2
CAS#	7782-41-4
Molecular Weight	37.996 g/mol
Melting point	−219°C
Boiling Point	−188.13°C
Solubility	Water
Density	1.517 at −188.13°C
Vapor pressure	760 mm Hg at 85 K
Source	https://pubchem.ncbi.nlm.nih.gov/compound/24524

Table 1.
Physical and chemical properties of fluoride.

concentrations and that progressively higher levels lead to increasing risks of skeletal fluorosis. This value is higher than that recommended for artificial fluoridation of water supplies for prevention of dental caries, which is usually 0.5–1.0 mg/L. WHO [74] recommends that, in setting a standard, Member States should consider drinking-watcr consumption and the intake of fluoride from other sources. Nevertheless, a content of 1 mg/l of fluoride ions is approximately the desirable concentration in the water supplied to the population to ensure optimal dental health [75]. However, several factors, including temperature, can influence this optimum value, which varies from one climatic region to another. It is therefore important to determine this optimal dose for each region depending on whether it is in a temperate zone or in a tropical zone [76]. Dean [77] has shown that the optimum concentration of fluorine as a function of the ambient temperature is 1.0–1.2 mg/l.

The optimal dose of fluoride in drinking water is defined as the amount of fluoride which decreases the prevalence of dental caries with the absence of significant fluorosis [78–80]. Fluorosis is the demineralization of tooth enamel by excessive fluoride ingestion during the years of tooth calcification [81]. This phenomenon, observed in children, can range from mild fluorosis to a severe manifestation Indeed, Dean [78] observed that 10% of children consuming water containing 1.0 mg/l of fluoride could develop benign fluorosis. It is reported in the literature that children living in the southwestern United States develop severe fluorosis, much more so than those living in the midwestern, while both groups are exposed to the supply systems. Water containing the same concentration of fluorine [82]. Other studies have suggested that the extremely high temperature of the southwest is a major factor contributing to the increase in demand for drinking water and the increase in severe and endemic dental fluorosis [80, 81, 82].

In Haiti, studies carried out on the water resources of the Center-Sud hydrographic region of Haiti (**Figure 2**), revealed fluorine concentrations between 0 and

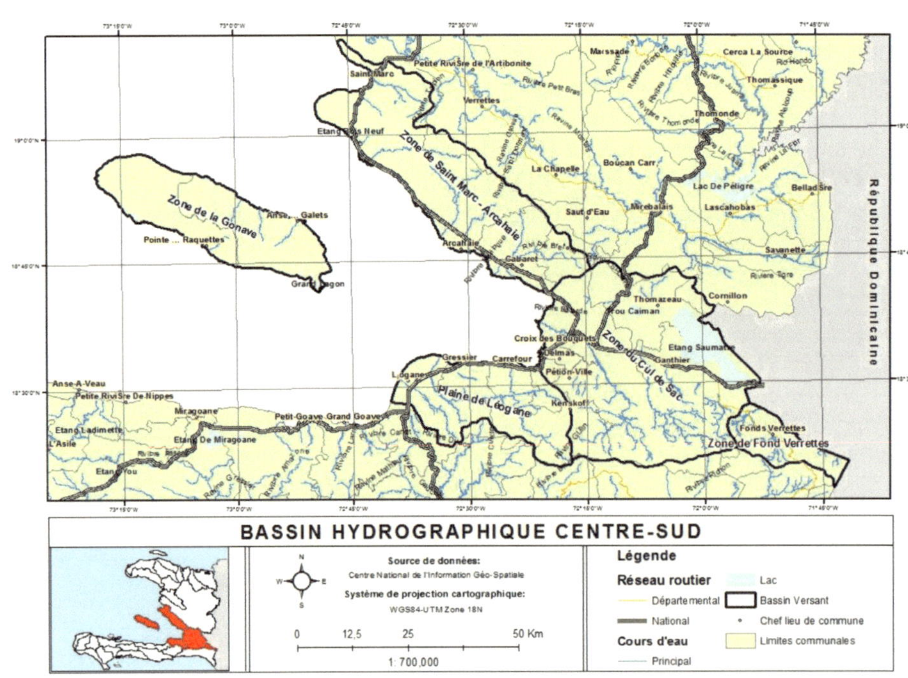

Figure 2.
Map of the "Centre-Sud" hydrographic region of Haiti.

2 mg/l [28, 83]. The various localities of this region are exposed to an average daily temperature ranging from 17 to 36° C.

These observations lead on the one hand to questioning the problems of dental caries and fluorosis from which the populations of the areas studied may suffer and, on the other hand, to determine the optimal dose of fluoride in water intended for human consumption. of the Center-South hydrographic region of the Republic of Haiti. Fluoride's exposure is a major public health problem particularly for children. Indeed, intake of high-water fluoride concentration during child's growth and development stages has been associated with mental and physical problems [84–86].

3.2 Water hardness and human health

Hardness is the traditional measure of the capacity of water to react with soap and describes the ability of water to bind soap to form lather, which is a chemical reaction detrimental to the washing process [87]. Water hardness results from the contact of groundwater with rock formations. It is the sum of the concentrations of dissolved polyvalent metal ions which Ca^{2+} and Mg^{2+} are predominant. The sources of the metallic ions are typically sedimentary rocks, and the most common are limestone ($CaCO_3$) and dolomite ($CaMg(CO_3)_2$) [66].

Ca and Mg are present as simple ions Ca^{2+} and Mg^{2+} with the Ca levels varying from tens to hundreds of mg/L and the Mg concentrations varying from units of tens of mg/L [88]. Magnesium is significantly less abundant than calcium in rocks and in most natural waters. In addition, magnesium concentrations are much lower in the water than calcium. They are generally less than 50 mg/L, although values higher or equal to 100 mg/L are stored particularly in cold climates [87]. The physical and chemical properties of Ca^{2+} and Mg^{2+} are presented in **Table 2**.

Hardness (in mg equivalent $CaCO_3$/L) can be determined by substituting the concentration of calcium and magnesium, expressed in mg/L, in the following equation [89]:

$$\text{Total hardness} = 2.497\left(Ca^{2+}, mg/L\right) + 4.118\left(Mg^{2+}, mg/L\right) \qquad (3)$$

Each concentration is multiplied by the ratio of the formula weight of $CaCO_3$ to the atomic weight of the ion; hence, the factors 2.497 and 4.118 are included in the hardness relation [89].

	Calcium	Magnesium
Molecular formula	Ca^{2+}	Mg
CAS#	7440-70-2	7439-95-4
Molecular Weight	40.08 g/mol	24.305 g/mol
Melting point	842°C	1100°C
Boiling Point	1484°C	651°C
Solubility	Water	Water
Density	1.54g/cm^3	1.738 at 20°C
Vapor pressure	10 mm Hg at 983°C	1 Pa at 428°C
Source	https://pubchem.ncbi.nlm.nih.gov/compound/5460341	https://pubchem.ncbi.nlm.nih.gov/compound/5462224

Table 2.
Physical and chemical properties of Ca^{2+} and Mg^{2+}.

Hardness is most expressed as milligrams of calcium carbonate equivalent per liter [90]. Water containing calcium carbonate at concentrations below 60 mg/l is generally considered as soft; 60–120 mg/l, moderately hard; 120–180 mg/l, hard; and more than 180 mg/l, extremely hard [91]. Although hardness is caused by cations, it may also be discussed in terms of carbonate (temporary) and non-carbonate (permanent) hardness [90].

Calcium and magnesium are essential for the human body [90]. They contribute to the formation and solidification of bones and teeth and play a role in the decrease of neuromuscular excitability, myocardial system, heart, and muscle contractility, intracellular information, transmission, and blood contractility [87, 88, 92]. They also play a major role in the metabolism of almost all cells of the body and interacts with many nutrients [93]. However, inadequate, or excess intake of either nutrient can result in adverse health consequences [90].

According to WHO [90] "*Inadequate intakes of calcium have been associated with increased risks of osteoporosis, nephrolithiasis (kidney stones), colorectal cancer, hypertension and stroke, coronary artery disease, insulin resistance and obesity. Most of these disorders have treatments, but not cures. Owing to a lack of compelling evidence for the role of calcium as a contributory element in relation to these diseases, estimates of calcium requirement have been made based on bone health outcomes, with the goal of optimizing bone mineral density.*

To a great extent, individuals are protected from excess intakes of calcium by a tightly regulated intestinal absorption and elimination mechanism through the action of 1,25-dihydroxyvitamin D, the hormonally active form of vitamin D. When calcium is absorbed more than need, the excess is excreted by the kidney in healthy people who do not have renal impairment" [90].

Magnesium is the fourth most abundant cation in the body and the second most abundant cation in intracellular fluid [90]. In the cardiovascular system, magnesium is the candidate element. It plays an important role as a cofactor and activator of more than 300 enzymatic reactions including glycolysis, ATP metabolism, transport of elements such as Na, K and Ca through membranes, synthesis of proteins and nucleic acids, neuromuscular excitability and muscle contraction [94]. That can have hand in various mechanism where the main is the calcium antagonist effect which can be direct or indirect [95].

Low magnesium levels are associated with endothelial dysfunction, increased vascular reactions, elevated circulating levels of C-reactive protein (a proinflammatory marker that is a risk factor for coronary heart disease) and decreased insulin sensitivity. Low magnesium status has been implicated in hypertension, coronary heart disease, type 2 diabetes mellitus and metabolic syndrome. Magnesium deficiency has been implicated in the pathogenesis of hypertension, with some epidemiological and experimental studies demonstrating a negative correlation between blood pressure and serum magnesium levels. However, data from clinical studies have been less convincing [90].

Indeed, water hardness has become an important public excess health issue [96]. Kobayaski [97] showed a relationship between water hardness and the incidence of vascular diseases. The scientific literature reported the existence of a relationship between cardiovascular disease mortality and water hardness [98–100]. Miyake and Iki [101] observed a lack of association between water hardness and coronary heart diseases mortality in Japan. Nonetheless, many studies covering many countries suggest such a correlation and geochemically it is worthy of serious study [88]. Based on available information in the literature on the association of water hardness and the incidence of cardiovascular diseases (CVD), Eisenberg [102] considered that Mg seems to be the basic element. Indeed, extremely hard natural water with $CaCO_3$ concentration higher than 200 mg/l with a magnesium concentration lower than 7 mg/l may affect various organs including the cardiovascular physiology [87].

In Haiti, studies on the spring waters used to supply a part of the population of the Metropolitan Area of Port-au-Prince (MAPP), the most important urban area of the country, showed a total hardness greater than 200 mg/l, with magnesium concentration less than 7 mg/l [29]. In addition, magnesium concentrations ranging from 5.58 to 6.9 mg/l have been measured in groundwater in the metropolitan area of Port-au-Prince [103]. Drinking water low in Mg significantly increases the likelihood of cardiovascular mortality [104]. Catling et al., [105] found significant evidence of an inverse association between magnesium levels in drinking water and cardiovascular mortality following a meta-analysis of case control studies. In Haiti, cardiovascular disease (CVD) is now the leading cause of adult mortality in Haiti [106, 107].

3.3 Groundwater pollution by heavy metals and human health

Metals are natural constituents of the Earth's crust. The distribution and fate of metals in the environment is governed by their properties and the influence of environmental factors [108]. In environmental compartments, heavy metals constitute an ecological and human health concern since heavy metals are not degraded biologically like certain organic pollutants [109]. Metals exert biological effects that can be beneficial or harmful. Many metals such as Fe, Cu, Co, Mn, Zn, and Cr are essential for humans, and deficiency states with clinical abnormalities have been identified [27, 108, 110]. Other metals such as Hg, Pb, Cd, and As are not known to be essential for any animals [110]. Essential elements can also cause toxic effects at high doses.

In Haiti, heavy metals (lead, chromium, and nickel) have been measured in groundwater [27]. The physical and chemical properties of these heavy metals are presented in **Table 3**.

3.3.1 Effects of chromium on human health

Chromium is one of the heavy metals considered a major pollutant. It has been widely used in industrial processes for leather tanning, dyes and paint preparation,

	Chromium	Lead	Nickel
Molecular formula	Cr	Pb	Ni
CAS#	7440-47-3	7439-92-1	7440-02-0
Molecular Weight	51.996 g/mol	207 g/mol	58.693 g/mol
Melting point	1907°C	327.4°C	1455°C
Boiling Point	2642°C	1740°C	2730°C
Solubility	Water	-	Water
Density	7.14	11.34 g/cm^3	8.9 g/cm^3
Vapor pressure	1 mmHg at 2941° F	1.77 mm Hg at 1000°C	1 mm Hg at 1810°C
Source	https://pubchem.ncbi.nlm.nih.gov/compound/23976	https://pubchem.ncbi.nlm.nih.gov/compound/5352425	https://pubchem.ncbi.nlm.nih.gov/compound/935

Table 3.
Physical and chemical properties of chromium, lead and nickel.

textile manufacturing, paper mills, wood preservation, stainless steel production, and photography [111]. Chromium exists in several oxidation states. The most stable and common forms are trivalent chromium, Cr(III), and hexavalent chromium, Cr(VI), which exhibit contrasting biochemical properties and toxicokinetics [112, 113]. Cr(III) compounds occur naturally in the form of oxides, hydroxides or sulfates, and they are nutritionally necessary to humans for glucose, fat and protein metabolism [114]. In contrast, Cr(VI) compounds are mainly anthropogenic and highly toxic; its mutagenic and carcinogenic nature and high oxidation state enhances its ability to move into living cells [114]. Cr(III) and Cr(VI) interchangeability depends on their concentration in solution, pH, the redox potential (Eh) of the medium, and the presence or absence of a strong oxidant or reductant [111, 115].

The toxicity of chromium is directly dependent on the valence state, with hexavalent chromate Cr(VI) and trivalent chromate Cr(III) being of the greatest interest [112]. Oral bioavailability varies with valence state, with Cr(VI) being more readily absorbed. Cr(VI) can be broken down into Cr(III) within the acidic environment of the stomach [111]. Acute exposure to chromium is indicated by immediate irritation of the eye, nose, throat, and respiratory tract, which results in burning, congestion, epistaxis, and cough. Ulceration, bleeding, and erosion of the nasal septum mark chronic exposure. Cough, chest pain, dyspnea, and chromium-induced asthma indicate exposure to soluble chromium products [113]. If chronic exposure is suspected, in conjunction with weight loss, cough, and hemoptysis, this suggests the development of bronchogenic carcinoma. Dermatological manifestations include painless, slow-healing ulceration of the fingers, knuckles, and forearms. Ingestion is marked by nausea, vomiting, abdominal pain, prostration, and death associated with uremia [114].

3.3.2 Effects of lead on human health

Drinking water is one of the major sources of human exposure to lead [115]. Lead particularly targets the nervous system, blood, and kidney [116]. Many studies found associations between low level environmental Pb exposure and chronic kidney disease, a general term for heterogeneous disorders affecting the structure and function of the kidney (CKD) [117, 118]. Long-term lead exposure may generate irreversible functional and morphological renal changes [119], distal motor neuropathy and possibly seizures and coma [120]. Infants and small children are more sensitive to the effects of lead, which moreover is transported through the placenta to the foetus [121]. Lead accumulation in fetuses and small children might cause developmental disruption in terms of neurological impairment characterized by a decrease of cognitive faculties, which can be reversible or not, evaluated by psychomotor tests such as the verbal IQ (Intellectual Quotient) test [27, 109]. The period when IQ is most affected is from birth to about 4 years of age [122].

Scientific literature on lead water pollution reports "Lead remains a problem in drinking water in many parts of the world, with millions of properties served by distribution systems containing lead components. Strong links have been established between human exposure to lead and health effects in both adults and children. As a result, the allowable levels of lead indrinking water have generally become lower. Implementation of these regulations is difficult with the controls available. Future recommendations for aspiring to zero lead in drinking water are: (i) improving sampling, monitoring and modeling; (ii) Wider application of short-term pointof- use devices; (iii) replacement of all lead pipes and plumbing through applicable regulations and increased awareness public" [123–126].

3.3.3 Effects of nickel on human health

Nickel is insoluble in water. However, when it is in the form of exceptionally fine particles, it ionizes as Ni (II) in water and in body fluids such as blood. During oral exposure, the major effects observed are the death of a child after ingestion of 570 mg of nickel/kg [127] and intestinal disorders such as nausea, abdominal cramps, and diarrhea [128]. Immunological, hematological, hepatic, renal, genotoxic effects on embryonic development and reproduction have been reported depending on the route of entry into the body [129].

4. Conclusion

The aim of this study is: (i) to analyze the contribution of geological factors and anthropogenic actions in the alteration of water quality in Port-au-Prince. The toxicology of chemicals of three heavy metal (chromium, lead, and nickel) and fluoride, substances detected in groundwater and tap water, has been reviewed. The information available on the effects of the selected heavy metals highlights major chemical risks, particularly for children, relating to Pb (II), Cr (III), Cr (VI) and Ni (II) contained in the groundwater were also characterized [27]. The level of pollution of underground water resources in the metropolitan area of Port-au-Prince does not only require the application of an approach based on water treatment processes. It also reflects the need to approach the issue of the quality of water intended for human consumption in this urban space based on a transdisciplinary approach based on the theories of medical geology and the approach. One Health. Indeed, the level of organic and mineral pollution of these resources can compromise the rare efforts made to achieve the SDGs, more particularly the 3, 6, 11, 13. The results available in the literature and used in the context of this work clearly indicate the existence of chronic toxicities of trace heavy metals (Cr, Pb, Ni), fluoride and hardness of drinking water on the human organism and on kidney tissues. In the future, it will be necessary to initiate research work on the combined effects of these substances from observations on laboratory animals and then proceed to modeling to finally arrive at an understanding of certain interactions that may exist between these pollutants.

Acknowledgements

The authors are thankful to the "One Health" University Space of Quisqueya University, FOKAL-Open Society Foundation Haiti, the Agence universitaire de la Francophonie (AUF), the Representation of the Institute for Research for Development (IRD) in Mexico, Cuba, and Haiti, the SCAC (Service for Cooperation and Cultural Action) of the French Embassy in Haiti, and the AOG (Association communautaire paysanne des Originaires de Grande Plaine) for their support in carrying out this work.

Author details

Alexandra Emmanuel[1,2] and Evens Emmanuel[1,3]*

1 Groupe Haïtien d'Études et de Recherche en Environnement et Santé (GHERES), Pétion-Ville, Haiti

2 Association Haïtienne Femmes, Science et Technologie, Port-au-Prince, Haiti

3 Université Quisqueya, Laboratoire Santé-Environnement (LS-E), Port-au-Prince, Haiti

*Address all correspondence to: evens.emmanuel@gmail.com

References

[1] Kılıç, Z.(2020). The importance of water and conscious use of water. Int J Hydro. 4(5):239–241. DOI: 10.15406/ijh.2020.04.00250

[2] Calderon R. L. (2000). The epidemiology of chemical contaminants of drinking water. Food and chemical toxicology, 38, S13-S20. doi:10.1016/S0278-6915(99)00133-7

[3] Ghernaout, D., & Elboughdiri, N. (2020). Disinfection By-Products: Presence and Elimination in Drinking Water. Open Access Library Journal, 7 (2), 1–27. doi:10.4236/oalib.1106140

[4] Hamidin, N., Yu, Q. J., & Connell, D. W. (2008). Human health risk assessment of chlorinated disinfection by-products in drinking water using a probabilistic approach. Water research, 42(13), 3263–3274. doi:10.1016/j.watres.2008.02.029

[5] Krasner, S. W., McGuire, M. J., Jacangelo, J. G., Patania, N. L., Reagan, K. M., & Aieta, E. M. (1989). The occurrence of disinfection by-products in US drinking water. Journal-American Water Works Association, 81(8), 41–53. doi:10.1002/j.1551-8833.1989.tb03258.x

[6] Fuge, R., Andrews, M.J. (1988). Fluorine in the UK environment. Environ Geochem Health 10, 96–104. doi:10.1007/BF01758677

[7] Pitter, P. (1985). Forms of occurrence of fluorine in drinking water. Water Research, 19(3), 281–284. doi:10.1016/0043-1354(85)90086-7

[8] Deshmukh, A. N., Wadaskar, P. M., & Malpe, D. B. (1995). Fluorine in environment: A review. Gondwana Geol. Mag, 9, 1–20.

[9] Levallois, P., Barn, P., Valcke, M., Gauvin, D., & Kosatsky, T. (2018). Public health consequences of lead in drinking water. Current environmental health reports, 5(2), 255–262. doi:10.1007/s40572-018-0193-0

[10] Hayes, C. R., & Skubala, N. D. (2009). Is there still a problem with lead in drinking water in the European Union? Journal of Water and Health, 7 (4), 569–580. doi:10.2166/wh.2009.110

[11] EFSA Panel on Contaminants in the Food Chain (CONTAM). (2014). Scientific Opinion on the risks to public health related to the presence of chromium in food and drinking water. EFSA Journal, 12(3), 3595.

[12] Zhitkovich, A. (2011). Chromium in drinking water: sources, metabolism, and cancer risks. Chemical research in toxicology, 24(10), 1617-1629.doi. 10.1021/tx200251t

[13] World Health Organization. (2020). Chromium in Drinking-water (No. WHO/HEP/ECH/WSH/2020.3). World Health Organization.

[14] Schroeder, H. A., & Vinton JR, W. H. (1962). Hypertension induced in rats by small doses of cadmium. American Journal of Physiology-Legacy Content, 202(3), 515–518. doi:10.1152/ajplegacy.1962.202.3.515

[15] Gonzalez, S., Lopez-Roldan, R., & Cortina, J. L. (2013). Presence of metals in drinking water distribution networks due to pipe material leaching: a review. Toxicological & Environmental Chemistry, 95(6), 870–889. doi:10.1080/02772248.2013.840372

[16] Kumar, M., & Puri, A. (2012). A review of permissible limits of drinking water. Indian journal of occupational and environmental medicine, 16(1), 40. DOI: 10.4103/0019-5278.99696

[17] Giammarino, M., & Quatto, P. (2015). Nitrates in drinking water:

relation with intensive livestock production. Journal of preventive medicine and hygiene, 56(4), E187.

[18] Sjerps, R. M., Kooij, P. J., van Loon, A., & Van Wezel, A. P. (2019). Occurrence of pesticides in Dutch drinking water sources. Chemosphere, 235, 510–518. doi:10.1016/j.chemosphere.2019.06.207

[19] Griffini, O., Bao, M. L., Barbieri, C., Burrini, D., & Pantani, F. (1997). Occurrence of pesticides in the Arno river and in potable water—a survey of the period 1992–1995. Bulletin of environmental contamination and toxicology, 59(2), 202–209.

[20] Wasana, H. M., Aluthpatabendi, D., Kularatne, W. M. T. D., Wijekoon, P., Weerasooriya, R., & Bandara, J. (2016). Drinking water quality and chronic kidney disease of unknown etiology (CKDu): synergic effects of fluoride, cadmium and hardness of water. Environmental geochemistry and health, 38(1), 157–168. DOI 10.1007/s10653-015-9699-7

[21] Wasana, H. M., Perera, G. D., Gunawardena, P. D. S., Fernando, P. S., & Bandara, J. (2017). WHO water quality standards Vs Synergic effect (s) of fluoride, heavy metals and hardness in drinking water on kidney tissues. Scientific Reports, 7(1), 1–6. DOI: 10.1038/srep42516

[22] Brown, K. G., & Ross, G. L. (2002). Arsenic, drinking water, and health: a position paper of the American Council on Science and Health. Regulatory Toxicology and Pharmacology, 36(2), 162–174. doi:10.1006/rtph.2002.1573

[23] He, J., & Charlet, L. (2013). A review of arsenic presence in China drinking water. Journal of hydrology, 492, 79–88. doi:10.1016/j.jhydrol.2013.04.007

[24] Nriagu, J. O. (1988). A silent epidemic of environmental metal poisoning? Environmental pollution, 50 (1–2), 139–161.

[25] Bowen, H. J. M. (1979). Environmental chemistry of the elements. New York: Academic Press. 333.

[26] Fifi, U., Winiarski, T., & Emmanuel, E. (2013). Assessing the mobility of lead, copper and cadmium in a calcareous soil of Port-au-Prince, Haiti. International journal of environmental research and public health, 10(11):5830–5843. doi: 10.3390/ijerph10115830

[27] Emmanuel, E., Pierre, M.G., Perrodin, Y. (2009). Groundwater contamination by microbiological and chemical substances released from hospital wastewater: Health risk assessment for drinking water consumers. Environ. Int., 35, 718–726. doi:10.1016/j.envint.2009.01.011

[28] Emmanuel, E., Fanfan, P. N., Louis, R., & Michel, G. A. (2002). Détermination de la dose optimale de fluor de l'eau destinée à la consommation humaine de la région hydrographique Centre-Sud de la république d'Haïti. Cahiers d'études et de recherches francophones/Santé, 12 (2), 241–245.

[29] TRACTEBEL (1998). Définition des périmètres de protection pour les sources exploitées par la CAMEP. Bruxelles: Tractebel Development, 235 p.

[30] Schwartzbord, J. R., Emmanuel, E., & Brown, D. L. (2013). Haiti's food and drinking water: a review of toxicological health risks. Clinical Toxicology, 51(9), 828–833. doi:10.3109/15563650.2013.849350

[31] Butterlin, J. (1960) Géologie générale de la République d'Haïti. Institut des Hautes Etudes de l'Amérique Latine, Paris, p. 194.

[32] Finkelman, R. B., Centeno, J. A., & Selinus, O. (2005). The emerging medical and geological association. Transactions of the American Clinical and Climatological Association, 116, 155.

[33] Mercier, M. (2002). Johannesbourg 2002: vers le développement durable?

[34] Gérin, M. (2003). Avant propos. In. Gérin M, Gosselin P, Cordier S, Viau C, Quénel P, Dewailly E. Environnement et santé publique. Fondements et pratiques. Edisem, Éditions Tec & Doc, 2003, 1023 p. ISBN: 2-89130-193-5 (Edisem). ISBN: 2-7430-0603-X (Tec & Doc).

[35] Abenhaim, L. (2003). Préfaces. In. Gérin M, Gosselin P, Cordier S, Viau C, Quénel P, Dewailly E. Environnement et santé publique. Fondements et pratiques. Edisem, Éditions Tec & Doc, 2003, 1023 p. ISBN: 2-89130-193-5 (Edisem). ISBN: 2-7430-0603-X (Tec & Doc).

[36] National Research Council. (1983). Risk Assessment in the Federal Government: Managing the Process. Washington, DC: National Academy Press. 191 p.

[37] Groten, J. P. (2000). Mixtures and interactions. Food and Chemical Toxicology, 38, S65-S71.

[38] Bliss, C. I. (1939). The toxicity of poisons applied jointly 1. Annals of applied biology, 26(3):585–615. doi: 10.1111/j.1744-7348.1939.tb06990.x

[39] Plackett, R. L., & Hewlett, P. S. (1948). Statistical aspects of the independent joint action of poisons, particularly insecticides: I. the toxicity of a mixture of poisons. Annals of applied biology, 35(3):347–358. doi: 10.1111/j.1744-7348.1948.tb07379.x

[40] Plackett, R. L., & Hewlett, P. S. (1952). Quantal responses to mixtures of poisons. Journal of the Royal Statistical Society: Series B (Methodological), 14 (2):141–154. doi:10.1111/j.2517-6161.1952.tb00108.x

[41] Fox, M. A., Tran, N. L., Groopman, J. D., & Burke, T. A. (2004). Toxicological resources for cumulative risk: an example with hazardous air pollutants. Regulatory Toxicology and Pharmacology, 40(3), 305–311. doi: 10.1016/j.envint.2018.03.026

[42] US EPA, 2003. The Feasibility of Performing Cumulative Risk Assessments for Mixtures of Disinfection By-products in Drinking Water. National Center for Environmental Assessment, Cincinnati, OH. EPA/600/R-03/051.

[43] US EPA, 2003. Framework for Cumulative Risk Assessment. Risk Assessment Forum, Washington, DC.

[44] U.S. EPA. (2000). Supplementary guidance for conducting health risk assessment of chemical mixtures. U.S. EPA (United States Environmental Protection Agency's), Risk Assessment Forum. Washington, DC. EPA/630/R-00/002.

[45] Villanueva, C. M., Cordier, S., Font-Ribera, L., Salas, L. A., & Levallois, P. (2015). Overview of disinfection by-products and associated health effects. Current environmental health reports, 2 (1), 107–115. doi:10.1007/s40572-014-0032-x

[46] Li, X. F., & Mitch, W. A. (2018). Drinking water disinfection byproducts (DBPs) and human health effects: multidisciplinary challenges and opportunities. doi:10.1021/acs.est.7b05440

[47] Feron, V. J., & Groten, J. P. (2002). Toxicological evaluation of chemical mixtures. Food and chemical toxicology, 40(6), 825–839. doi:10.1016/S0278-6915(02)00021-2

[48] Ministère de la Santé Publique et de la Population (MSPP) et Organisation Mondiale de la Santé OMS (1998). Analyse de la situation sanitaire – Haïti. Port-au-Prince: Imprimerie Henri Deschamps Port-au-Prince.

[49] Lombart, M., Pierrat, K., & Redon, M. (2014). Port-au-Prince: un «projectorat» haïtien ou l'urbanisme de projets humanitaires en question. Cahiers des Amériques latines, 2014 (75), 97–124.

[50] Fifi, U., Winiarski, T., Emmanuel, E. (2010). Impact of surface runoff on the aquifers of Port-au-Prince, Haiti. In.: Eddie N. Laboy-Nieves, Matheus Goosen and Evens Emmanuel (Editors). Environmental and Human Health: Risk Management in Developing Countries. p. 123-140. CRC Press. Taylor and Francis Group.

[51] Saade L. 2006. Act together for an effective management of the drinking water services and sanitation in Haiti. United Nations, Economic Commission for Latin America and the Caribbean. Mexique, 44 p.

[52] Kreft, S., Eckstein D., Melchior I. (2017). Global Climate Risk Index 2017, Who Suffers Most from Extreme Weather Events? Weather-related Loss Events in 2015 and 1996 to 2015, Bonn, Allemagne, Germanwatch, 31 p.

[53] Simonot, M. (1982). Les ressources en eau souterraine de la région de Port-au-Prince. Situation actuelle et recommendation. Port-au-Prince: PNUD (Programme des Nations Unies pour le Développement). 52 p.

[54] Desreumaux, C. (1987). Contribution à l'étude géologique des régions centrales et méridionales d'Haïti, (Grandes Antilles) du Crétacé à l'Actuel. Thèse de doctorat de l'Université de Bordeaux I. Bordeaux. 424 p.

[55] Maurasse F. (1990). New data on the stratigraphy of the southern penisula of Haïti. In: Actes du 1er Colloque sur la géologie d'Haïti, Port-au-Prince.

[56] Denić-Jukić, V., & Jukić, D. (2003). Composite transfer functions for karst aquifers. Journal of hydrology, 274(1–4), 80–94. doi:10.1016/S0022-1694(02)00393-1

[57] Emmanuel, E., Angerville, R., Joseph, O., Perrodin, Y. (2007). Human health risk assessment of lead in drinking water: a case study from Port-au-Prince, Haiti. International journal of Environment and pollution, 31(3–4), 280–291.

[58] Damiani, C., Balthazard-Accou, K., Clervil, E., Diallo, A., Da Costa, C., Emmanuel, E., Totet, A., & Agnamey, P. (2013). Cryptosporidiosis in Haiti: surprisingly, low level of species diversity revealed by molecular characterization of Cryptosporidium oocysts from surface water and groundwater. Parasite (Paris, France), 20, 45. doi:10.1051/parasite/2013045

[59] Gonfiantini, R., et Simonot, M. (1989). Isotopic study of the groundwater of the flatland of Cul-de-Sac, Republic of Haiti (No. IAEA-TECDOC–502).

[60] UNDP. (2015). 2030 Agenda for Sustainable Development - Sustainable Development Goals. United Nations. https://www.undp.org/content/dam/undp/library/corporate/brochure/SDGs_Booklet_Web_En.pdf.

[61] Guterres, A. (2017). The Sustainable Development Goals Report 2017. United Nations. https://www.un.org/development/desa/publications/sdg-report-2017.html.

[62] Ramirez-Mendoza, R. A., Morales-Menendez, R., Melchor-Martinez, E. M., Iqbal, H. M., Parra-Arroyo, L., Vargas-Martínez, A., & Parra-Saldivar, R. (2020). Incorporating the sustainable

development goals in engineering education. International Journal on Interactive Design and Manufacturing (IJIDeM), 14(3), 739–745. doi:10.1007/s12008-020-00661-0

[63] TWAS (2016). Science Policy. United Nations Secretary-General's Scientific Advisory Board. The world Academy of Science (TWAS). https://twas.org/united-nations-secretary-generals-scientific-advisory-board (2016) [Accessed June 15, 2019].

[64] United Nations (2008) Contributing to One World, One Health: A strategic framework for reducing risk of infectious diseases at the animal-human-ecosystem interface. FAO/OIE/WHO/UNICEF/UNSIC/World Bank. Available: http://un-influenza.org/files/OWOH_14Oct08.pdf.

[65] Mazet, J. A., Clifford, D. L., Coppolillo, P. B., Deolalikar, A. B., Erickson, J. D., Kazwala, R. R. (2009). A "one health" approach to address emerging zoonoses: the HALI project in Tanzania. PLoS Med, 6(12), e1000190. doi:10.1371/journal.pmed.1000190

[66] Desjardins, R. (1988). Le traitement des eaux. 2éme edition revue. Montreal: École Polytechnique de Montréal, 304 p. ISBN: 2-553-00211-5.

[67] IPCS. (2002). Fluorides. Geneva, World Health Organization, International Programme on Chemical Safety (Environmental Health Criteria 227). http://www.inchem.org/documents/ehc/ehc/ehc227.htm.

[68] O'Mullane DM, Baez RJ, Jones S, Lennon MA, Petersen PE, Rugg-Gunn AJ, et al. (2016). Fluoride and oral health. Community Dent Health. 33(2): 69–99. Doi:10.1922/CDH_3707O'Mullane31

[69] Indermitte, E., Saava, A., & Karro, E. (2009). Exposure to high fluoride drinking water and risk of dental fluorosis in Estonia. International journal of environmental research and public health, 6(2):710–721. DOI: 10.3390/ijerph6020710

[70] Edmunds M., Smedley P. (2005) Fluoride in natural waters. In.: Selinus O., Alloway J. B., Centeno A. J., Finkelman B. R., Fuge R., Lindh U., Smedley P. Essentials of Medical Geology. London: Elsevier Academic Press, pp. 301–329. ISBN: 0-12-636341-2.

[71] Chandra, S., Thergaonkar, V. P., Sharma, R. (1981). Water quality and dental fluorosis. Indian journal of public health, 25(1), 47–51.

[72] WHO (2019). Preventing disease through healthy environments: inadequate or excess fluoride: a major public health concern (No. WHO/CED/PHE/EPE/19.4. 5). World Health Organization. https://apps.who.int/iris/bitstream/handle/10665/329484/WHO-CED-PHE-EPE-19.4.5-eng.pdf

[73] WHO (2017). Guidelines for drinking-water quality, 4th edition incorporating the first addendum. Geneva, World Health Organization, pp. 370–373 https://apps.who.int/iris/bitstream/handle/10665/254637/9789241549950-eng.pdf.

[74] RGNDWM. (1993). Prevention and control of fluorisis, health aspects. Vol. I. New Delhi: Rajiv Gandhi national drinking water mission (RGNDWM). 125 p.

[75] Sawyer, CN., McCarty, P. (1967). Chemistry for Sanitary Engineers, McGraw-Hill Series in Sanitary Science and water Engineering. New York: McGraw-Hill. 455 p.

[76] Yam, A. A., Dioufndiaye, M., Badiane, M., & Sawadogo, G. (1995). Détermination de la dose optimale de fluor dans l'eau de boisson au Sénégal.

TSM. Techniques sciences méthodes, génie urbain génie rural, (6), 488-490.

[77] Dean, H.T. (1936). Chronic endemic dental fluorisis (Mottled Enamel). Jour Amer Medical Assn. 107: 1269–1272.

[78] Dean, H.T. (1941). Domestic water and dental caries. A study of 2,832 white children aged 12-14 years of eight suburban Chicago communities, including L. acidophilus studies of 1,761 children. Public Health Repts. 56: 761–792.

[79] Dean, H.T., Arnold, F.A. Jr., Elvove, E. (1942. Domestic water and dental caries. V. additional studies of the relation of fluoride in domestic waters to dental caries experience in 4 4,25 white children aged 12-14 years of 13 cities in 4 States. Public Health Repts. 57: 1155–1171.

[80] Lalumandier, J.A., Jones, J.L. (1999). Fluoride concentrations in drinking water. Jour Amer Water Works Assn. 91: 42–51.

[81] Galagan, D.J., Lamson, G.G. (1953). Climate and endemic dental fluorisis. Public Health Repts. 68: 497–508.

[82] Szpunar, S.M., Burt B.A. (1987). Trends in the prevalence of dental fluorisis in the United States: a review. Jour Public Health Dentistry. 47: 71–79.

[83] Angeville, R., Emmanuel, E., Nelson, J., Saint-Hilaire, P. (1999). Evaluation of the fluorine concentration in the water resources of hydrographic area "Centre-Sud" of Haiti. Proceedings of 8th annual CWWA and 4th AIDIS Region 1 conference, Jamaica. CDROM.

[84] Wang, S. X., Wang, Z. H., Cheng, X. T., Li, J., Sang, Z. P., Zhang, X. D., Wang, Z. Q. (2007). Arsenic and fluoride exposure in drinking water: children's IQ and growth in Shanyin county, Shanxi province, China. Environmental health perspectives, 115 (4), 643–647. doi: 10.1289/ehp.9270

[85] Saxena, S., Sahay, A., & Goel, P. (2012). Effect of fluoride exposure on the intelligence of school children in Madhya Pradesh, India. Journal of neurosciences in rural practice, 3(2), 144. Doi: 10.4103/0976-3147.98213

[86] Seraj, B., Shahrabi, M., Shadfar, M., Ahmadi, R., Fallahzadeh, M., Eslamlu, H. F., & Kharazifard, M. J. (2012). Effect of high-water fluoride concentration on the intellectual development of children in makoo/iran. Journal of Dentistry (Tehran, Iran), 9 (3), 221.

[87] Rubenowitz-Lundin, E., & Hiscock, K. M. (2013). Water hardness and health effects. In: Essentials of Medical Geology. Springer, Dordrecht, p. 337–350.

[88] Eaton, A. D., Clesceri, L. S., Rice, E. W., Greenberg, A. E., & Franson, M. A. H. (2005). Standard methods for the examination of water and wastewater. Washington D.C.: American public health association, 1015.

[89] Freeze, R.A., Cherry, J.A. (1979). Groundwater. Englewood Cliff: Prentice Hall. 604 p.

[90] WHO (2011). Hardness in Drinking-water. Background document for development of WHO Guidelines for Drinking-water Quality. Geneva: World Health Organization, WHO Press. 19 p. WHO/HSE/WSH/10.01/10/Rev/1.

[91] McGowan, W., & Harrison, J. F. (2000). Water processing: residential, commercial, light industrial. Lisle, IL, Water Quality Association.

[92] Baker, S.B., Worthley, L.I.G. (2002). The essentials of calcium, magnesium, and phosphate metabolism: part I. Physiology. Critical care resuscitation. 4: 301–306.

[93] Bootman M.D., Collins T.J., Peppiatt C.M., Prothero L.S., MacKenzie L., De Smet P., Travers M., Tovey S.C., Seo J.T., Berridge M.J., Ciccolini F., Lipp P. 2001. Calcium signalling—an overview. Semin Cell Dev Biol 12: 3–10.

[94] Kožíšek, F. (2003). Health significance of drinking water calcium and magnesium. National Institute of Public Health, 29, 9285–9286.

[95] Berthollet A. (2003). Le magnésium: un nutriment important. Forum Med Suisse. 27: 638–640.

[96] Emmanuel, E., Simon, Y., and Joseph, O. (2013). Characterization of hardness in the groundwater of Port-au-Prince. An overview on the health significance of magnesium in the drinking water. Aqua-LAC, 5(2), 35–43.

[97] Kobayashi J. 1957. On geographical Relations Between the Chemical Nature of River Water and Death Rate from Apoplexy, Berich. Ohara Inst. Landwirtsh. biol.11: 12–21.

[98] Schroeder, H. A. (1960). Relations between hardness of water and death rates from certain chronic and degenerative diseases in the United States. Journal of Chronic Diseases, 12 (6), 586–591.

[99] Sharett, A.R. (1979) The role of chemical constituents of drinking water in cardiovascular diseases. Am J Epidemiol 110:401–419.

[100] Masironi, R., & Shaper, A. G. (1981). Epidemiological studies of health effects of water from different sources. Annual review of nutrition, 1 (1), 375–400.

[101] Miyake, Y., & Iki, M. (2004). Lack of association between water hardness and coronary heart disease mortality in Japan. International journal of cardiology, 96(1), 25–28.

[102] Eisenberg, M. J. (1992). Magnesium deficiency and sudden death. American Heart Journal. 124(2): 544–549. doi: 10.1016/0002-8703(92) 90633-7

[103] Emmanuel, E. (2004). Évaluation de risques sanitaire et écotoxicologiques liées aux effluents hospitaliers, thèse de l'Institut National des Sciences Appliquées de Lyon, Université de Lyon, France. p. 259

[104] Kozisek, F. (2020). Regulations for calcium, magnesium or hardness in drinking water in the European Union member states. Regulatory Toxicology and Pharmacology, 112, 104589. doi: 10.1016/j.yrtph.2020.104589

[105] Catling, L. A., Abubakar, I., Lake, I. R., Swift, L., & Hunter, P. R. (2008). A systematic review of analytical observational studies investigating the association between cardiovascular disease and drinking water hardness. Journal of water and health, 6(4), 433–442. doi:10.2166/wh.2008.054

[106] Roth, G. A., Johnson, C., Abajobir, A., Abd-Allah, F., Abera, S. F., Abyu, G., Ukwaja, K. N. (2017). Global, regional, and national burden of cardiovascular diseases for 10 causes, 1990 to 2015. Journal of the American College of Cardiology, 70(1), 1–25. doi: 10.1016/j.jacc.2017.04.052.

[107] Lookens, J., Tymejczyk, O., Rouzier, V., Smith, C., Preval, F., Joseph, I., McNairy, M. (2020). The Haiti cardiovascular disease cohort: study protocol for a population-based longitudinal cohort. BMC Public Health, 20(1), 1–11. doi:10.1186/s12889-020-09734-x

[108] Emmanuel, A., & Simon, Y. (2018). Environmental lead exposure and its impact on the health of children, pregnant women, and the general population in Haiti. Haïti Perspectives, 6(3):5–11.

[109] Emmanuel, E., Angerville, R., Joseph, O., & Perrodin, Y. (2007). Human health risk assessment of lead in drinking water: a case study from Port-au-Prince, Haiti. International journal of Environment and pollution, 31(3–4): 280–291.

[110] Caussy, D., Gochfeld, M., Gurzau, E., Neagu, C., & Ruedel, H. (2003). Lessons from case studies of metals: investigating exposure, bioavailability, and risk. Ecotoxicology and environmental safety, 56(1):45–51. doi: 10.1016/S0147-6513(03)00049-6

[111] El Nemr, A., Khaled, A., Abdelwahab, O., & El-Sikaily, A. (2008). Treatment of wastewater containing toxic chromium using new activated carbon developed from date palm seed. Journal of Hazardous Materials, 152(1), 263–275. doi: 10.1016/j.jhazmat.2007.06.091

[112] McGrath SP, Smith S. 1990. Chromium and nickel. In: Alloway BJ, editor. Heavy metals in soils. New York, USA): John Wiley & Sons, Inc. p 125–150.

[113] Cervantes, C., Campos-García, J., Devars, S., Gutiérrez-Corona, F., Loza-Tavera, H., Torres-Guzmán, J. C., & Moreno-Sánchez, R. (2001). Interactions of chromium with microorganisms and plants. FEMS microbiology reviews, 25(3), 335–347. doi: 10.1111/j.1574-6976.2001.tb00581.x

[114] Agency for Toxic Substance and Disease Registry [ATSDR]. (2000). Toxicological profile for chromium. Atlanta, Georgia, USA: U.S. Department of Health and Human Services. 461 p.

[115] Tadesse I, Isoaho SA, Green FB, Puhakka JA. 2006. Lime enhanced chromium removal in advanced integrated wastewater pond system. Bioresource Technology 97: 529–534.

[116] Académie des Sciences. (1998). Contamination des sols par les éléments traces: les risques et leur gestion. Rapport No 42. Paris: Lavoisier Tec& Doc. 440 p.

[117] Robson, M. (2003). Methodologies for assessing exposures to metals: human host factors. Ecotoxicology and Environmental Safety, 56(1), 104–109. doi:10.1016/S0147-6513(03)00054-X

[118] Lewis R. Metals. In: Ladou J, editor. Occupational and environmental medicine. New York: McGrawHill; 1997. p. 405–439. (Chapter 27).

[119] Fertmann, R., Hentschel, S., Dengler, D., Janßen, U., & Lommel, A. (2004). Lead exposure by drinking water: an epidemiologial study in Hamburg, Germany. International journal of hygiene and environmental health, 207(3):235–244. doi:10.1078/1438-4639-00285

[120] INERIS (Institut National de l'Environnement Industriel et des Risques). Plomb et ses dérivés, in Fiche de données toxicologiques et environnementales des substances chimiques. Paris: INERIS; ERIS-DRC-01-25590-ETSC-Api/SD-N 00df257, 90 p.

[121] Ab Latif Wani, A. A., & Usmani, J. A. (2015). Lead toxicity: a review. Interdisciplinary toxicology, 8(2):55. DOI:10.1515/intox-2015-0009

[122] Needleman, H. (2004). Lead poisoning. Annu. Rev. Med., 55:209–222. doi:10.1146/annurev.med.55.091902.103653

[123] Christensen, J. M. (1995). Human exposure to toxic metals: factors influencing interpretation of biomonitoring results. Science of the total environment, 166(1–3):89–135. doi: 10.1016/0048-9697(95)04478-J

[124] Cleymaet, R., Collys, K., Retief, D. H., Michotte, Y., Slop, D., Taghon, E., Coomans, D. (1991). Relation between

lead in surface tooth enamel, blood, and saliva from children residing in the vicinity of a non-ferrous metal plant in Belgium. Occupational and Environmental Medicine, 48(10):702–709. doi:10.1136/oem.48.10.702

[125] Watt, G. C. M., Britton, A., Gilmour, H. G., Moore, M. R., Murray, G. D., & Robertson, S. J. (2000). Public health implications of new guidelines for lead in drinking water: a case study in an area with historically high water lead levels. Food and Chemical Toxicology, 38, S73-S79. doi:10.1016/S0278-6915(99)00137-4

[126] Jarvis, P., & Fawell, J. (2021). Lead in drinking water–an ongoing public health concern? Current Opinion in Environmental Science & Health, 100239. doi:10.1016/j.coesh.2021.100239

[127] Daldrup, T., Haarhoff, K., & Szathmary, S. C. (1983). Fatal nickel sulfate poisoning. Beitrage zur gerichtlichen Medizin, 41, 141–144.

[128] Sunderman Jr, F. W., Hopfer, S. M., Sweeney, K. R., Marcus, A. H., Most, B. M., & Creason, J. (1989). Nickel absorption and kinetics in human volunteers. Proceedings of the Society for Experimental Biology and Medicine, *191*(1), 5–11. doi:10.3181/00379727-191-42881

[129] Agency for Toxic Substances and Disease Registry (ATSDR). Toxicological Profile for Nickel. Altanta, GA: U.S. Department of Health and Human Services; 1993. http://www.atsdr.cdc.gov.

Chapter 11

Microplastics and Environmental Health: Assessing Environmental Hazards in Haiti

Daphenide St. Louis, Ammcise Apply, Daphnée Michel and Evens Emmanuel

Abstract

Microplastics (MP) refer to all plastic particles that are less than 5 mm in size. Over the past decades, several studies have highlighted the impact of microplastics (MP) on living organisms. In addition to being pollutants themselves, these synthetic polymers also act as vectors for the transport of various types of chemicals in natural ecosystems. MP has been ubiquitously detected in a wide range of shapes, polymers, sizes and concentrations in marine water, freshwater, agroecosystems, atmospheric, food and water environments. Drinking water, biota, and other remote places. According to the World Bank, over 80% of the world's marine litter is plastic and the concentration of litter on Caribbean beaches is often high, with a high presence of single-use plastics and food containers. In its work, the World Health Organization (WHO) suggests an in-depth assessment of microplastics present in the environment and their potential consequences on human health, following the publication of an analysis of the state of research on microplastics in drinking water. It also calls for reducing plastic pollution to protect the environment and reduce human exposure. In Haiti, the bay of Port-au-Prince is the natural receptacle of all the urban effluents generated by human activities in the Metropolitan Zone. This urban wastewater carries household waste, sludge from pit latrines and sewage, industrial wastewater which largely contributes to the pollution of the bay. Furthermore, 1,673,750 tonnes per year of household waste, including 93,730 tonnes of plastic waste, are not collected. What are the environmental dangers represented by the MP contained in those wastes for living organisms in exposed tropical ecosystems? The purpose of this paper is: (i) to do a bibliographical review of the physical and chemical properties, as well as the toxicological profile of MP, (ii) to identify the environmental hazards associated with MP contained in urban waste in the metropolitan area of Port-au-Prince.

Keywords: microplastics, wastes, physical and chemical characteristics, natural ecosystems, fate, environmental hazards

1. Introduction

Synthetic polymers appeared at the end of the nineteenth century around the 1860s, but it was not until after World War II that the "rise of plastics" really began [1].

Plastic has become one of the most ubiquitous materials since its inception as a phenol-formaldehyde resin (i.e., bakelite) [2]. Basically, plastic was designed to improve the conditions of human life, but today it is becoming a real environmental concern [1].

Nowadays, plastic is ubiquitous in all environmental compartments (air, water, and soil) [3]. Simonneau et al., [4] report that rain and snow contain a significant number of MP, invisible to the naked eye and less than 5 mm in size. The presence of MP in soil ecosystems has been detected [5, 6]. Scientific literature reports the environmental occurrence of MP in surface waters [7], coastal sediments [8], beach sands [9], freshwater sediments [10], and deep-sea environments [11]. Indeed, the intensive exploitation of plastic associated with poor performance of waste management systems, including end-of-life collection and capture, have resulted in a massive accumulation of plastic waste in the environment [12]. The release of plastic materials into the environment is recognized as an important pollution related issue [13–15].

The proliferation of MP in the environment causes serious pollution all over the world [16]. According to their characteristics, namely, synthetic materials with a high content of polymers, solid particles, less than 5 mm, insoluble in water, and not degradable, they are easily introduced into the environment and persist there due to their low solubility [17]. Food chains are subject to significant pollution from the release of hydrophobic organic chemicals [18–22]. Being present in different aquatic ecosystems (surface water, oceans, estuarine waters, etc.), organisms are directly or indirectly exposed to microplatiscs [17]. Scientific literature reports negative impacts of microplastics on benthic organisms [23, 24]. The toxic effects of these pollutants have been studied on the feeding habits, growth and reproductive systems of several aquatic species [25–29]. Human beings are therefore exposed through the consumption of seafood, fish and crustaceans [30].

The purpose of this paper is: (i) to do a bibliographical review of the physical and chemical properties, as well as the toxicological profile of MP, (ii) to identify the environmental hazards associated with MP contained in urban waste in the metropolitan area of Port-au-Prince.

2. Methodology

Scientific and technical information from several world-wide documentation databases was used. Academic social networks, scientific databases such as Google Scholar, PubMed, academia.edu, researchgate.net, academic presses (springer.com, sciendirect.com, Wiley Online Library, ACS Publications, etc.) were consulted in this way as electronic data available on the sites of certain research universities. The search equations launched on the various sites consulted were implemented from the crossing of the following keywords: "Microplastics", "Microplastics (and) definition", "Microplastics (and) plastics", "Microplastics (and) thermodynamics", "Microplastics (and) Epidemiology", "Microplastics (and) physical and chemical properties", "Toxicological profile of microplastics", "Microplastics (and) Human health effects" , "Microplastics (and) Environment" , "Microplastics (and)) partition coefficient" , "Microplastics (and) Haiti", "Haiti (and) solid waste" , "Fate and Microplastics" , "Microplastics (and) Ocean" , etc.

The results obtained have been the subject of a critical examination. Each article read, referred the authors of this study for the reading of another article cited in the list of his references. We considered articles that were published from 2005 to 2021. The number of times cited (citations analysis).

3. Definition, composition, and physical and chemical characteristics of plastics

The term plastic refers to "a material which contains as an essential ingredient a high polymer and which, at some stage of its transformation into finished products, can be shaped by flow," [31]. However, elastomeric materials (also shaped by flow) are generally not considered plastics [32, 33].

Plastics are mainly produced from non-renewable substances, extracted from petroleum and natural gas [1, 34, 35], or renewable like sugar cane, starch, or vegetable oil or even of mineral origin like salt [36]. The evolution of plastic, correlated with its major strengths, makes it a substitute material, to the detriment of metals, for example [37]. Thus, the increase in plastic, and its multiple applications, place it at the forefront of market share, ahead of traditional materials [38].

The International Organization for Standardization (ISO) [31] recommends the use of the term "macromolecule" for individual molecules, the term "polymer" being reserved for a substance consisting of macromolecules, further stipulating that the term "high polymer" or more generally "polymer" denotes a product consisting of molecules characterized by a large number of repeats of one or more species of atoms or groups of atoms (constitutional units), linked in sufficient quantity to lead to a set of properties which hardly vary with the addition or elimination of a single or a small number of constituent motifs [31]. The denomination of "plastics" comes from the characteristic plasticity property of many polymer materials which can be deformed at will under the effect of temperature (the notion of temperature is relative here: certain plastics are deformable at room temperature) [39]. Thus, most of the plastic materials placed on the market result from complex formulation steps intended to give the macromolecules the desired properties of use. Adjuvants such as stabilizers and additives will be used to limit the degradation of the chains under the effect of heat, radiation, abrasion (antioxidants, mineral fillers, etc.) and give them specific properties (plasticizers, dyes, flame retardants, reinforcements ...) [39].

A main classification of plastics is based on the durability or non-durability of their shapes, or whether they are thermosets or thermoplastics [40]. According to Plastics Europe [36], plastics can be classified into various types. A typology of plastic as well as their applications and benefits are published on the website of this institution, which is an association of plastic manufacturers in Europe (**Table 1**).

3.1 Microplastics

Jiang et al. [40] note that the degradation of plastic waste generates microplastic (MP) or nanoplastic particles (NP); this division is based on the diameter of the plastic fragments or particles, MP being less than 5 mm in diameter and NP being 1 to 100 or 1000 nm in diameter [40]. The scientific literature on the diameter of plastic particles provides several information and divisions of microplastics. Arthur et al. [41] report when it was reported in 2004, the term microplastics was used to describe fragments of plastic approximately 20 μm in diameter. However, while these early reports referred to truly microscopic particles, they did not provide a specific definition of microplastic. In 2008, the United States National Oceanographic and Atmospheric Agency (NOAA) hosted the first International Microplastics Workshop in Washington and, as part of that meeting, formulated a broader working definition to include all particles. Less than 5 mm in diameter [41]. Other authors consider that particles>5 mm are macroplastics, mesoplastics 5 to>1 mm, microplastics 1 mm to>0.1 μm and nanoplastics as 0.1 μm [5].

Plastics	Description
Bio-based plastics	*Bio-based plastics are made in whole or partially from renewable biological resources. For example, sugar cane is processed to produce ethylene, which can then be used to manufacture polyethylene. Starch can be processed to produce lactic acid and subsequently polylactic acid (PLA).*
Biodegradable plastics	*Biodegradable plastics are plastics degraded by microorganisms into water, carbon dioxide (or methane) and biomass under specified conditions. To guide consumers in their decision-making and give them confidence in a plastic's biodegradability, universal standards have been implemented, new materials have been developed, and a compostable logo has been introduced.*
Engineering plastics	*Engineering plastics exhibit higher performance than standard materials, making them ideal for tough engineering applications. They have gradually replaced traditional engineering materials such as wood or metal in many applications because, not only do they equal or surpass them in their weight/strength ratio and other properties, but they are also much easier to manufacture, especially in complicated shapes.*
Epoxy resins	*Epoxy resins have been around for more than 50 years and are one of the most successful of the plastics families. Their physical state can be changed from a low viscosity liquid to a high melting point solid, which means that a wide range of materials with unique properties can be made. In the home, you'll find them in soft-drinks cans and special packaging, where they are used as a lining to protect the contents and to keep the flavor in. They are also used as a protective coating on everything from beds, garden chairs, office and hospital furniture, to supermarket trolleys and bicycles. They are also used in special paints to protect the surfaces of ships, oil rigs and wind turbines from bad weather.*
Expanded polystyrene	*Expanded polystyrene, or EPS, is widely used commodity polymer. It has been a material of choice for more than 50 years because of its versatility, performance, and cost effectiveness. It is widely used in many everyday applications, such as fish boxes, bicycle helmets and insulation material.*
Fluoropolymers	*Fluoropolymers are renowned for their superior non-stick properties associated with their use as a coating on cookware and as a soil and stain repellent for fabrics and textile products. They also contribute to significant advancement in areas such as aerospace, electronics, automotive, industrial processes (chemical and power sectors, including renewable energy), architecture, food and pharma and medical applications. The most well-known member of Fluoropolymers is PTFE (polytetrafluoroethylene).*
Polyolefins	*Polyolefins are a family of polyethylene and polypropylene thermoplastics. They are produced mainly from oil and natural gas by a process of polymerization of ethylene and propylene respectively. Their versatility has made them one of the most popular plastics in use today.*
Polystyrene	*Polystyrene is a synthetic polymer made from styrene monomer which is a liquid petrochemical. It is a thermoplastic polymer which softens when heated and can be converted via semi-finished products such as films and sheets, into a wide range of final articles.*
Polyurethanes	*Polyurethane (PUR) is a resilient, flexible, and durable manufactured material. There are various types of polyurethanes, which look and feel quite different from each other. They are used in a broad range of products. In fact, we are surrounded by polyurethane-containing products in every aspect of our everyday lives. While most people are not overly familiar with polyurethanes because they are generally 'hidden' behind covers or surfaces made of other materials, it would be hard to imagine life without them.*
Polyvinyl chloride	*Polyvinyl chloride (PVC) was one of the first plastics discovered and is also one of the most extensively used. It is derived from salt (57%) and oil or gas (43%). It is the world's third-most widely produced synthetic plastic polymer, after polyethylene and polypropylene. PVC comes in two basic forms: rigid (sometimes abbreviated as RPVC) and flexible.*
Thermoplastics	*Thermoplastics are defined as polymers that can be melted and recast almost indefinitely. They are molten when heated and harden upon cooling. When frozen, however, a thermoplastic becomes glass-like and subject to fracture. These characteristics, which lend the material its name, are reversible, so the material can be reheated, reshaped, and frozen repeatedly. As a result, thermoplastics are mechanically recyclable. Some of the most common types of thermoplastic are polypropylene, polyethylene, polyvinylchloride, polystyrene, polyethylenetheraphthalate and polycarbonate.*

Table 1.
Type of plastics [plastic Europe – Online].

Microplastics samples are usually sorted into different shapes according to observed morphology. The Joint Group of Experts on the Scientific Aspects of Marine Environmental Protection (GESAMP) [42] recommends five general categories of recommends, including fragment, foam, film, line, and pellet. **Figure 1** presents the standardized size and color sorting system (SCS) for categorizing microplastics [43]. It is recommended the original data in these finer subdivisions with the recognition that subdivisions can be combined for ease of harmonizing and comparing data [42].

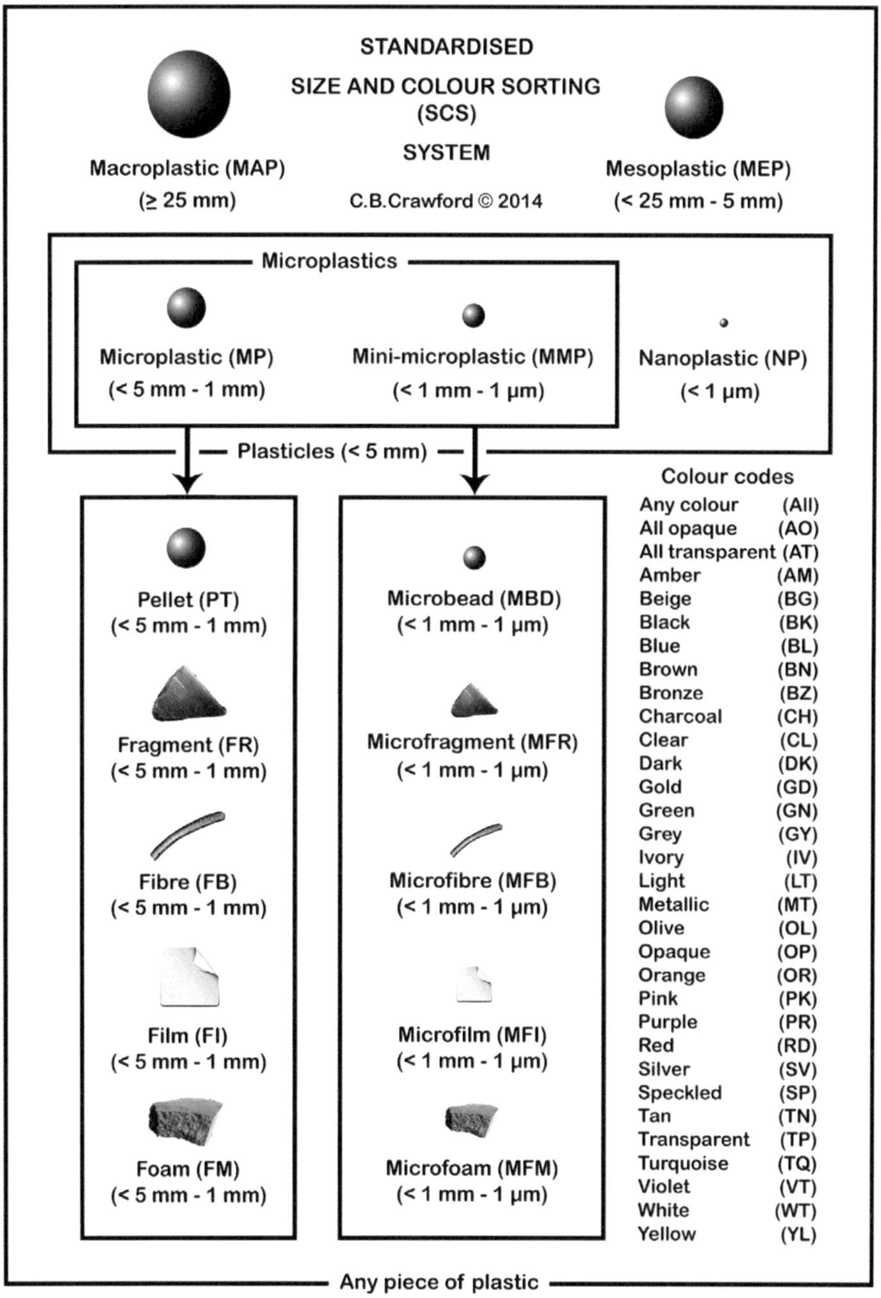

Figure 1.
The standardized size and color sorting (SCS) system [43].

According to Crawford et al. [43], the SCS system generates unique codes to process microplastic abundance data, requiring an efficient categorization system. **Table 2** presents a categorization of plastic according to size, while the **Table 3** gives the categorization of microplastics according to morphology.

There are many hundreds of different types of polymer and mixtures of polymer in commercial production, but the market is dominated by: polyethylene (as both

Category	Abbreviation	Size	Size definition
Macroplastic	MAP	≥25 mm	Any piece of plastic equal to or larger than 25 mm in size along its longest dimension
Mesoplastic	MEP	<25 mm–5 mm	Any piece of plastic less than 25 mm–5 mm in size along its longest dimension
Plasticle	PLT	<5 mm	All pieces of plastic less than 5 mm in size along their longest dimension
Microplastic	MP	<5 mm–1 mm	Any piece of plastic less than 5 mm–1 mm in size along its longest dimension
Mini-microplastic	MP	<1 mm–1 μm	Any piece of plastic less than 1 mm–1 μm in size along its longest dimension
Nanoplastic	NP	<1 μm	Any piece of plastic less than 1 μm in size along its longest dimension

Table 2.
Categorization of pieces of plastic based on size [43].

Abbreviation	Type	Size	Definition
PT	Pellet	<5 mm–1 mm	A small spherical piece of plastic less than 5 mm to 1 mm in diameter
MBD	Microbead	<1 mm–1 μm	A small spherical piece of plastic less than 1 mm to 1 μm in diameter
FR	Fragment	<5 mm–1 mm	An irregular shaped piece of plastic less than 5 mm to 1 mm in size along its longest dimension
MFR	Microfragment	<1 mm–1 μm	An irregular shaped piece of plastic less than 1 mm to 1 μm in size along its longest dimension
FB	Fiber	<5 mm–1 mm	A strand or filament of plastic less than 5 mm to 1 mm in size along its longest dimension
MFB	Microfibre	<1 mm–1 μm	A strand or filament of plastic less than 1 mm to 1 μm in size along its longest dimension
FI	Film	<5 mm–1 mm	A thin sheet or membrane-like piece of plastic less than 5 mm to 1 mm in size along its longest dimension
MFI	Microfilm	<1 mm–1 μm	A thin sheet or membrane-like piece of plastic less than 1 mm to 1 μm in size along its longest dimension
FM	Foam	<5 mm–1 mm	A piece of sponge, foam, or foam-like plastic material less than 5 mm to 1 mm in size along its longest dimension
MFM	Microfoam	<1 mm–1 μm	A piece of sponge, foam, or foam-like plastic material less than 1 mm to 1 μm in size along its longest dimension

Table 3.
Categorization of microplastics based on morphology [43].

Polymers	Abbreviation	CAS #	Molecular formula	2D Structure
Polyethylene	PE	9002-88-4	$(C_2H_4)_n$	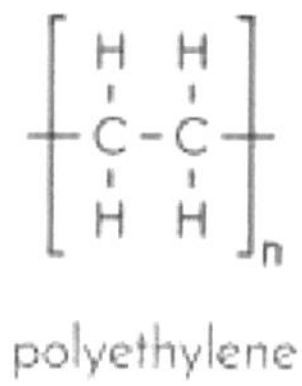
Polypropylene	PP	9003-07-0	$(C_3H_6)_n$	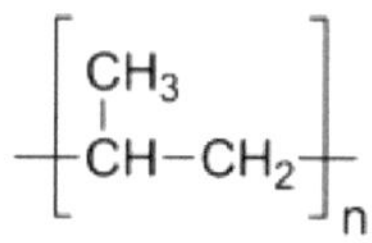
Expanded polystyrene	EPS	9003-53-6	$(C_8H_8)_n$	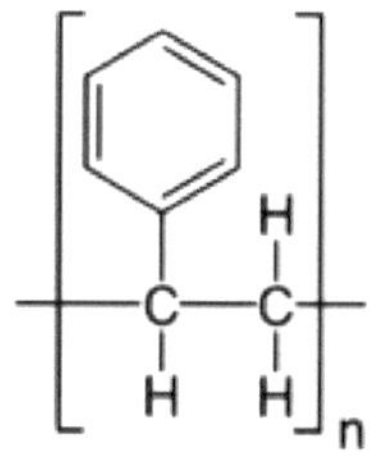
Polyethylene Terephthalate	PET	25038–59-9	$(C_{10}H_8O_4)_n$	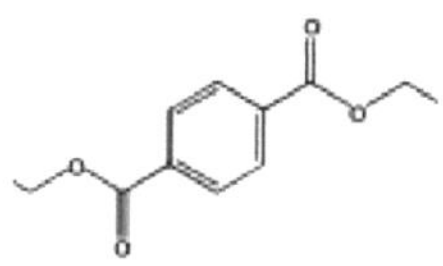
Polymethylmethacrylate	PMMA	9011-14-7	$[(CH_2C(CH_3)(CO_2CH_3)]_n$	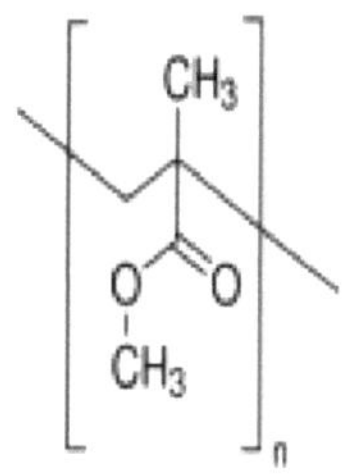
Polyetrafluoroethylene	PTFE	9002-84-0	$(CF_2CF_2)_n$	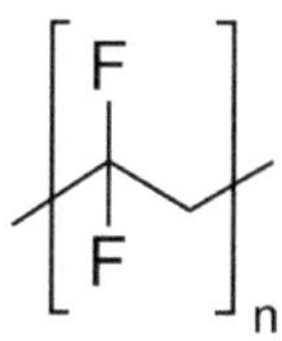
Polyamide (nylon)	PA	63428–84-2	C$_{23}$H$_{26}$N2O4	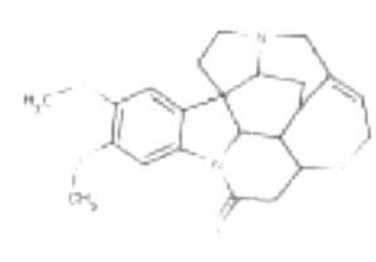
Polyurethane	PU	9009-54-5	$C_3H_8N_2O$	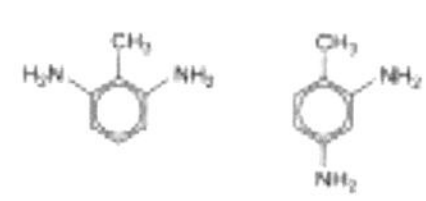

Table 4.
Main polymers found in microplastics [32].

high-density HDPE, and low-density LDPE), polypropylene (PP), polyvinyl chloride (PVC), polyurethane (PUR), polystyrene (PS), and polyethylene terephthalate (PET). These six polymers make up about 80% of plastics production and are likely to form a large proportion of most marine litter (GESAMP, 2019). The most common human-produced and petroleum-derived polymers found in microplastics are listed in **Table 4**.

According to Lambert, et al. [16], "Microplastic" is an umbrella term that covers many particle shapes, sizes, and polymer types, and as such the physical and chemical properties of environmental microplastics will differ from the primary microbeads commonly used for ecotoxicity testing. In the **Figure 2** is presented the physical and chemical properties of MP, by concentrating particle size, particle shape, surface area and crystallinity, as well as chemical composition, while considering the type of polymer, additive compounds, and changes in surface properties) [16].

3.2 Legal and regulatory framework on MP

Microplastics are subdivided into two groups: primary microplastics and secondary microplastics [26]. The distinction between primary and secondary microplastics is based on whether the particles were originally manufactured to be that size (primary) or whether they have resulted from the breakdown of larger items (secondary) [44]. It is a useful distinction because it can help to indicate potential sources and identify mitigation measures to reduce their input to the environment. Primary microplastics include industrial 'scrubbers' used to blast clean surfaces, plastic powders used in molding, micro-beads in cosmetic formulation, and plastic nanoparticles used in a variety of industrial processes [44, 45]. In addition, spherical or cylindrical virgin resin pellets, typically around 5 mm in diameter, are widely used during plastics manufacture and transport of the basic resin 'feedstock' prior to production of plastic products. Secondary microplastics result from the fragmentation and weathering of larger plastic items. This can happen during the use phase of products such as textiles, paint, and tires, or once the items have been released into the environment [44]. The rate of fragmentation is controlled by several factors [46].

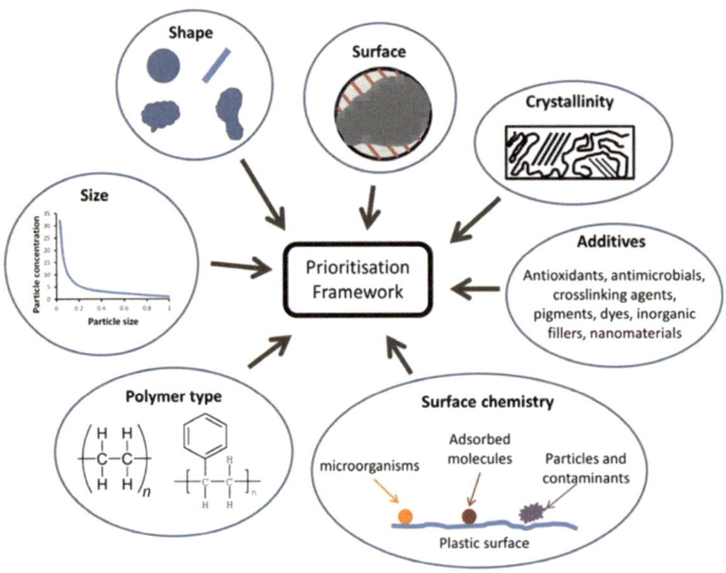

Figure 2.
Different microplastic physical and chemical properties to be considered in a prioritization framework [16].

Plastics can be lost to the environment across their entire value chain [47], which creates different opportunities (and challenges) to prevent leakage into technical and natural systems [48]. In this context, it is useful to frame the separate but interconnected issues of plastic pollution, which are nestled into one another [47]. A list of microplastic sources entering the environment is presented in **Figure 3**.

Some sources and pathways are interconnected (e.g., mechanical stress, plastic waste, plasticulture) and some sources are stand-alone (e.g., primary microplastics in products, targeted applications, or transportation losses), but collectively all sources are part of the puzzle of how microplastic enters the environment.

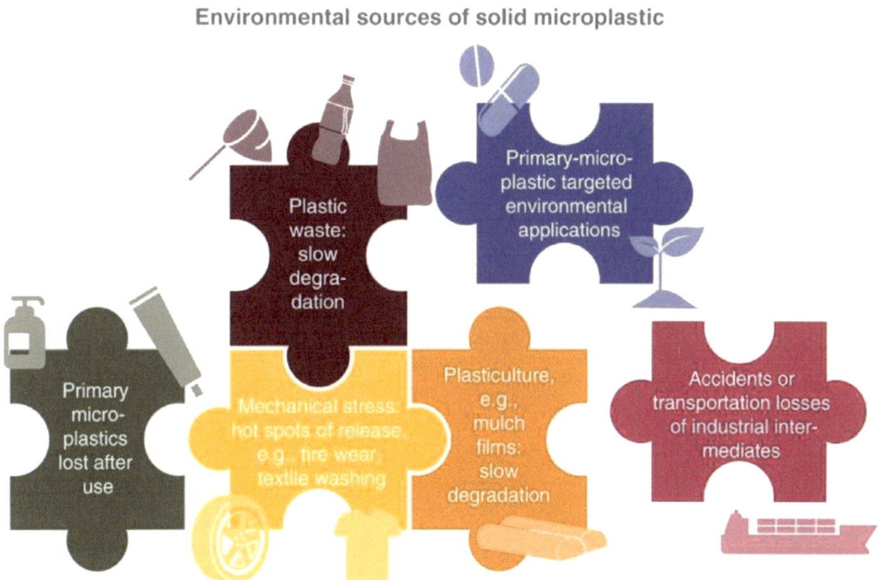

Figure 3.
Environmental sources of pollution by microplastic [47].

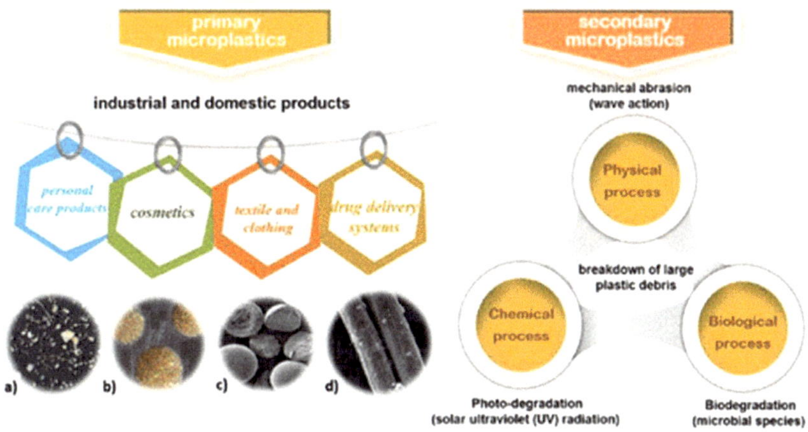

Figure 4.
Sources of microplastics in natural ecosystems [50]: (a) different color and shaped microplastics collected from seawater, shorelines, or marine sediments; (b) photomicrographs of the microplastics in facial cleansers; (c) scanning electron microscopy image of microbeads found in cosmetics; and (d) scanning electron microscopy image of a typical fiber from fabric [50].

Microplastics in the environment are generally supposed to be a heterogeneous aggregate of particles, which can be of both primary and/or secondary origins. However, whatever the group to which they belong, depending on their physical and chemical properties, the size and shape of the particles, the crystallinity, the surface chemistry and the composition of the polymers and additives, the toxicity of microplastics can be crucial for the environment [49]. In a critical review on the sources and instruments of microplastics in marine ecosystems, Wang & al [50] present a figure in which the landbased origins of primary and secondary MP are well explained (**Figure 4**).

Although there is no specific international marine legislation regarding microplastics so far, many proactive countermeasures have been taken – voluntary or legally binding practices at international, regional, and national levels [47]. Indeed, the available literature on marine pollution reports the existence of three global international conventions that deal with the problem of plastic waste in the marine environment at the beginning of the 1970s: (i) the United Nations Convention (UN) on the Law of the Sea [51], (ii) the International Convention for the Prevention of Pollution from Ships (1973) as amended by the Protocol of 1978

International instruments	Period	Specific contents
United Nations Convention on the Law of the Sea	1982	Part XII (Articles 192–237): protection and control of marine pollution from sea−/ land-based sources
MARPOL 73/78	1973	Annex V prohibits "the disposal into the sea of all plastics, cargo residues, fishing gear including but not limited to synthetic ropes, synthetic fishing nets and plastic garbage bags". (revised in 2011 and come into force in 2013)
London Convention	1972	To prevent the "deliberate disposal at sea of wastes and other matter from vessels, aircraft and other structures, including the vessels themselves". (Annex I, paragraph 2)
London Protocol	1996	To prohibit the dumping of any wastes or other matter including the export of waste to countries for dumping and incineration at sea except for the materials listed in Annex I. (Article 4.1.1, 5 and 6)
Basel Convention	1989	Include plastic waste and microplastics issues into the Basel Convention workstream at COP 13 (Plastic waste in Annex II Y 46 (Household wastes) and Annex VIII (Non-hazardous wastes))
United Nations Environment Programme – Regional Seas Programme and Global Programme of Action	2003	Regional activities in 12 regional seas
Manila Declaration	2012	Prevent marine litter from land-based sources and agree to establish a Global Partnership on Marine Litter (GPML)
G7 Summit	2014	G7 Marine Litter Action Plan
G20 Summit	2017	G20 Marine Litter Action Plan
United Nations Environment Assembly (UNEA) I	2014	Resolutions 1/6: put forward the issue of "Marine plastic debris and microplastics".
UNEA II	2016	Resolutions 2/11: measures to reduce marine plastic litter and microplastics
UNEA III	2017	Resolutions 3/7: combating the spread of marine plastic litter and microplastics.

Table 5.
Overview of current legislation, regulations and instruments related to microplastics [50].

(MARPOL 73/78) [52] and (iii) the Convention for the Prevention of Pollution by Dumping of Wastes and Other Matter (London Convention or LC, 1972) [53].

Table 5 shows an overview of current legislation, regulations and instruments related to microplastics. Considering the abundance of microplastics in the environment, their ability to absorb pollutants, their impact on living organisms, the health and environmental authorities in several countries have applied the precautionary principle by adopting a legal framework on MP. However, uncertainties and gaps in the evidence regarding the effects of microplastics on the environment and on human health prevent the adoption of more restrictive measures, with the precautionary principle - in line to the World Trade Organization (WTO) obligations on international trade - only playing a minor role [54]. Available information on current regional and national instruments related to microplastics is discussed in Wang & al. [50].

4. Impact of microplastics on living organisms in natural ecosystems

The global plastics production has increased from 1.5 million tons in the 1950s to 335 million tons in 2016, with plastics discharged into virtually all components of the environment [55]. The MPs present in the environment result from the successive breakdown of larger plastic pieces or from the direct input of micro- and nano-sized particles used in various industries and products available to consumers [56]. Indeed, during their production, industrial and domestic use, and after such processes, a considerable part of the plastics produced globally end up in the environment. Moreover, Plastics rarely biodegrade but through different processes they fragment into microplastics and nanoplastics, which have been reported as ubiquitous pollutants in all marine environments worldwide [55]. In fact, plastics represent one of the fastest-growing portions of the urban waste contributing to environmental contamination and pollution, with plastic debris accounting for approximately 60–80% of all marine litter, reaching 90–95% in some areas [55, 57–59].

4.1 Environmental occurrence

According to Lambert et al. [5] "Upon their release to the environment MPs are transported and distributed to various environmental compartments. The distances that an individual item will travel depends on its size and weight. Lightweight materials can be readily transported long distances via a windblown route or carried by freshwater to eventually accumulate in the oceans. During heavy rainfall events, roadside litter can be washed into drains and gullies, and, where the topography is favorable for it, can be carried to the sea". **Figure 5** shows a conceptual model illustrating degradation pathways for polymer materials [5].

Once in the environment MPs are degraded through abiotic or biotic factors working together or in sequence; these processes cause the polymer matrix to disintegrate, resulting in the formation of fragmented particles of various sizes and leached additives [5]. According to Lambert et al. [5] "there is a broad literature dealing with the degradation of various polymer types under various conditions. Most of these studies were performed in the laboratory and had a major focus on samples exposed to high-energy UV irradiation".

In the environment, MPs constitute a matrix of pollutants, composed of several monomers and polymers (PE, PP, EPS, PET, PMMA, PTFE, PA, PU, etc.), metal catalysts, additives: phthalates, retardants. Flame, bisphenols A and F, etc.), loading materials (talc, Ti dioxide), adsorbed environmental pollutants (organic and

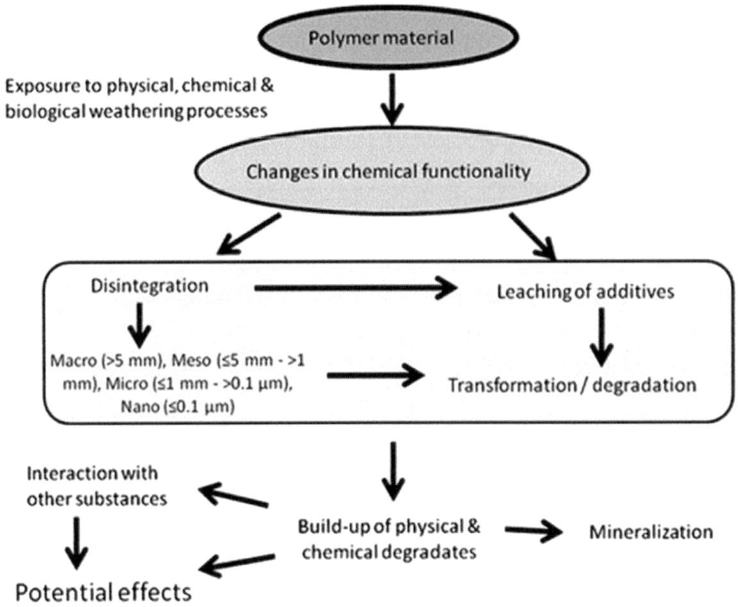

Figure 5.
Conceptual model illustrating degradation pathways for polymer materials [5].

inorganic, pathogenic agents, etc. The exposure of living organisms to MPs leads to consider the interactions between the combined effects of different pollutants. The characterization of exposure to microplastics will depend on: (i) the number of particles; (ii) size distribution, shape, surface properties, polymer composition and particle density; (iii) the duration of the exposure; (iv) the kinetics of absorption and desorption of contaminants, vis-à-vis the plastic and the organism; and (v) the biology of the organism [44].

4.2 Environmental effects

Microplastics have been detected in sediments, surface waters, estuarine and marine waters [60–62]. The negative effects of microplastics on algae, mussels, fish, and other organisms have been the subject of several studies and have shown [20, 63–66]. Given the difficulty for large filter-feeding organisms (fins, whales, ..) and zooplankton to differentiate between microplastics and food itself [27, 67], cellular intoxication has been documented by ingestion by inadvertently adhered microplastics with other pollutants [26, 25]. Flame retardants (chemicals derived from plastics) have been found in birds [29] and phthalates in whales and filter-feeding sharks [27]. Microplastics can affect growth and reproduction in daphnids [28].

Alimba and Faggio [55] observed effects of MPs on marine vertebrates and invertebrates, including asphyxiation by drowning, restricted diet and increased starvation, skin abrasions and skeletal injuries (which are the basis of intestinal mucosal damage, morbidity, and mortality), oxidative stress, altered immunological responses, genomic instability, endocrine disruption, neurotoxicity, reproductive abnormalities, embryotoxicity and transgenerational toxicity [55].

Present in an environment, MPs can mimic the natural food sources of living species [5]. 135 species of marine vertebrates and 8 species of invertebrates susceptible to entanglement, and 111 species of seabirds have been identified, among others, among the species that ingest plastic objects [67]. Other studies have shown that MPs wrapping loops are a threat to sea lions in California and fur seals in Australia, respectively [68, 69]. Plastic bags have been identified as the main type of debris ingested by sea turtles [70]. **Figure 6** shows a conceptual model illustrating the potential effects produced during the degradation of polymer-based materials [5].

4.3 Potential effects of microplastics on human health

The primary route of human exposure to MPs is the ingestion of foodstuffs, in particular seafood which has ingested microplastics [30], processed commercial fish [71], sea salt [72], honey [73], beer, food components [73]. Most of these food products are sometimes contaminated by the presence of impurities in processing materials and contaminants in packaging [74]. The second route of exposure is inhalation of air and dust containing MPs [30]. Due to their nutritional value, seafood plays an important role in human nutrition. Indeed, the consumption of seafood represents 6.7% of all protein and about 17% of animal protein in 2015 [75]. The risk of exposure is therefore great and increases with small fish eaten whole [46].

Several studies have highlighted the evidence for the presence of microplastics in several commercial aquatic species such as mussels, oysters, crabs, sea cucumbers and fish [76–78]. The results of this work suggest that humans are exposed to microplastics through their diet and the presence of microplastics in seafood could pose a threat to food safety [76]. The potential accumulation of microplastics in the food chain, especially in fish and shellfish (species of mollusks, crustaceans, and echinoderms) could have consequences for the health of human consumers [44]. In this trophic context, the fate and toxicity of microplastics in humans constitutes a major lack of knowledge which deserves special attention. The potential

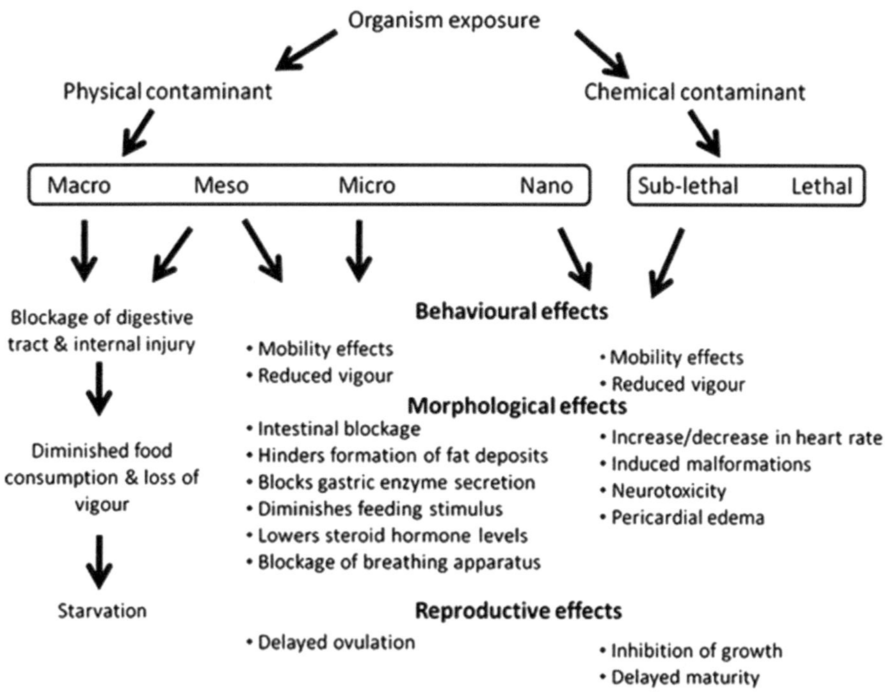

Figure 6.
Conceptual model illustrating the potential effects produced during the degradation of polymer-based materials [5].

accumulation of microplastics in food chains, particularly in fish and crustaceans (mollusks, crustaceans, and echinoderms), appears to be the main source of human exposure to microplastics [44]. Contamination of food products with MP could have consequences for the health of human consumers. In this trophic context, the fate and toxicity of microplastics in humans constitutes a major lack of knowledge which deserves special attention.

The translocation of microplastics from the intestine to the circulatory system and various tissues and cells in humans has been studied by several authors [44]. Indeed, Hussain et al. [79] have shown the absorption of PE particles captured in the lymph and the circulatory system from the gastrointestinal tract. Exposure of human macrophages to fluorescent microspheres of PS (1, 0.2 and 0.078 μm), demonstrated particle capture driven by non-endocytic processes (diffusion or adhesive interactions) [44].

5. Waste management, environmental pollution, microplastics and loss of biodiversity in Port-au-Prince

5.1 The issue of solid waste in Port-au-Prince

Urban cleanliness and its variations over time reflect the aspects of each civilization, [...], the capacity of societies to legislate, to mobilize techniques and to organize the complexity of urban services [80]. In developing countries (DCs), however, the issue of urban cleanliness a priori highlights the weakness of urban managers and institutions in terms of their capacity to manage the growing and very heterogeneous flow of waste produced [81].

In Port-au-Prince, the capital of Haiti, solid waste management is practiced in a context of rapid population growth and extreme urban poverty [82]. Indeed, urban cleanliness and its variations over time highlight a clear discrepancy between the objective of the waste management service (making and maintaining the city clean) and the realities on the ground. The combination of the low rate of garbage collection and high human densities accentuates unsanitary conditions in the city and represents a risk factor not only in terms of human health but also of the environment. Also, vacant spaces, voids in the urban fabric of Port-au-Prince very quickly become public landfill spaces [81]. In this urban space, notes Lacour [83], urban cleanliness is established in the mix of most urban waste management systems where state and private services coexist, as well as public funds and international funding, through development organizations. In addition, the negative impacts (pollution, nuisance, proliferation of rodents and insects, risk of disease, etc.), linked to the size, nature, and unsuitable management methods of organic waste (landfill with other categories, combustion, etc.), are generally very pronounced [83].

The characteristics of the waste management system in Haiti have been defined as follows [84]:

- "At source, the general behavior tends to immediately remove unsorted waste. Consequently, the nearest (common) public space becomes the preferred outlet. This reflex is particularly predominant in rural and peri-urban areas and the precarious neighborhoods of so-called "low-standing" urban areas.

- The existence of an informal circuit, said to be rather pragmatic, compensates for the absence of an institutional waste management service in rural areas or the dysfunction of this service in urban areas. This circuit is characterized by a pre-collection by voluntary contribution, an individual (rural and peri-urban) or private (urban "medium standing" and "high standing") collection, waste disposal in non-dedicated spaces (vacant lots, gullies, etc.) spontaneously transformed into wild dumps.

- The total absence of a landfill site that meets environmental standards, in terms of waste categorization, development work for the control of discharges and the recovery of leachate and biogas, odor management, animal control, etc.

- The practices of recycling organic waste, by feeding pets and livestock (free and rope) are quite frequent at the level of pre-collection and collection points.

- The lack of information relating to the deposits of waste, in terms of their masses, their compositions and their bio-physico-chemical characteristics, through the seasons and rural, peri-urban and urban spaces, constitutes an obstacle to the implementation, the monitoring and anticipation of management strategies" [84].

5.2 The issues of plastic waste and microplastics in Port-au-Prince

According to the World Bank (2019) [85], in the Caribbean and elsewhere in the world, marine pollution is linked to poor waste management on land: illegal dumping, open burning or dumping of waste in streams. In addition, the quantity of plastics reaches a concentration of 200,000 pieces of debris per square kilometer in the northeast of the Caribbean. In this region of the world, about 85% of wastewater is discharged into the ocean without having been previously treated; and, in island countries more particularly - Bahamas, Greater Antilles (Cuba, Dominican Republic, Haiti, Jamaica and Puerto Rico) and Lesser Antilles - approximately 52% of households are not connected to sewers. However, 14 Caribbean countries (more than a third) have banned single-use plastic bags and / or styrofoam containers (**Figure 7**).

In Haiti, the government issued on August 9, 2012, a decree prohibiting the production, import, marketing, and use, in any form whatsoever, of polyethylene bags and expanded polystyrene objects (PSE or PS or Styrofoam) for single food

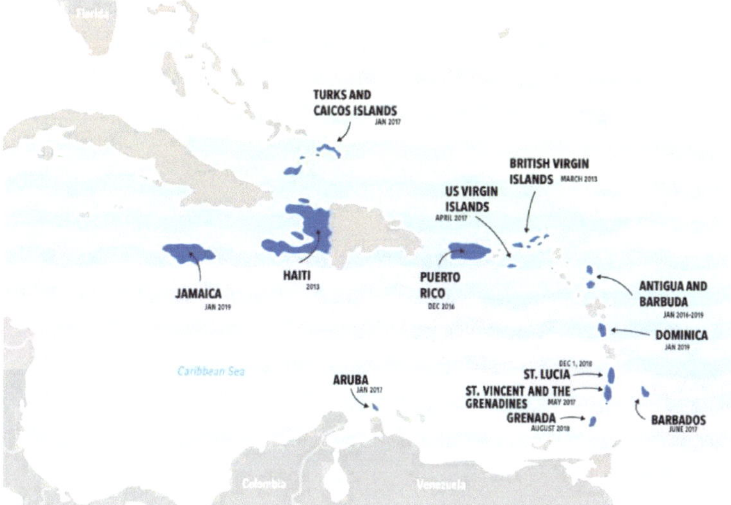
TURKS AND CAICOS ISLANDS
JAN 2017
BRITISH VIRGIN ISLANDS
MARCH 2013
US VIRGIN ISLANDS
APRIL 2017
HAITI
2013
JAMAICA
JAN 2019
PUERTO RICO
DEC 2016
ANTIGUA AND BARBUDA
JAN 2016-2019
DOMINICA
JAN 2019
Caribbean Sea
ARUBA
JAN 2017
DEC 1, 2018
ST. LUCIA
ST. VINCENT AND THE GRENADINES
MAY 2017
GRENADA
AUGUST 2018
BARBADOS
JUNE 2017
Colombia
Venezuela

Figure 7.
Caribbean countries that have banned single-use plastic bags and/or expanded polystyrene containers [85].

use, such as trays, trays, bottles, sachets, cups and plates. On July 10, 2013, a second decree was issued to ban once again "the importation, production or sale of expanded polystyrene articles for food use". In support of the second decree, the ministries of the Environment, Justice and Public Security, Trade, and Industry as well as Economy and Financc announced in a note published in January 2018 that brigade's specialists will be deployed on the territory to force the application of the said decree.

To better approach the problem of plastic and microplastic waste management in Port-au-Prince, it is important to look at the waste management system. In Haiti, the National Solid Waste Management Service (*Service National de Gestion des Résidus Solides* (SNGRS)). This public institution has the status of an autonomous body, and an authority which extends over the entire territory of the country.

In the agglomeration of Port-au-Prince, there is a single space that has been officially designated to receive any type of waste. Due to the insufficient capacity of public actors to collect all waste, it ends up in different types of space according to different logics [86]. The uncontrolled presence of waste induces a certain number of potential nuisances. It is therefore necessary to consider the health risk classically associated with waste [87], as a vector of pathology and contamination of natural resources [86]. Beyond the environmental dangers generated by chemical substances and pathogenic microorganisms present in solid waste, the latter not only obstruct traffic routes, but are also a source of flooding by blocking irrigation canals and gullies (**Figure 8**).

Port-au-Prince's marine ecosystem is liable to suffer locally profoundly serious damages caused by the direct discharge of urban effluents [88]. Indeed, the discharge of contaminants in natural ecosystems, by example water bodies pose a significant concern to water quality and to the health of aquatic organism because of not only the varied types of pollutants that impact these systems, also because of the many ways pollutants can affect the health of aquatic organism [89].

With the tropical temperature of Haiti and the average daily duration (12 hours / day), the plastics present in the urban water canals could degrade more quickly by generating microplastics. Their discharge in the bay of Port-au-Prince exposes this ecosystem to environmental dangers [90], that of pollutants contained in wastewater, and that of climatic hazards, in particular the acidification of the oceans. The stress of benthic organisms (coral reefs, bivalves) should then be observed and monitored.

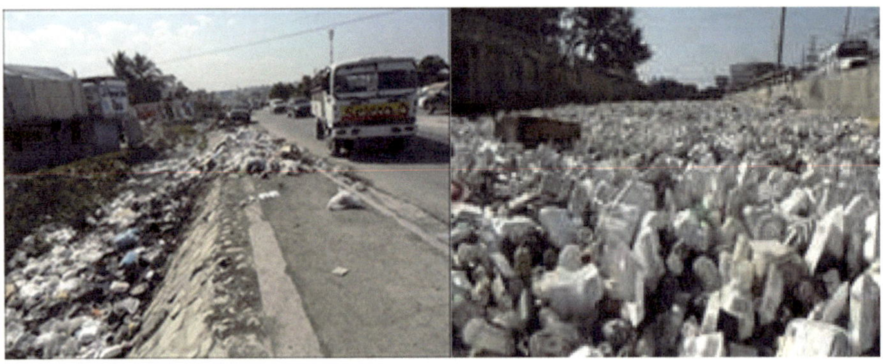

Figure 8.
Uncontrolled presence of waste in public spaces in Port-au-Prince. (left illustration - unauthorized deposit of household waste along a road [86]. Right illustration - unauthorized deposit of PSE or PS or Styrofoam waste in the largest urban water collector in Port-au-Prince).

6. Conclusion

The presence of microplastics in the environment first and foremost generates environmental health hazards, which need to be increasingly identified and assessed. Most of the research in the field of environmental pollution from microplastics has been carried out on aquatic ecosystems. There then arises the need to initiate research programs on terrestrial ecosystems.

The future of MPs in the environment represents real research challenges. Indeed, there is a lack of knowledge at the local and national level of the different flows. At the global level, the toxicological reference values have not yet been obtained. Human dose–response relationships need to be investigated on the basis of still possible animal species exposures.

The field of environmental assessment of MPs, in the Caribbean for example, a priori calls for transdisciplinary approaches. Indeed, this region of the world, thanks to its tropical climate and the Caribbean Sea, makes tourism one of its main development niches. Pollution from plastic waste exposes its economy to a risk of economic imbalance. In the case of Haiti, beyond the urgent need to review its public policies in terms of urban water and solid waste management, the pollution of ecosystems by MPs highlights the need to initiate real research work. in the field of marine ecotoxicology.

Acknowledgements

The authors are thankful to the "One Health" University Space of Quisqueya University, FOKAL-Open Society Foundation Haiti, the Agence universitaire de la Francophonie (AUF), the Representation of the Institute of Research for Development (IRD) in Mexico, Cuba, and Haiti, the SCAC (Service de Coopération et d'Action Culturelle) of the France Embassy in Haiti, and the AOG (Association Communautaire Paysanne des Originaires de Grande Plaine), for their support in carrying out this study.

Author details

Daphenide St. Louis[1,2,3], Ammcise Apply[1,2,4], Daphnée Michel[1,2,3] and Evens Emmanuel[3,4*]

1 Faculté des Sciences de la Santé, Programme de Maîtrise en Santé Publique, Université Quisqueya, Port-au-Prince, Haiti

2 Association Haïtienne Femmes, Science et Technologie (AHFST), Port-au-Prince, Haiti

3 Équipe de Recherche sur la Santé-Environnement (Ci-devant Laboratoire Santé-Environnement (LS-E)), Université Quisqueya, Port-au-Prince, Haiti

4 Équipe de recherche sur Changements Climatiques (ERC2), Université Quisqueya, Port-au-Prince, Haiti

*Address all correspondence to: evens.emmanuel@uniq.edu.ht

References

[1] Bissagou Koumba, G. (2018). Fragmentations chimique et physique de plastiques et microplastiques en eau douce sous irradiation UV-visible (Doctoral dissertation, Clermont Auvergne).

[2] American Chemical Society. (2013). The bakelizer. American Chemical Society: Washington, DC, USA.

[3] Achouri, S. (2020). Les microplastiques dans les rivières et eaux de surfaces, exploration des méthodes d'échantillonnages et analyses en laboratoire: préparation à une application à l'exutoire de deux stations d'épurations Arlon et Libramont. https://matheo.uliege.be/handle/2268.2/10115

[4] Simonneau, A., Allen, D., Le Roux, G. (2019). Des contaminants venus d'ailleurs. Microscoop: Un regard sur les laboratoires en Centre Limousin Poitou-Charentes (CNRS), CNRS. https://hal-insu.archives-ouvertes.fr/insu-02299176

[5] Lambert, S., Sinclair, C.J., Boxall, A. B.A. (2014). Occurrence, degradation, and effects of polymer-based materials in the environment. Rev. Environ. Contam. Toxicol. 227:1–53. https://doi.org/10.1007/978-3-319-01327-5_1

[6] Mougin, C. (2019, June). Etat de l'art des impacts écotoxicologiques des microplastiques sur les écosystèmes terrestres. In Séminaire de la Fédération Ile de France de Recherche sur l'Environnement. HAL Id: hal-02788504 https://hal.inrae.fr/hal-02788504

[7] Faure, F., Saini, C., Potter, G., Galgani, F., De Alencastro, L. F., & Hagmann, P. (2015). An evaluation of surface micro-and mesoplastic pollution in pelagic ecosystems of the Western Mediterranean Sea. Environmental Science and Pollution Research, 22(16), 12190-12197. https://doi.org/10.1007/s11356-015-4453-3

[8] Browne, M. A., Dissanayake, A., Galloway, T. S., Lowe, D. M., & Thompson, R. C. (2008). Ingested microscopic plastic translocates to the circulatory system of the mussel, *Mytilus edulis* (L.). Environmental science & technology, 42(13), 5026-5031. https://doi.org/10.1021/es800249a

[9] Liebezeit, G., & Dubaish, F. (2012). Microplastics in beaches of the East Frisian islands Spiekeroog and Kachelotplate. Bulletin of environmental contamination and toxicology, 89(1), 213-217. DOI: 10.1007/s00128-012-0642-7

[10] Castañeda, R. A., Avlijas, S., Simard, M. A., & Ricciardi, A. (2014). Microplastic pollution in St. Lawrence river sediments. Canadian Journal of Fisheries and Aquatic Sciences, 71(12), 1767-1771. https://doi.org/10.1139/cjfas-2014-0281

[11] Woodall, L. C., Sanchez-Vidal, A., Canals, M., Paterson, G. L., Coppock, R., Sleight, V., ... & Thompson, R. C. (2014). The deep sea is a major sink for microplastic debris. Royal Society open science, 1(4), 140317. https://doi.org/10.1098/rsos.140317

[12] Francois, G., Stéphane, B., Guillaume, D., Pascale, F., Emmanuelle, C., Jeff, G., ... & Alexandra, H. (2020). Pollution des océans par les plastiques et les microplastiques. Pollution of oceans by plastics and microplastics. Techniques de l'Ingenieur. https://hal.archives-ouvertes.fr/hal-03067254/document

[13] Sutherland, W.J., Clout, M., Cote, I. M., Daszak, P., Depledge, M.H., Fellman, L., Fleishman, E., Garthwaite, R., Gibbons, D.W., De Lurio, J., Impey, A.J., Lickorish, F., Lindenmayer, D., Madgwick, J., Margerison, C., Maynard, T., Peck, L.S., Pretty, J., Prior, S.,

Redford, K.H., Scharlemann, J.P.W., Spalding, M., Watkinson, A.R. (2010). A horizon scan of global conservation issues for 2010. Trends Ecol. Evol. 25:1–7.

[14] UNEP. (2011). UNEP Year book 2011: Emerging Issues in Our Global Environment. United Nations Environment Programme (UNEP). Division of Early Warning, & Assessment UNEP/Earthprint. 2011.

[15] Lambert, S., & Wagner, M. (2016). Characterisation of nanoplastics during the degradation of polystyrene. Chemosphere, 145, 265–268. https://doi.org/10.1016/j.chemosphere.2015.11.078

[16] Lambert, S., Scherer, C., & Wagner, M. (2017). Ecotoxicity testing of microplastics: Considering the heterogeneity of physicochemical properties. Integrated environmental assessment and management, 13(3), 470-475. https://doi.org/10.1002/ieam.1901

[17] Verschoor, A. J. (2015). Towards a definition of microplastics: Considerations for the specification of physico-chemical properties. RIVM Letter report 2015-0116. 42p.

[18] Bakir, A., O'Connor, I. A., Rowland, S. J., Hendriks, A. J., & Thompson, R. C. (2016). Relative importance of microplastics as a pathway for the transfer of hydrophobic organic chemicals to marine life. Environmental pollution, 219, 56-65. https://doi.org/10.1016/j.envpol.2016.09.046.

[19] Ma, Y., Huang, A., Cao, S., Sun, F., Wang, L., Guo, H., & Ji, R. (2016). Effects of nanoplastics and microplastics on toxicity, bioaccumulation, and environmental fate of phenanthrene in fresh water. Environmental Pollution, 219, 166-173. https://doi.org/10.1016/j.envpol.2016.10.061.

[20] Von Moos, N., Burkhardt-Holm, P., & Köhler, A. (2012). Uptake and effects of microplastics on cells and tissue of the blue mussel *Mytilus edulis* L. after an experimental exposure. Environmental science & technology, 46(20), 11327-11335. https://doi.org/10.1021/es302332w.

[21] Wang, J., Peng, J., Tan, Z., Gao, Y., Zhan, Z., Chen, Q., & Cai, L. (2017). Microplastics in the surface sediments from the Beijiang River littoral zone: composition, abundance, surface textures and interaction with heavy metals. Chemosphere, 171, 248-258. https://doi.org/10.1016/j.chemosphere.2016.12.074

[22] Wardrop, P., Shimeta, J., Nugegoda, D., Morrison, P. D., Miranda, A., Tang, M., & Clarke, B. O. (2016). Chemical pollutants sorbed to ingested microbeads from personal care products accumulate in fish. Environmental science & technology, 50(7), 4037-4044. https://doi.org/10.1021/acs.est.5b06280

[23] Besseling, E., Wegner, A., Foekema, E. M., Van Den Heuvel-Greve, M. J., & Koelmans, A. A. (2013). Effects of microplastic on fitness and PCB bioaccumulation by the lugworm *Arenicola marina* (L.). Environmental science & technology, 47(1), 593-600. https://doi.org/10.1021/es302763x

[24] Syberg, K., Khan, F. R., Selck, H., Palmqvist, A., Banta, G. T., Daley, J., ... & Duhaime, M. B. (2015). Microplastics: addressing ecological risk through lessons learned. Environmental toxicology and chemistry, 34(5), 945-953. https://doi.org/10.1002/etc.2914

[25] Chua, E. M., Shimeta, J., Nugegoda, D., Morrison, P. D., & Clarke, B. O. (2014). Assimilation of polybrominated diphenyl ethers from microplastics by the marine amphipod, *Allorchestes compressa*. Environmental science & technology, 48(14), 8127-8134. https://doi.org/10.1021/es405717z

[26] Cole, M., Lindeque, P., Halsband, C., & Galloway, T. S. (2011). Microplastics as contaminants in the marine environment: a review. Marine pollution bulletin, 62(12), 2588-2597. https://doi.org/10.1016/j.marpolbul.2011.09.025

[27] Fossi, M. C., Coppola, D., Baini, M., Giannetti, M., Guerranti, C., Marsili, L., ... & Clò, S. (2014). Large filter feeding marine organisms as indicators of microplastic in the pelagic environment: the case studies of the Mediterranean basking shark (*Cetorhinus maximus*) and fin whale (*Balaenoptera physalus*). Marine environmental research, 100, 17-24. https://doi.org/10.1016/j.marenvres.2014.02.002

[28] Besseling, E., Wang, B., Lürling, M., & Koelmans, A. A. (2014). Nanoplastic affects growth of *S. obliquus* and reproduction of *D. magna*. Environmental science & technology, 48(20), 12336-12343. https://doi.org/10.1021/es503001d

[29] Tanaka, K., Takada, H., Yamashita, R., Mizukawa, K., Fukuwaka, M. A., & Watanuki, Y. (2013). Accumulation of plastic-derived chemicals in tissues of seabirds ingesting marine plastics. Marine pollution bulletin, 69(1-2), 219-222. https://doi.org/10.1016/j.marpolbul.2012.12.010

[30] Smith, M., Love, D. C., Rochman, C. M., & Neff, R. A. (2018). Microplastics in seafood and the implications for human health. Current environmental health reports, 5(3), 375-386. https://doi.org/10.1007/s40572-018-0206-z.

[31] ISO. (2013). ISO 472: Plastics - vocabulary. International Organization for Standardization (ISO). https://www.iso.org/obp/ui/#iso:std:iso:472:ed-4:v1:en

[32] AFWE (2017). Intentionally added microplastics in products. Envrionment Agency Austria. Final report. Report.

[33] Wu, D., Qian, X., & Shen, J. (2017). Macromolecular reorganization as a basis for converting cellulosic hydrogels into sustainable plastics. *BioResources*, *12* (4), 6902-6903.

[34] Asamany, E. A., Gibson, M. D., & Pegg, M. J. (2017). Evaluating the potential of waste plastics as fuel in cement kilns using bench-scale emissions analysis. *Fuel*, *193*, 178-186. https://doi.org/10.1016/j.fuel.2016.12.054

[35] Thompson, R. C., Swan, S. H., Moore, C. J., & Vom Saal, F. S. (2009). Our plastic age. *Phil. Trans. R. Soc. B.* 364:1973–1976 doi:10.1098/rstb.2009.0054

[36] Plastics Europe. (2019). Plastics–the facts: an analysis of European plastics production, demand, and waste data. *Plastics Europe, Brussels. https://www.plasticseurope.org/application/files/1115/7236/4388/FINAL_web_version_Plastics_the_facts2019_14102019.pdf*

[37] Gilbert, M. (2017). Plastics materials: Introduction and historical development. In.*Brydson's plastics materials.* pp.1-18. Butterworth-Heinemann. https://doi.org/10.1016/B978-0-323-35824-8.00001-3

[38] Duval, C. (2009). *Matières plastiques et environnement-2e éd.: Recyclage. Biodégradabilité. Valorisation*. Dunod.

[39] Hamaide, T. (2008). Quelques idees a propos de l'enseignement de la chimie macromoleculaire. *Actualite Chimique*, 319:15-23. https://www.lactualitechimique.org/Quelques-idees-a-propos-de-l-enseignement-de-la-chimie-macromoleculaire

[40] Jiang, B., Kauffman, A. E., Li, L., McFee, W., Cai, B., Weinstein, J., ... & Xiao, S. (2020). Health impacts of environmental contamination of micro- and nanoplastics: a review. *Environmental health and preventive*

medicine, *25*(1), 1-15. https://doi.org/10.1186/s12199-020-00870-9

[41] Arthur. C., Baker. J, Bamford H., (2009). Proceedings of the international research workshop on the occurrence, effects and fate of microplastic marine debris. NOAA Technical Memorandum NOS-OR&R-30.

[42] GESAMP (2019). Guidelines or the monitoring and assessment of plastic litter and microplastics in the ocean (Kershaw P.J., Turra A. and Galgani F. editors), (IMO/FAO/UNESCOIOC/UNIDO/WMO/IAEA/UN/UNEP/UNDP/ISA Joint Group of Experts on the Scientific Aspects of Marine Environmental Protection). Rep. Stud. GESAMP No. 99, 130p.

[43] Crawford, C. B., Quinn, B., Crawford, C. B., & Quinn, B. (2017). Microplastic identification techniques. *Microplastic Pollutants, 1st ed.; Crawford, CB, Quinn, B., Eds*, 219-267. https://doi.org/10.1016/B978-0-12-809406-8.00010-4

[44] GESAMP (2015). Sources, fate and effects of microplastics in the marine environment: a global assessment. (Kershaw, P. J., ed.). (IMO/FAO/UNESCO-IOC/UNIDO/WMO/IAEA/UN/UNEP/UNDP. Joint Group of Experts on the Scientific Aspects of Marine Environmental Protection). Rep. Stud. GESAMP No. 90, 96 p. http://www.gesamp.org/publications/reports-and-studies-no-90.

[45] Frias, J. P. G. L., & Nash, R. (2019). Microplastics: finding a consensus on the definition. *Marine pollution bulletin*, *138*, 145-147. https://doi.org/10.1016/j.marpolbul.2018.11.022

[46] GESAMP (2016). Sources, fate and effects of microplastics in the marine environment: part two of a global assessment. (Kershaw, P.J., and Rochman, C.M., eds). (IMO/FAO/UNESCO-IOC/UNIDO/WMO/IAEA/UN/UNEP/UNDP. Joint Group of Experts on the Scientific Aspects of Marine Environmental Protection). Rep. Stud. GESAMP No. 93, 220 p. http://www.gesamp.org/publications/microplastics-in-the-marineenvironment-

[47] Mitrano, D. M., & Wohlleben, W. (2020). Microplastic regulation should be more precise to incentivize both innovation and environmental safety. *Nature communications*, *11*(1), 1-12. https://doi.org/10.1038/s41467-020-19069-1

[48] Ryberg, M. W., Hauschild, M. Z., Wang, F., Averous-Monnery, S. & Laurent, A. (2019). Global environmental losses of plastics across their value chains. Resour. Conserv. Recycling 151, 104459.

[49] Liu, F. F., Liu, G. Z., Zhu, Z. L., Wang, S. C., & Zhao, F. F. (2019). Interactions between microplastics and phthalate esters as affected by microplastics characteristics and solution chemistry. *Chemosphere*, *214*, 688-694. https://doi.org/10.1016/j.chemosphere.2018.09.174

[50] Wang, J., Zheng, L., & Li, J. (2018). A critical review on the sources and instruments of marine microplastics and prospects on the relevant management in China. *Waste Management & Research*, *36*(10), 898-911. https://doi.org/10.1177/0734242X18793504

[51] UNCLOS. (1982). United Nations Convention on the Law of the Sea. Concluded at Montego Bayon 10 December 1982. https://www.un.org/Depts/los/convention_agreements/texts/unclos/unclos_f.pdf

[52] IMO (1978). International Convention for the Prevention of Pollution from Ships, 1973, as modified by the Protocol of 1978 relating thereto (MARPOL 73/78). International Maritime Organization (IMO). https://www.imo.org/fr/About/Conventions/

Pages/International-Convention-for-the-Prevention-of-Pollution-from-Ships-(MARPOL).aspx

[53] Farnelli, G. M., & Tanzi, A. (2017). Convention on the Prevention of Marine Pollution by Dumping of Wastes and Other Matter 1972 and 1996 Protocol. In *Elgar Encyclopedia of Environmental Law* (pp. 175-183). Edward Elgar Publishing Limited. https://doi.org/10.4337/9781783477210.V.16

[54] Kentin, E., & Kaarto, H. (2018). An EU ban on microplastics in cosmetic products and the right to regulate. *Review of European, Comparative & International Environmental Law*, *27*(3), 254-266. https://doi.org/10.1111/reel.12269

[55] Alimba, C. G., & Faggio, C. (2019). Microplastics in the marine environment: current trends in environmental pollution and mechanisms of toxicological profile. *Environmental toxicology and pharmacology*, *68*, 61-74. https://doi.org/10.1016/j.etap.2019.03.001

[56] Peixoto, D., Pinheiro, C., Amorim, J., Oliva-Teles, L., Guilhermino, L., & Vieira, M. N. (2019). Microplastic pollution in commercial salt for human consumption: A review. *Estuarine, Coastal and Shelf Science*, *219*, 161-168. https://doi.org/10.1016/j.ecss.2019.02.018

[57] Moore, C.J. (2008). Synthetic polymers in the marine environment: a rapidly increasing, long-term threat. Environ. Res. 108, 131–139. https://doi.org/10.1016/j.envres.2008.07.025.

[58] Qiu, Q., Tan, Z., Wang, J., Peng, J., Li, M., Zhan, Z. (2016). Extraction, enumeration and identifification methods for monitoring microplastics in the environment. Estuar. Coast Shelf Sci. 176, 102–109. https://doi.org/10.1016/j.ecss.2016.04.012.

[59] Wang, Y., Zhang, D., Zhang, M., Mu, J., Ding, G., Mao, Z., Cao, Z., Jin, Y., Cong, Y., Wang, L., W, Z., Wang, J. (201. Effects of ingested polystyrene microplastics on brine shrimp, Artemia. Environ. Pollut. 244, 715 722. https://doi.org/10.1016/j.envpol.2018.10.024.

[60] Li, X., Yin, P., & Zhao, L. (2016). Phthalate esters in water and surface sediments of the Pearl River Estuary: distribution, ecological, and human health risks. *Environmental Science and Pollution Research*, *23*(19), 19341-19349.. https://doi.org/10.1007/s11356-016-7143-x

[61] Turner, A., & Rawling, M. C. (2000). The behaviour of di-(2-ethylhexyl) phthalate in estuaries. *Marine Chemistry*, *68*(3), 203-217. https://doi.org/10.1016/S0304-4203(99)00078-X

[62] Zeng, F., Cui, K., Xie, Z., Liu, M., Li, Y., Lin, Y., ... & Li, F. (2008). Occurrence of phthalate esters in water and sediment of urban lakes in a subtropical city, Guangzhou, South China. *Environment International*, *34*(3), 372-380. https://doi.org/10.1016/j.envint.2007.09.002

[63] Green, D. S., Boots, B., O'Connor, N. E., & Thompson, R. (2017). Microplastics affect the ecological functioning of an important biogenic habitat. *Environmental science & technology*, *51*(1), 68-77. https://pubs.acs.org/doi/abs/10.1021/acs.est.6b04496

[64] Lagarde, F., Olivier, O., Zanella, M., Daniel, P., Hiard, S., & Caruso, A. (2016). Microplastic interactions with freshwater microalgae: hetero-aggregation and changes in plastic density appear strongly dependent on polymer type. *Environmental pollution*, *215*, 331-339. https://doi.org/10.1016/j.envpol.2016.05.006

[65] Setälä, O., Fleming-Lehtinen, V., & Lehtiniemi, M. (2014). Ingestion and

transfer of microplastics in the planktonic food web. *Environmental pollution*, *185*, 77-83. https://doi.org/10.1016/j.envpol.2013.10.013

[66] Cole, M., Lindeque, P., Fileman, E., Halsband, C., Goodhead, R., Moger, J., & Galloway, T. S. (2013). Microplastic ingestion by zooplankton. *Environmental science & technology*, *47* (12), 6646-6655. https://pubs.acs.org/doi/abs/10.1021/es400663F

[67] Laist DW (1987) Impacts of marine debris: entanglement of marine life in marine debris including a comprehensive list of species with entanglement and ingestion records. In: Coe JM, Rogers DB (eds) Marine debris —sources, impacts and solutions. Springer, New York, pp 99–139

[68] Hanni KD, Pyle P (2000) Entanglement of pinnipeds in synthetic materials at south-east Farallon Island, California, 1976–1998. Mar Pollut Bull 40(12):1076–1081

[69] Page B, McKenzie J, McIntosh R, Baylis A, Morrissey A, Calvert N, Haase T, Berris M, Dowie D, Shaughnessy PD, Goldsworth SD (2004) Entanglement of Australian sea lions and New Zealand fur seals in lost fishing gear and other marine debris before and after government and industry attempts to reduce the problem. Mar Pollut Bull 49(1–2):33–42

[70] Bugoni L, Krause L, Petry MV (2001) Marine debris and human impacts on sea turtles in southern Brazil. Mar Pollut Bull 42(12):1330–1334

[71] Lusher, A., Hollman, P., & Mendoza-Hill, J. (2017). *Microplastics in fisheries and aquaculture: status of knowledge on their occurrence and implications for aquatic organisms and food safety*. FAO.

[72] Yang, D., Shi, H., Li, L., Li, J., Jabeen, K., & Kolandhasamy, P. (2015). Microplastic pollution in table salts from China. *Environmental science & technology*, *49*(22), 13622-13627.

[73] Liebezeit, G., & Liebezeit, E. (2013). Non-pollen particulates in honey and sugar. *Food Additives & Contaminants: Part A*, *30*(12), 2136-2140.

[74] Liebezeit, G., & Liebezeit, E. (2014). Synthetic particles as contaminants in German beers. *Food Additives & Contaminants: Part A*, *31*(9), 1574-1578.

[75] FAO. (2000). The State of the World's Fisheries and Acquaculture. *Rome: Food*.

[76] Van Cauwenberghe, L. & Janssen, C. R. (2014). Microplastics in bivalves cultured for human consumption. Environmental Pollution, 193 (0):65-70.

[77] De Witte, B., Devriese, L., Bekaert, K., Hoffman, S., Vandermeersch, G., Cooreman, K. & Robbens, J. (2014). Quality assessment of the blue mussel (*Mytilus edulis*): Comparison between commercial and wild types. Marine Pollution Bulletin, 85 (1):146-155.

[78] Leslie, H. A., van Velzen, M. J. M., Vethaak, A. D (2013) Microplastic survey of the Dutch environment. Novel data set of microplastics in North Sea sediments, treated wastewater effluents and marine biots. Amsterdam, The Netherlands: IVM Institute for Environmental Studies, Final report R-13/11.

[79] Hussain, N., V. Jaitley and A. T. Florence (2001). 'Recent advances in the understanding of uptake of microparticulates across the gastrointestinal lymphatics. Advanced Drug Delivery Reviews 50(1-2): 107-142.

[80] Berdier, C., Deleuil, J.-M. (2002). Promenade Historique dans le système

Ville-Déchet. In Botta H., Berdier C., Deleuil J.-M. (Dir), Enjeux de la propreté urbaine. Lausanne: Presses polytechniques et universitaires romandes. pp.11-16.

[81] Bras, A. (2010). Éléments pour une définition de la problématique de la propreté urbaine en Haïti: le cas de Port-au-Prince (Doctoral dissertation, thèse de doctorat, Université Quisqueya & INSA de Lyon).

[82] Bras, A., Berdier, C., Emmanuel, E., & Zimmerman, M. (2009). Problems and current practices of solid waste management in Port-au-Prince (Haiti). Waste Management, 29(11), 2907-2909. https://doi.org/10.1016/j.wasman.2009.07.015

[83] Lacour, J. (2012). Valorisation de résidus agricoles et autres déchets organiques par digestion anaérobie en Haïti (Doctoral dissertation, thèse de doctorat, Université Quisqueya & INSA de Lyon).

[84] Bras A. et Lacour J. Gestion des déchets solides à Port-au-Prince. Conjonction, 2009, vol., n° 221-222, pp. 79-96.

[85] Diez, S. M., Patil, P. G., Morton, J., Rodriguez, D. J., Vanzella, A., Robin, D., ... & Corbin, C. (2019). Marine Pollution in the Caribbean: Not a Minute to Waste (No. 135647, pp. 1-102). The World Bank.

[86] Popescu, R., Durand, M., & d'Ercole, R. (2014). La gestion des déchets post-catastrophe à Port-au-Prince: entre relégation et proximité. EchoGéo, (30).

[87] Ngo, C., Regent, A., (2008). Déchets, effluents et pollution, impacts sur l'environnement et la santé. Paris, Dunod, 178 p.

[88] Adams, S.M. and Greeley, M.S. (2000). Ecotoxicological indicators of water quality using multi-response indicators to assess the health of aquatic ecosystems. Water, Air and Soil Pollution 123:103-115.

[89] Emmanuel E., Lacour J., Balthazard-Accou K., & Joseph O. (2009a). Ecological hazards assessment of heavy metals and nutrients containing in urban effluents on bay ecosystems of Port-au-Prince (Haiti). AQUA-LAC. Journal of the International Hydrological Programme for Latin America and Caribbean, UNESCO, 1, 1.

[90] Emmanuel, E., Balthazard-Accou, K., & Joseph, O. (2009b). Impact of urban wastewater on biodiversity of aquatic ecosystems. Environmental Management, Sustainable Development and Human Health. In: Laboy-Nieves EN, Schaffner FC, Abdelhadi AH and Goosen MFA, editors. Environmental Management, Sustainable Development and Human Health. Taylor and Francis Group, London UK, 399-422.

Chapter 12

A Review of Alternative Marine Fuels

Şevket Süleyman İrtem

Abstract

Today, ships navigating all around the world are not allowed to emit SO_x more than 0.5%. Same regulation for nitrogen has already come into force. More and more nations are becoming aware and concerned about the negative effects of climate change, whereas many countries are already feeling the effects of harmful greenhouse gas emissions. Therefore, the world's fleet needs a new fuel types, which are alternative to conventional petroleum-based ship fuels. Benefits such as low sulphur standards accompany all alternative fuel options. As will be discussed further in Section 2, there are challenges and limitations associated with CO_2 emissions along with benefits. The review of the literature and field shows that the impact of these current choices on the management and environments is still not bright enough, although each alternative has consisted entirely different effects in their body and each alternative pose specific risks to the environment, crew, management and port states. This chapter gives a review on the impact of each alternative fuels on the environment. In addition, the chapter touches upon handling of risks associated with alternative fuels and technologies.

Keywords: Global Warming, Alternative fuels, Shipping, Emissions, LNG, HFO, Methanol, Greener Shipping

1. Introduction

An ocean-going vessel has been thought of as a critical factor in the transportation of the goods all around the world throughout the history. As a political goal of the regions, the financial growth has been maintained since the industrial revolution. However, these rapid changes are having a severe effect on the environment. The consumption of the combustible and flammable elements has significantly accelerated with the increase in international trade. Air pollution and its impact on the environment have been a subject of research since the 1850s. Emission from factories and transportation vessels is a significant area of interest within the field of climate. In the new global economy, the environment has become a central issue for human health. Previous studies have reported that the leading cause of some of diseases is industrialization and transportation. For example, respiratory tract diseases such as asthma, trachea, bronchioles, alveoli, pleura, apnea are increasingly recognized as a serious, worldwide public health concern [1]. Alternatives to current oils are becoming an instrument in the transportation sector. Recent evidence suggests that it is required an alteration from fuel oil to Liquefied Natural Gas (LNG) or Methanol due to the limited sources and the adverse effects of the emissions on the human health and environment [2]. Investigating zero emission is a continuing concern within environmental science. The sections below provide an understanding of each alternative fuels such as a LNG, a Liquefied Petroleum Gas (LPG), a methanol, a Heavy Fuel Oil (HFO) with scrubber technology based on the literature and Authors' technical visits some shipping companies.

2. Liquified Natural Gas (LNG)

In the management booklet of TarnTank, the significant information about LNG has been given. The information was given in the manual are listed below [3]:

LNG consists of methane (CH_4) and other substances. It's form can be changed by cooling down to −162°C at atmospheric pressure. By converting the gas form into the liquid form, the volume is reduced 600 times compare to gas form. This reduction makes it easier to transport and store. Typically, LNG tanks contain three times the capacity of an equivalent volume of heavy fuel oil. LNG also contains small quantities of nitrogen, ethane, propane, butane, and some other trace components, with the proportions varying according to the source of the LNG and how long it has been ageing. Cryogenic hazards could occur due to LNG, since it has a low temperature. Natural gas has a flammability range of between about 5% and 15% by volume when mixed with air. As an example, −187°C is a flashpoint. 530°C is autoignition degree means that natural gas is not readily ignited by hot surfaces – unlike marine gas and fuel oil, which can be readily ignited by hot surfaces such as unlagged exhaust systems, a primary cause of engine room fires. After the operations, some LNG can be trapped in the transfer line. If this amount meets with heat ingress, some local pressures can occur, and this high coefficient of volumetric expansion can cause pipe bursts as shown in **Figure 1**. This burst leads to the release of natural gas.

70 Bar (g) is the critical limit for the pipe structure. After one hour of the line, pressure reached 70 Bar, rupture of the pipework or equipment is highly likely. "Thermal relief valves" are being used to maintain release trapped gas or liquid. The first LNG fuel oil ship started to operate in 2000. Statistics dated first March 2018 showed that the number of LNG powered vessels reached to 121 whereas 127 new ship started to be built by shipyards [4]. In general, in a new ship construction, the highest cost of the investment belongs to engine compartments. Engines need to be modified or wholly renewed according to the fuel oils planning to be used onboard

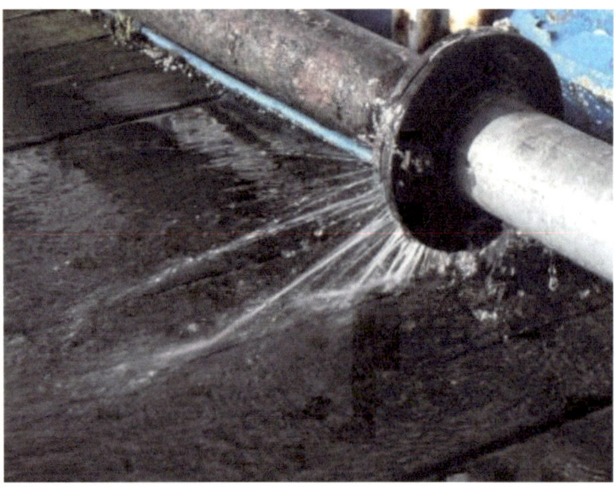

Figure 1.
Pipe burst due to the high coefficient of volumetric expansion.

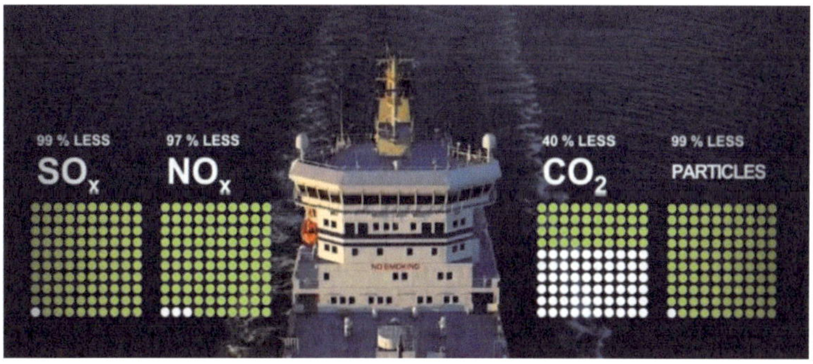

Figure 2.
Emission Decrements.

the vessels. A few former companies find the solution to use the hybrid fuel-powered engine. For instance, the MT TarnTank, which is LNG powered vessel, fuel gas supply system is designed for both the gas-fuelled engine and conventional type fuel engine. LNG powered engines are one of the most widely used groups of alternative fuel oil engines in Nordic countries. As the emissions shown in **Figure 2**., liquefied natural gas is very clean source. The releasing of SO_x is %99, NO_x %97 less than heavy fuel oils whereas CO_2 emission is high.

The energy density of liquefied natural gas is higher than heavy fuel oil. Despite its environment-friendly and efficacy, ship-owners suffer from several significant drawbacks: time loss to invest, spare parts, bunker supply, cost, educated crew to run this engine. By the help of IMO's regulations checklist shows the proper way for the bunkering operations of LNG. The main questions in the TarnTank Company checklist are about [3]; communication between the regulating authority, bunker deliverer and receiving vessel about safety and emergency response plans. Risk assessment forms are filled and discussed by each side, physical situation of the manifolds must be in operational range, LNG transfer profile (ratio/time) and vapour management schedule has been agreed upon, the receiving tank volume and temperature before bunkering must be within acceptable limits, temperature, pressure, methane number properties of the LNG must be acceptable, handling trapped volumes after an Emergency shutdown system for LNG bunkering – Electrostatic discharge (ESD) must be agreed upon, freeboards and the tidal and operational effects of the draft must be agreed, the ship must be ready for any shifting because of weather conditions, wavelength, wave height, wind speed, lightning is another critical point, the ships or other obstacles are essential in the Swinging Circle, cryogenic protection systems such as water curtains and insulated hose saddles must be compatible?, Safety zone should be established, Ship-Shore Connection box must be checked and ready to use. In the booklet, they call it as "Grounding and hose connection - a grounding cable from ship to quay must be connected and followed by bunker hose connection.", visual check must be done, stripping and purging, hoses must be drained before disconnection, disconnection of hoses and grounding.

3. Heavy Fuel Oil (HFO)

After the decisions of IMO, the debates and preparations for the new world combustion system had already started for decades. The industry intends to make investment decisions by the lights of the expert's predictions, but the experts do not have any specific clue about the future. Since ships were operating around the world, thus exploitation of the resources has been continuing making the prices of oil increase. However, what happened in 2015? The prices of oil fall dramatically from 120 USD/ton to 30 USD/ton against the market predictions [5]. In 2018, it was raising to 100USD/ton again, and the predictions were to reach 400 USD/ton. However, the other experts are expecting that the prices are going to fall again since the consumption of oil is decreasing.

The price of HFO is directly affected by the ship's operational costs since an average Panama Size ship consumes 24 ton in a voyage day. So, for the shipowners who are entirely in debt to banks with loans, this kind of investments are critically important. One prediction for the future is evident that half of the today's ship owners are going to bankrupt after 2020. HFO is still an option when the ship-owners and operators are concerned about the price increase and availability of complaint fuels but to be an alternative. HFO price graph is given in **Figure 3**. Scrubber technology makes HFO reasonable for managements which is installed by shipyards. To install this unit shown in **Figure 4**, significant investments must be paid [6]. An average Handymax ships conversion cost calculated as 6 million USD.

Current operational expenses such as sludge handlings, chemical consumables will go up by increased power consumption. In **Figure 5** the types of the scrubber technologies can be seen.

This scrubber technology, which is shown in **Figures 4** and **5**, can be adapted to new building vessels as well as currently navigating vessels.

In MS Fryken, a scrubber laboratory is carrying out experiments for Chalmers University. Obtained test results indicated so far that the scrubber technology has a potential to meet both 0.5% and 0.1% emission regulations. In **Figure 6**, we can see a closed-loop scrubber system. If in an open-loop system, the sea water is used to

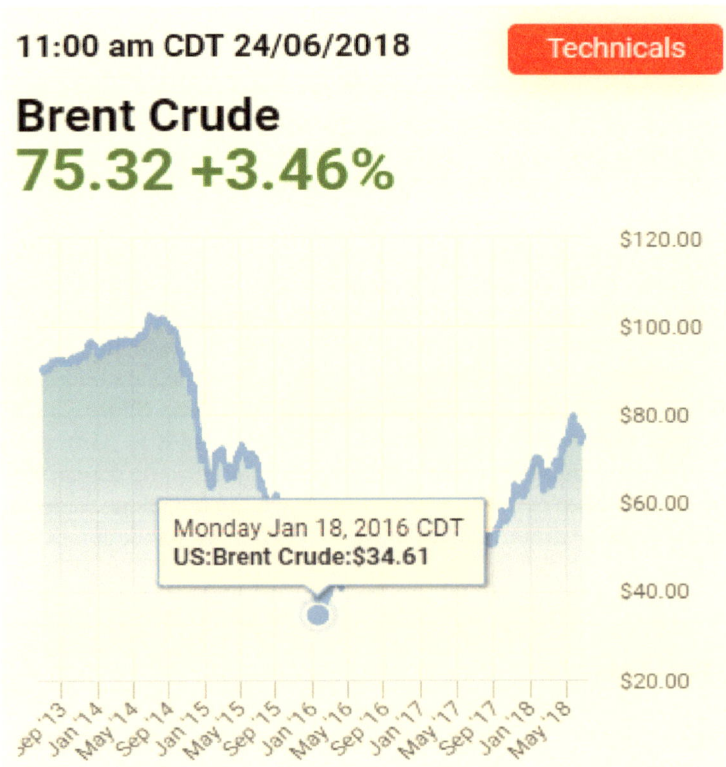

Figure 3.
Fuel Oil Prices last 15 years [5].

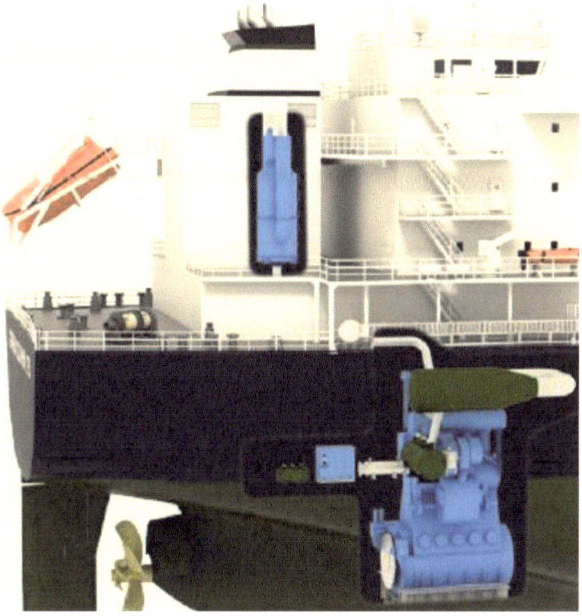

Figure 4.
Scrubber Unit [6].

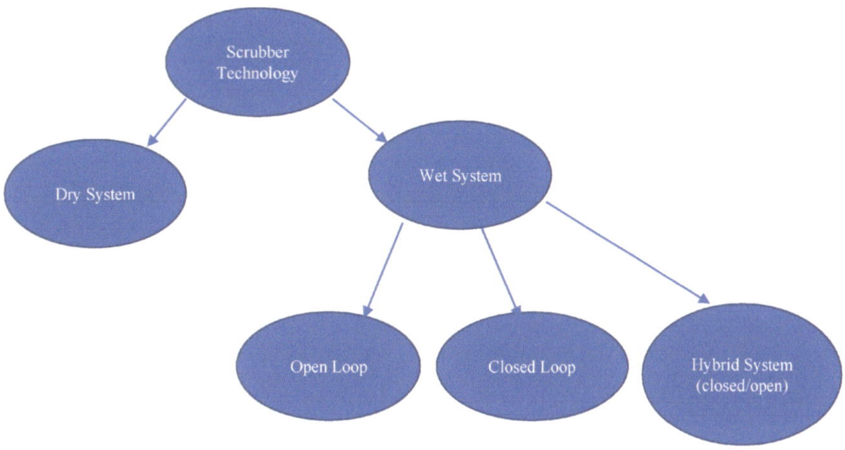

Figure 5.
Scrubber technology types.

wash out the SO_x in the exhaust, then in the closed-loop system uses chemicals such as caustic soda [8]. Closed loop scrubbers are installed on ships which are sailing in freshwaters [6].

In the open loop system, the used seawater discharge back to the sea. Discharging to the water in some locations is prohibited according to the MARPOL. Since the other ports will force the same regulations in the next years, a hybrid type of scrubbers is most likely to be used in many ships.

Current fuel type HFO has an extensive distribution network, and the engineers onboard are familiar with handling and operating the current fuel oil. The technical departments of the shipping companies work as an advisory team and technical problems in an average aged ship happen quite often. This advisory team is familiar with HFO and they can respond to any problems very promtly. Primarily by the

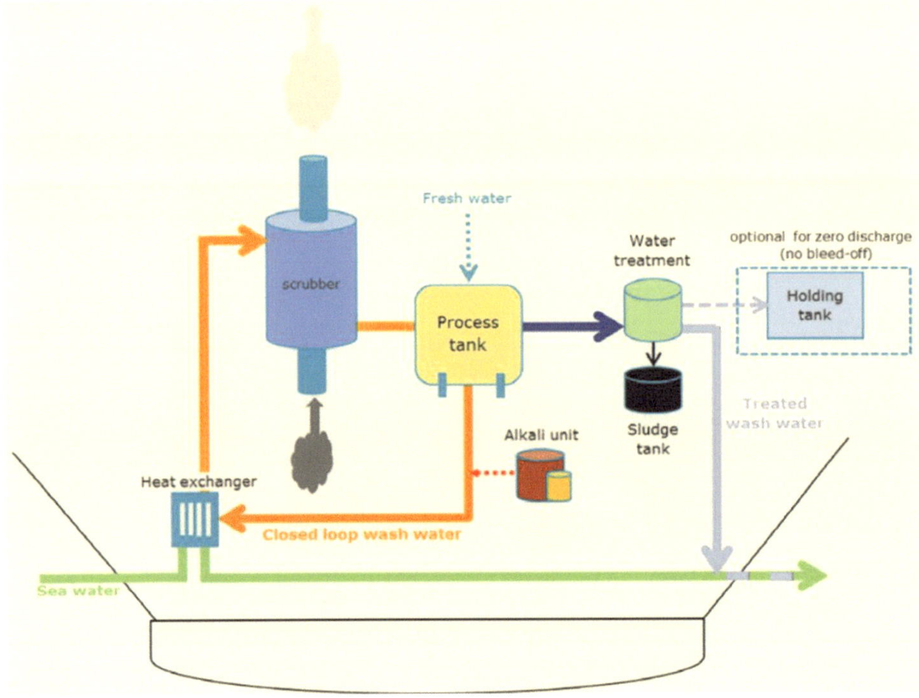

Figure 6.
Closed-Loop Scrubber [7].

influence of the technical department which consist of chief engineers, the shipping companies will insist on using HFO until it will disappear from the market. This prediction shows that the ships yards are going to be entirely busy with handling scrubber installations to meet the rising demand for scrubber technology.

Related to the safety domain, current HFO has its own risk inside. Currently, most of the ships in the market are using HFO and MGO as consumption. During the voyage in open seas, the engines use HFO, in the ports the generator runs by MGO, in the Sulphur Emission Control Area (SECA) areas they run with LSFO. Since the operating temperature is different (for example MGO is usually operated at 35C, and HFO is mostly at 135C), the risk of thermal shocks is highly possible during the oil change over. This shock may damage the structure of the pipeline and fuel systems [9].

4. Methanol

Methanol (CH_3OH) is the purest alcohol, consisting of a methyl group (CH_3) linked with a hydroxy group (OH). It boils at 65°C and solidifies at -94°C [10]. It has no colour and has an odour that is similar to ethyl alcohol. It consists of low carbon and high hydrogen contents. Methanol is the primary material of the derivatives of which is used to produce various compounds for daily living needs. For example, in building materials, perfumes, plastic bags, pharmaceuticals, paints, coatings. It is produced by natural gas, coal, biomass, bio-reshaping. Methanol can also be produced through gasification of coal and a cheap method with the widely available resource. The design and processing conditions may vary depending on the composition of the coal used as a feedstock. Methanol produced from coal has twice as high GHG (Green House Gas) as from natural gas. It can also be produced from virtually all biomass such as wood, algae, municipal and agricultural waste through gasification. As an example, black liquor from pulp industry can be gasified and used for methanol synthesis. The chemicals are recovered and reused. A plant at the Smurfit Kappa paper mill in Piteå, Sweden started to produce dimethyl ether in 2010. Diesel engines can be operated by dimethyl alcohol. With a volume of methanol, it is easy to reached the same energy level with 2,5 times larger volume of fuel oil. The flash point is low (11°C, 12°C) and guidelines are currently in the draft for incorporation into the International Maritime Organization's recently adopted International Code of Safety for Ships Using Gases or Other Low-Flashpoint Fuels (IGF Code). The risk and safety analysis carried out for the SPIRETH Project (Alcohol Spirits and Ethers as Marine Fuel), which was co-coordinated by SSPA and ScandiNAOS and tested methanol and DME as ship fuels, contributed to the development of the IGF code [11]. Pilot Methanol was initiated by JIP 6–7 to prove and showcase that methanol is an innovative, safe, and sustainable fuel for shipping. EU project aims to demonstrate methanol as a cost-effective, clean, and comfortable fuel alternative with an easy infrastructure implementation [12]. The Zero Vision Tool (ZVT) platform was focusing on the research of methanol usage, converting the MF Stena Germanica to be capable of running on methanol fuel, It is possible that more ships in the Stena Line Fleet would be converted to methanol ships to be operated in the Baltic and the North Sea.

5. Research results

HFO with scrubber, LNG and Methanol are the most excellent alternatives for the transformation of the industry. These three options are compared in the **Table 1**. According to todays and future expectations of price, infrastructure, regulation, availability, environmental impact, technology, capital and operational expenditures [13].

The technology used in the maritime industry has been bringing innovation to maintain safety and efficiency [14]. By this development, the data transfer between ship and shore became more available. More information onboard the vessels would help us to establish a higher degree of accuracy models.

Some machine learning tools were tested with real sample data from a ship which navigated from Norfolk to El Dekheila. The sample data used in the calculations are presented in **Table 5**.

In the pre-processing term for data cleaning, the columns "average speed, wind force, RPM, slip, swell" were selected to prevent overfittings of algorithms. Consequently, data science algorithms suit very well with these current sample data.

CRISP-DM "Cross-industry standard process for data mining" methodology which is given in **Figure 7** is one of the most common data science methodology [16]. When the procedure applied according to the CRISP-DM figure with the sample data, the model learned and predicted the columns successfully.

This model is based on correlations. Isabelle et al. (2013), draw our attention to the differences between correlation and causality, and difficulties of "Cause and Effect Experiment" [17].

By analysing data collected continuous data from onboard, it is possible to find causes of the events and prevent disasters as well as preventing climate changes, economic changes, epidemics, cancer. Ships are real-life laboratories for this methodology. Besides this, it proposes an evaluation methodology to take the right decision for company perspective.

Qualitative methods are mainly basing on expert's experience. However, when it comes to alternative fuel oils, the industry has not got enough experiences yet. We can say that; these qualitative methods are suitable for pre-AI shipping industry

	HFO- Scrubber	LNG	Methanol
Price	The price is expected to drop significantly due to low global demand.	The price level is competitive. With MGO and expected to be competitive with low-sulphur HFO. It is predicted that the competitiveness of LNG with scrubber high-sulphur HFO is also possible.	Since methanol is produced mainly from natural gas, its price is dependent on natural gas prices. The price of methanol can be lower in case of production from coal. However, the latter may have an adverse effect such as increased Green House Gas emissions. The production costs of methanol from hydrogen and CO_2 are higher than the costs of methanol synthesis methane.
Infrastructure	Well-developed infrastructure. It is uncertain whether in the future bunker suppliers will still be available at all geographical locations.	LNG in principle is available worldwide, and investments are underway to make LNG available to ships. LNG bunkering vessels, bunker truck and permanent bunker depot will continue to grow.	Truck or bunker vessels can accomplish the supply of methanol to ships. Stena Lines has developed a dedicated bunkering area in the port of Goteborg which includes a safety barrier to avoid problems associated with methanol leakage.
Regulation	The IMO MEPC limited the sulphur content of ship fuels to 0.5% worldwide and 0.1% in sulphur emission-controlled area. However, it is permissible to continue burning HFO and use scrubbers to clean the exhaust gas to achieve an equivalent level of sulphur emissions.	The IMO IGF came into force for the design and construction of LNG fuelled ships. Bunkering LNG fuelled ships are subject to national regulations. Some ports have established local rules for bunkering. Organisations such as ISO, IASC, SGMF developed requirements and guidelines for LNG bunkering.	The chapter for methanol in the IGF Code which is for all gas and other low flash point fuel ships is currently under development. Some other projects (i.e. SEDNA) are running to establish guidance for three bunkering processes; Truck to Ship, Shore to Ship and Ship to Ship. Also, class companies such as DNV GL has released rules for low flash point fuels that also includes methanol.
Availability	Available.	The production capacities of LNG have no limitations and are expected to increase.	In 2016 the global methanol demand was around 80 million tonnes.
Environmental Impact	Oil-based ship fuel has a more significant environmental effect than alternative fuels. The sulphur content, particle emissions, NO_x, CO_2 of even low sulphur ship fuels is much higher than of alternatives.	Natural gas from LNG is the cleanest fossil fuel available today. There are almost no SO_x emissions to it; particle emissions are very low, the NO_x emissions are lower than those of Marine Gas Oil (MGO) or Heavy Fuel Oil (HFO). Methane release must be considered.	With clean-burning methanol qualities as a marine fuel, methanol can reduce emissions of sulphur oxide by 99%, nitrogen oxide by up to 60%, particulate matter by 95%.

	HFO- Scrubber	LNG	Methanol
Technology	Scrubber technology is readily available to clean exhaust gases of oil-based ship fuels. In addition to scrubbers, selective catalytic reduction and exhaust gas system will be required to comply with NO_x emission limits.	Gas engines, gas turbines, LNG storage and processing systems have been available for land installations for decades. All above necessary process equipment are also commercially available.	There are two main engine options for the methanol-powered vessel: two-stroke diesel-cycle engine and four-stroke lean-burn Otto-cycle engine. The only single two-stroke diesel engine is currently commercially available.
CAPEX	The investment costs for scrubbers' range between \$650/kW (5000 kW engine) and \$100–\$150/kW (40,000 kW and larger engines)	The CAPEX is decreasing, as LNG technology is developing quite rapidly and the competition between suppliers is increasing. Compared to scrubber system with HFO the CAPEX cost for LNG is and continue to be higher.	The cost for installation of methanol systems onboards the vessels (e.g. internal combustion engine, fuel tanks, piping) is three times cheaper than the costs associated with LNG systems. No need for cryogenic temperatures and pressurized fuel tanks as in LNG.
OPEX	The operational costs of scrubbers are composed of the cost of maintenance and energy consumption (pumps, scrubbing unit to remove the SO_x from exhaust gases).	The OPEX cost for LNG systems onboard ships are almost the same as for conventionally fuelled system. However, the maintenance of gas burning engine in case of LNG used may be less expensive owing to its cleanliness.	The cost of OPEX is expected to be similar to that of oil-fuelled systems without scrubber technology. Also, the benefit can be gained, since some ports offer discounts to alternative fuelled ships.

Table 1.
Comparison of HFO - LNG- Methanol.

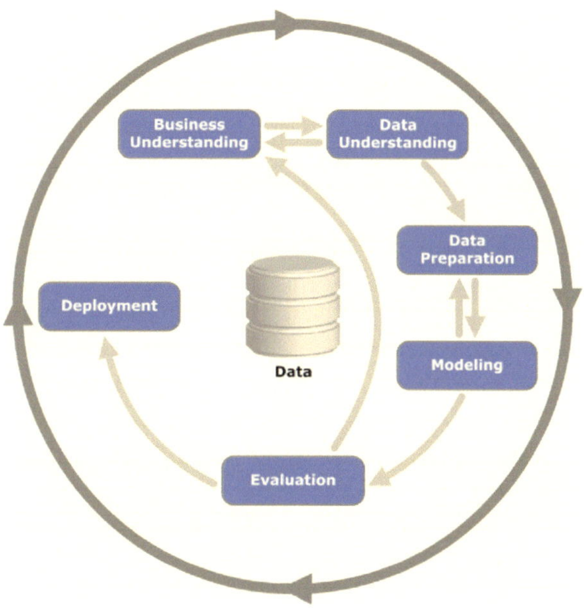

Figure 7.
CRISP-DM Process [15].

conditions. Today the shipping industry is living its technological age. The most significant benefit of this age is "being available of data transfers from ship to shore". With these advantages, we are going to find the opportunity to develop autonomous ships.

While the shipping industry is talking about autonomous ships, the rest of the industry has already started to use robots and artificial intelligence in the industrial activities. However, before the autonomous ships get into forced, we should find answers to these questions:

- Is it possible to collect any data for data mining application onboard the vessels?
- What can we use this data for?
- Is it possible to use these data to evaluate the risks of each type of oil?
- Is it possible to teach a machine by supplying the flowing data?
- Is it possible to develop a machine learning system which prevents accidents by prediction?
- We learn that to set a laboratory for "Cause and Effect Studies" is costly and has many other problems. How about onboard the ships?

In the current study, an empiric data mining and machine learning was applied to the real sample data from a vessel which is given in **Tables 2** and **3**.

Av. Speed	Wind Force	RPM	Slip	Swells
13.52	4	105.00	10.8	E
13.2696	6	104.80	12.3	E
13.4958	6	105.20	11.09	E
12.8652	5	106.50	14.69	W
12.75	6	107.56	17.85	W
13.0087	5	107.75	16.34	W
12.7958	7	107.88	17.82	W
12.2167	6	108.07	19.42	W
12.5609	6	107.55	19.07	W
13.1583	5	106.57	14.45	W
13.3042	3	105.21	14.00	W
13.4261	4	105.02	13.04	E
13.8917	4	106.19	9.38	E
13.3652	4	105.35	13.72	E
13.3792	1	105.35	12.84	E
13.3957	5	105.28	13.46	E
13.7125	4	105.43	12.38	E

Table 2.
*Extracted Voyage Data From **Table** 5.*

Correct classified: 2	Wrong classified: 4
Accuracy: 33,333%	Error: 66,667%
Cohen's kappa (κ) 0,2	

Table 3.
Accuracy rate.

When we look at the literature on data science methodology, we come across with different kind of analytics. Autonomous ships must use descriptive analytics that recognise the data, predict the data based on the description, then prescript the data and take action according to the traffic congestion found and predict the current condition from the history of the data. Prescriptive Analytic uses the results of the descriptive and predictive analytics. While descriptive analytics are evaluating the current data, Prescriptive Analytics examine the data and gives suggestion and takes the actions without a human. All the prescriptive systems are managed and run by machine without a human.

As an empirical application, the author used the data given in **Table 5** in order to predict the data shown in **Table 4**. The data in **Table 5** represents the real ship data collected from a voyage between Port of Norfolk to Port of El Dekheila during authors previous work experience with a largest shipping company in Turkey.

After performing following six-steps, the data presented in **Table 3** was achieved.

1. Excel reader

2. Statistics

3. Scatter Plot

4. Partitioning

5. Decision Tree Learner

6. Decision Tree Predictor Scorer

With the scorer node, the author checked the accuracy of the learner by prediction results.

Depending on the data's properties, the accuracy rate has been changing. In this data sets, the learner can predict the results with %33 accuracy. Healthier data and different partitioning tools can decrease this rate.

As we understand from the tree in **Figure 8** when the swell direction is from "N or north", the slip is going to be more than %14,5 which means that the consumption of the fuel oil and greenhouse gas emissions are going to increase.

By the help of this simple prediction model, the company can easily predict the engine slips from the up-to-date data getting from the ships. The distance of the

Row ID	RPM	Av. Sp	Wind F	Predicted slips
Row0	100	12	2	16.477
Row1	110	14	3	11.833
Row2	120	13	4	26.531

Table 4.
Predicted Slips.

DATE	NOON POSITION		SEA MILE	VOY TIME Steam	AV SP	REST DIST	COURE	WIND		SWELL	SEA		TEMP	SEA TEMP	RPM	slip %	TIME ZONE	DAILY FUEL OIL CONSUMPTION			REST OIL			ENGINE DISTANCE	FRESH WATER		
	LAT	LON	Nm.	h.m	Knt	Nm.		DIR	FORCE	DIR&FOR	DIR	FORCE						IFO	MDO	L/O	oil1	oil2	oil3		REST	Eva	CONSUMP
5/31/2013	**COSP 1600 LT**					**5269.4**											GMT-4	**1293.2**	**130.1**	**55560**	**14600**	**39560**	**1400**		**380**		
01.06.2013	36 04N	070 42 W	270.40	20.00	13.52	4999.00	067	SW-6	4	E-2M	E	3	22	21	105.00	10.76	GMT-4	31.2	1.5	**250**	14600	39310	1400	303.0	370	0	10.00
02.06.2013	38 48 N	064 19 W	305.20	23.00	13.27	4693.80	090	WSW - 2	6	SE-3M	E	5	23	18	104.80	12.30	GMT-3	35.0	1.7	**295**	14600	39015	1400	348.0	372	19.1	17.10
03.06.2013	38 48 N	057 23 W	323.90	24.00	13.50	4369.90	090	WSW - 2	6	SE-2M	SE	5	25	23	105.20	11.09	GMT-3	36.5	1.8	**310**	14600	38705	1400	364.3	384	22	10.00
04.06.2013	38 48 N	051 03 W	295.90	23.00	12.87	4074.00	090	ENE-8	5	W-2M	NW	4	18	20	106.50	14.69	GMT-2	35.0	1.7	**295**	14600	38410	1400	346.8	390	23	17.00
05.06.2013	37 50 N	044 43 W	306.00	24.00	12.75	3768.00	103	ENE-8	6	WNW-2/ 3M	WNW	5	19	20	107.56	17.85	GMT-2	36.5	1.8	**315**	14600	38095	1400	372.5	400	20	10.00
06.06.2013	36 40 N	038 39 W	299.20	23.00	13.01	3468.80	103	NE-8	5	W-2/3M	W	5	20	21	107.75	16.34	GMT-1	35.0	1.7	**305**	14600	37790	1400	357.7	416	20	4.00
07.06.2013	35 29 N	032 31 W	307.10	24.00	12.80	3161.70	103	NNE-6	7	W-3M	W	6	18	20	107.88	17.82	GMT-1	36.5	1.8	**315**	14600	37475	1400	373.7	427	21	10.00
08.06.2013	34 17 N	026 56 W	293.20	24.00	12.22	2868.50	085	NE-6	6	W-4/5M	W	5	23	20	108.07	19.42	GMT-1	36.5	1.8	**308**	14600	37167	1400	363.8	440	20	7.00
09.06.2013	34 44 N	021 07 W	288.90	23.00	12.56	2579.60	085	NNE-6	6	WNW- 2/3 M	NW	5	23	20	107.55	19.07	GMT 0	35.0	1.7	**300**	14600	36867	1400	357.0	456	19	3.00
10.06.2013	35 14 N	014 45 W	315.80	24.00	13.16	2263.80	085	NNE	5	NNW - 1M	NW	4	21	20	106.57	14.45	GMT 0	36.5	1.8	**312**	14600	36555	1400	369.1	460	21	17.00
11.06.2013	35 44 N	008 20 W	319.30	24.00	13.30	1944.50	085	NNW-6	3	WNW-1M	WNW	2	20	20	105.21	14.00	GMT 0	36.5	1.8	**313**	14600	36242	1400	371.3	460	20	20.00
12.06.2013	36 23 N	002 00 W	308.80	23.00	13.43	1635.70	081	W-5	4	E - 0.5M	E	3	22	21	105.02	13.04	GMT 1	35.0	1.7	**298**	14600	35944	1400	355.1	450	4	14.00
13.06.2013	37 05 N	004 51 E	333.40	24.00	13.89	1302.30	086	SW - 4	4	E-1M	E	4	25	22	106.19	9.38	GMT 1	36.5	1.8	**311**	14600	35633	1400	367.9	431	0	19.00
14.06.2013	37 08 N	011 10 E	307.40	23.00	13.37	994.90	109	E-8	4	E-1M	E	3	24	22	105.35	13.72	GMT 2	35.0	1.7	**298**	14600	35335	1400	356.3	424	0	7.00
15.06.2013	35 14 N	017 23 E	321.10	24.00	13.38	673.80	111	CALM	CALM	E-1M	E	CALM	25	22	105.35	12.84	GMT 2	36.5	1.8	**310**	14600	35025	1400	368.4	414	0	10.00

DATE	NOON POSITION		SEA MILE	VOY TIME	AV SP	REST DIST	COURE	WIND		SWELL	SEA		TEMP	SEA TEMP	RPM	slip %	TIME ZONE	DAILY FUEL OIL CONSUMPTION			REST OIL			ENGINE DISTANCE	FRESH WATER		
				Steam																							
	LAT	LON	Nm.	h.m	Knt	Nm.		DIR	FORCE	DIR&FOR	DIR	FORCE						IFO	MDO	L/O	oil1	oil2	oil3		REST	Eva	CONSUMP
16.06.2013	33 30 N	023 10 E	308.10	23.00	13.40	365.70	111	NW-6	5	E-1M	E	4	28	23	105.28	13.46	GMT 3	35.0	1.7	**299**	14600	34726	1400	356.0	405	0	9.00
17.06.2013	31 25 N	029 12 E	329.10	24.00	13.71	36.60	111	NW-6	4	E-1M	E	3	26.5	23	105.43	12.38	GMT 3	36.5	1.8	**316**	14600	34410	1400	375.6	393	0	12.00
TOTAL VALUE			5232.80	397.00	13.18	36.60									106.16	14.27		604.70	29.60	5150				6106.5		209.10	196.10
																		688.50	100.500	50410.0				359.2		12.30	11.54
																		36.56	1.79	311.34							

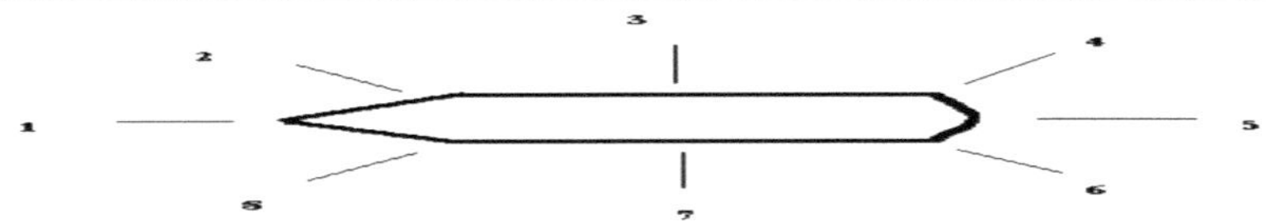

Table 5.
Navigation Data from Norfolk to El Dekheila.

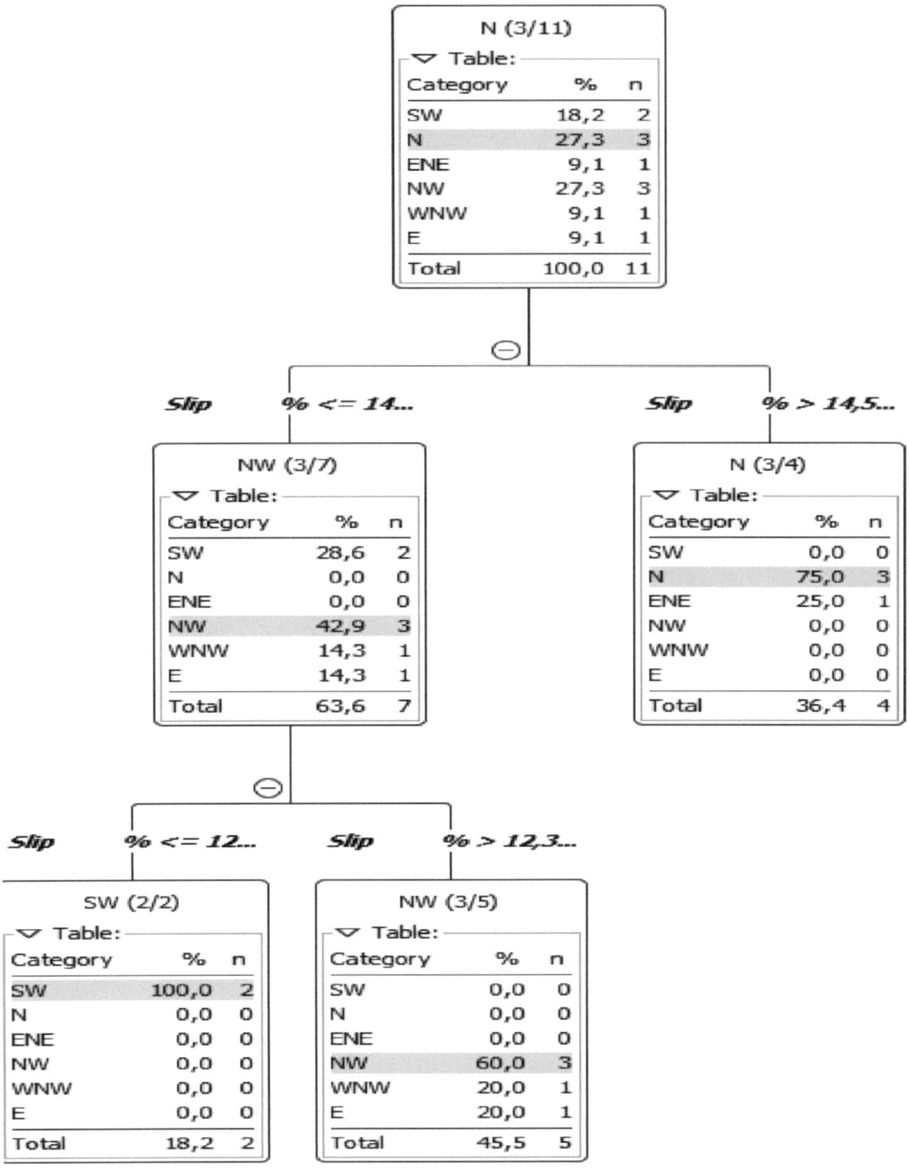

Figure 8.
Decision Tree Results.

ship movement by one complete rotation of the propeller or the propeller pitch is calculated by shipyard and written in the "ship's manual". Engine distance is calculated by multiplying the propeller pitch to propeller distances. For a certain time period the ship movement distance can be calculated by engine distance. But in reality, engine distance can vary due to weather conditions such as wind, current and swells directions, fouling on the ship's hull, etc. Therefore, the observed distance might be less or more than engine distance.

Slip is a rate of the difference between the engine distance and observed distance. The simple formulation showed below:

$$\text{Slip} = 100 \times \frac{\text{Engine Distance} - \text{Observed Distance}}{\text{Engine Distance}} \qquad (1)$$

If this machine learning model can be fed by long term data, the engine performance under the same sea conditions can be predicted. In **Table 4**, the actual slip rates predicted by the model. The daily slip, from the noon reports which is daily given by ship captain, can be compared with the actual slip. In that way, by comparing the daily slip with actual slip, potential problems associated with ship performance could be spotted. Since there is not enough chief engineers who have experiences with alternative fuel powered vessels, this kind of machine learning algorithms is going to accelerate the experience accumulation in the technical department of the companies. Shipping market could be ready for an engine evolution, but the industry has not enough well-experienced engineers for this conversion.

If we can use the algorithms efficiently and feed the machine learning by real ship data, the developing models can be trained and after be used to give predictions and suggestion in a short time as well as well-experienced engineers working at ocean-going vessels. By intensive use of algorithms, the market can close the gap of the well-experienced engineers on alternative fuel powered engine.

Table 6 was generated to demonstrate what kind of element can affect the bunkering operations. From the study visit to industry, some parameters were found. During the fuel transfer, there are many parameters which can affect the soundness of the operation;

- Illumination of the work area
- Sea condition
- Wind Force
- Tank pressure of
    - Ship Tank
    - Bunker Tank
    - Line
    - Manifold
- Density
- Temperature of
    - Weather
    - Ship Tank
    - Bunker Tank
    - Line
    - Manifold
- Capacity
    - Ship tank
    - Bunker tank (rest)

Sea Condition	Work day of assigned Crew	Wind Force	Illumination	Ship Tank Temperature °C	Ship Tank Pressure MPa (abs)	Density t/m3	Bunker Tank Temperature °C	Bunker Tank Pressure bar (abs)	Ship tank available (rest) capacity	Bunker Tank rest capacity	Rest M3/ 315 M3 capacity *100	Line Pressure MPa (abs)	Line Temperature °C	The temperature at manifold ° C	The pressure at the manifold bar (rel)	Transfer rate M3 (per hour)	Leakage
6		4	enough		0.1												Y
2		2	not enough	−187.0	0.4		−187.0						−187.0	−187.0			N
6		6			0.48												Y
3		2		−163	0.5												N
6		6		−162.5								7.00					
5		5															
7		7			0.75												
6		6															
6		6		530.00			530.00						530.00	530.00			
5		5															
3		3				0.5											
4		4															
4		4															
4		4															
1		1															
5		5															
4		4															

Table 6.
ML Alternative Fuel Powered Vessels Data Table for ML Applications.

- Transfer rate per hour
- Working day of the assigned crew since embarked onboard

These parameters are dynamic and thus frequently change due to inherent nature of the water. During the bunkering, assigned personnel observes the changes. Here, we should bear in mind the associated human errors. **Table 6** presents mentioned above main parameters that affect the bunkering operations.

By the use of ML algorithms, the shipping industry can learn about alternative fuels more and more in the future, and the **Table 6** is most likely to expand with new columns.

6. Conclusions

Notably, the sulphur limit for automotive diesel is much lower than that for ship fuel. Across Europe, it is at 0,001%, 100 to 500 times below the 2020 limit for shipping. Therefore, it is most likely that the shipping industry will still be under scrutiny regarding the sulphur limits in marine fuels. The International Maritime Organization (IMO) has already taken steps to limit the sulphur content of ship fuels to 0.5% worldwide from 1st January 2020. The IMO has recently adopted an ambitious target to reduce GHG emission by 50% or from 940 mton (in 2008) to 470 mton (in 2050). This will serve as a driving force in introducing a broader range of environmentally friendly fuels, propulsion solutions and energy efficiency measures. This study has reviewed selected alternative ship fuels such as LNG, methanol and compared these fuels against heavy fuels oil with scrubbers in **Table 1** in terms of risks, price, infrastructure, regulations, availability of fuels, their environmental impacts, technologies required, capital expenditure (CAPEX), Operational expenditure (OPEX).

According to available research and information, LNG is the cleanest of fossil fuels which can satisfy the demand of shipping industry for years to come. However, it is not totally carbon free. For example, the release of unburned methane (so-called methane slip) could reduce the benefit of LNG over HFO. The prices of LNG on the market are comparable to the process of HFO. The price of methanol production also depends on which type of resource (e.g. natural gas, coal, biomass) is used as a feedstock. However, the prices of methanol are higher when compared to LNG and HFO. Although this methanol is gaining interest in the market because of its sulphur free and it, therefore, has the potential to meet the current 0.1% SO_x emission in the Control Area requirements. Safety requirements for methanol as low flash point fuel must be followed according to existing rules, eg. IGF Code, which is still being expanded and developed by the IMO.

Being critical can also mean looking for reasons why we should not just accept big risk prediction as being binominal. By generating a prediction model which is fed by all aspects that leads to unwanted results such as fuel leakage, grounding, fire etc. a pre-notification system can be developed as in **Figure 9**. To establishing the similar model to the bunkering operations of alternative fuel oils, **Table 6** was generated. When we investigate the result of intended model what we are going to predict is binominal which means this model predicts the existence of leakage by answering “yes or no”. However, it is highly possible that the methodology of the model can be extended toward answers which give possibility. By adding the possibility to the answers, the results are going to be more meaningful.

The wellness of the crew onboard is also another critical issue. Today’s shipping industry is on the way to autonomous, and most of the inventions brought

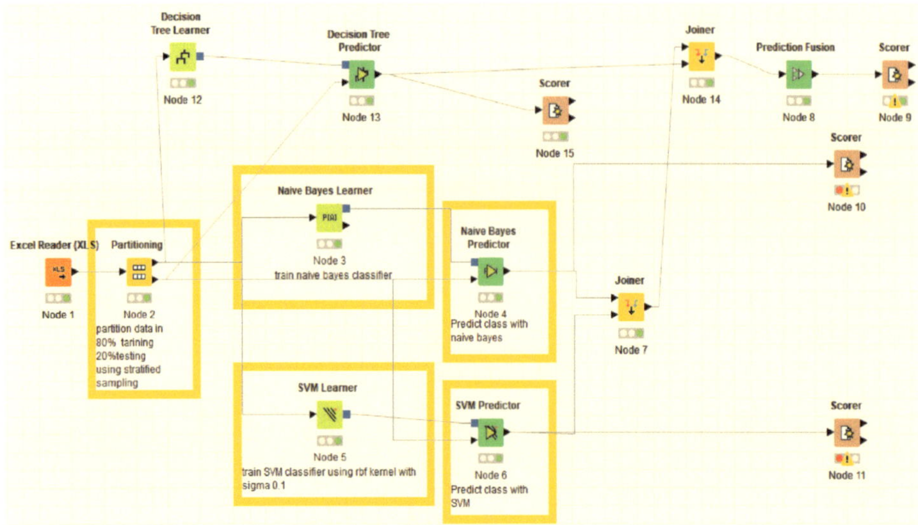

Figure 9.
Comparison with Decision Tree Naive Bayes and SVM Learner.

simplicity to onboard. By the time this easiness coming, most of the ship operators take advantages by reductions of the numbers of the crew onboard. While technological development has led to higher efficiency in maritime industry, some tasks, e.g. maintenance of the equipment or machinery, have not been affected by technical development and must still be handled manually in an often time-consuming manner [18]. Due to reduced staffing, these tasks must now be carried out by fewer employees. Lundh and her colleagues found that many engine room engineers reported using unauthorised shortcuts to be able to handle these tasks under time pressure [19]. These unauthorised shortcuts increase risks onboard the vessels. Briefly, the wellness of the crew must also be reflected in **Table 6** and algorithms.

Moreover, the ergonomy of the engine room is also essential for the shipping. For example, the study carried out by Lundh and her colleagues showed that the design of the engine control room and engine room is crucial for how different tasks are performed. According to this study, the design which does not support operational procedures, can induce an increased risk of exposure to hazardous substances and the engine crew members becoming injured [18].

Author details

Şevket Süleyman İrtem
Burdur Mehmet Akif Ersoy University, Burdur, Turkey

*Address all correspondence to: sevketirtem@gmail.com

References

[1] Garantziotis S, Schwartz DA. Ecogenomics of respiratory diseases of public health significance. *Annual Review of Public Health* 2010; 31: 39.

[2] Soner O, Akyuz E, Celik M. A Maritime Research Concept through Establishing Ship Operational Problem Solution (Shipos) Centre via Information Technologies Integrated with or/Ms. *Procedia - Social and Behavioral Sciences* 2015; 195: 2796–2803.

[3] Tärntank Ship Management AB. *Lng Powered Vessel Manual*. 2018.

[4] Methanex Corporation. About Methanol, https://www.methanex.com/about-methanol/methanol-marine-fuel (2017).

[5] James Stafford. Brent Crude Oil Market, https://oilprice.com/oil-price-charts/46 (2018).

[6] DNV GL. *GLOBAL SULPHUR CAP 2020*. 2016. Epub ahead of print 2016. DOI: 1267709.

[7] DNV GL Maritime Academy. *GLOBAL SULPHUR CAP 2020 Know the different choices and challenges for on-time compliance*. 2016. Epub ahead of print 2016. DOI: 1267709.

[8] King O. Finding the right fit, https://safety4sea.com/dnv-gl-explains-why-to-invest-in-scrubbers/ (2016).

[9] DNV GL. *Preparing For Low Appendix Sulphur Limits 2015*. 2015.

[10] Britannica TE of E. Methanol, https://www.britannica.com/science/methanol (2019, accessed April 25, 2021).

[11] Ellis J. Methanol as an alternative fuel for smaller vessels, https://www.sspa.se/alternative-fuels/methanol-alternative-fuel-smaller-vessels (2018, accessed June 15, 2018).

[12] Zero Vision Tool. ZVT Projects, http://www.zerovisiontool.com/projects (2017, accessed March 3, 2018).

[13] DNV GL. *Assessment of Selected Alternative Fuels and Technologies*. 2018.

[14] Man Y, Lützhöft M, Costa NA, et al. Gaps between users and designers: A usability study about a tablet-based application used on ship bridges. *Advances in Intelligent Systems and Computing* 2018; 597: 213–224.

[15] Kenneth Jensen. CRISP-DM Process Diagram, https://commons.wikimedia.org/wiki/File:CRISP-DM_Process_Diagram.png (accessed April 25, 2021).

[16] IBM Corporation. *IBM SPSS Modeler CRISP-DM Guide Product Information*. 2016.

[17] Guyon I. Cause-Effect Pairs Challenge. In: *Cause-Effect Pairs Challenge*. 2013.

[18] Lundh M, Lützhöft M, Rydstedt L, et al. Working conditions in the engine department - A qualitative study among engine room personnel on board Swedish merchant ships. *Applied Ergonomics* 2011; 42: 384–390.

[19] Lundh M, Rydstedt LW. A static organization in a dynamic context - A qualitative study of changes in working conditions for Swedish engine officers. *Applied Ergonomics* 2016; 55: 1–7.

Chapter 13

Vector-Borne Diseases and Climate Change in the Environmental Context in Haiti

Ketty Balthazard-Accou, Max François Millien, Daphnée Michel, Gaston Jean, David Telcy and Evens Emmanuel

Abstract

Climate change is one of the main challenges facing many countries, particularly developing countries, because of its negative impact on their various ecosystems and their socio-economic development, which very often leads them down a slow descent into poverty. This is because climate change can manifest itself in different forms such as climate variability and extreme events (droughts, epidemics, floods, storms and hurricanes), which can affect biodiversity and cause many human and animal diseases and deaths. In fact, the evolution of ecosystems is dependent on climate and environmental change and appears to be closely associated with many emerging or re-emerging diseases. In general, the ecosystems considered to be most exposed to climate change are those located in and around the intertropical convergence zone in particular. They are believed to be closely linked to the occurrence of several emerging diseases, particularly vector-borne diseases. For years, the Republic of Haiti has been experiencing the adverse effects of these global changes with a marked disruption of its rainfall pattern and prolonged periods of drought as well as a pronounced increase in temperatures even in high altitude areas. Although there is evidence that climate change is increasing the frequency of vector-borne diseases and may contribute to increasing the virulence of their pathogens, there are very few studies conducted in Haiti on the relationship between climate change and vector-borne diseases. The purpose of this chapter is to define the interrelationships between climate change and vector-borne diseases in Haiti by identifying avenues of research to better understand the effects of climate change on public health and to make appropriate recommendations to decision-makers to ensure proper management.

Keywords: Climate change, Vector-Borne Diseases, Ecosystems, Environmental Factors, Public Health, Ecological Sanitation (Haiti)

1. Introduction

Global warming is a serious threat to humanity [1]. At the global level, warming trends have not ceased to manifest. As evidence of this, global annual air temperature increased by nearly 1°C between 1880 and 2017 [2] and the years 2015 to 2017 are considered to have been the warmest of all previous years within this period [3]. Moreover, the last three decades have been warmer than any previous decade since

1850 [4]. Long-term changes in temperature and precipitation are often accompanied by heat waves and intense rainfall, increasing the risk of flooding [5], mainly in countries in the Caribbean region such as Haiti.

Climate change is often described as one of the most pressing environmental challenges we face worldwide [6]. The latest report of the Intergovernmental Panel on Climate Change (IPCC) has confirmed that climate is being affected by human activities and has also highlighted that this has multiple impacts on human and animal health. Indeed, the work of the IPCC puts into perspective the weight of industrialization in climate disruption through significant greenhouse gas emissions. These actions are responsible for extreme hydrometeorological phenomena (droughts and floods), which can cause multiple cases of death and emergence of pathologies in living beings. Climatic disturbances are also at the origin of many infectious diseases, among which vector-borne diseases transmitted by hematophagous arthropods such as dengue fever, Zika, chikungunya and malaria.

Climate change is a major threat to Haiti, even though it contributes very little to the phenomenon. Like the countries of Latin America and the Caribbean, the Republic of Haiti has been suffering for years from the adverse effects of global changes with a marked disruption in the rainfall pattern, the occurrence of prolonged periods of drought and a pronounced warming of temperature and air. As agricultural productivity continues to decline, water resource management is becoming increasingly difficult. The upward trending emergence of vector-borne diseases such as dengue, Zika and chikungunya inoculated by invasive species of mosquitoes was observed in 2015. In the context of global climate change, dengue is considered one of the important diseases because of its high social impact recorded over the last three decades in the humid tropical world, with a risk of expansion into the temperate zone. According to the World Health Organization [7], dengue is the most important neglected disease today. Although it is reported that climate change is affecting the occurrence of infectious diseases, particularly vector-borne diseases, there have very few studies conducted in Haiti on the interrelationships between climate and vector-borne diseases. The purpose of this chapter is to define the interrelationships between climate change and vector-borne diseases in Haiti while conceptualizing the research in order to make the appropriate recommendations for their mitigation and the protection of public health. This chapter is divided into five sections:

- Climate Change and Environmental Degradation at a Glance: Global and Haitian Climate Change and Environmental Degradation;
- Impact of Climate Change and Environmental Change on Health;
- Elements of Epidemiology of Vector-Borne Diseases in Haiti
- Climate change and global health approach;
- Methods to combat climate change and vector-borne diseases

2. Climate change and environmental degradation

2.1 Main characteristics of climate change

According to the IPCC Third Assessment Report, the global average surface air temperature is projected to increase by 1.4 to 5.8°C by 2100 [8], with significant impacts on all elements of the global climate system. In addition, the fifth report published in 2014 also reveals that all physical and biological systems on all continents and in virtually all oceans will be affected by temperature increases due to climate change [9]. Therefore, changes in climatic conditions and induced effects such as rainfall variability, temperature, humidity affect the human and ecological systems of the planet. However, rising temperatures and increased drought periods generally lead to new challenges that are very difficult for a developing country to overcome.

The IPCC [10] predicts that climate change will affect coastal areas in a variety of ways and indicates that current changes in temperature and precipitation are likely to increase the frequency of life-threatening events. Changes in climate variability will also have consequences for human health. Climate variables such as temperature and precipitation have a major impact on the hydrological cycle and changes in these variables will alter runoff and evaporation patterns and the amount of water stored in soils and aquifers. They could also degrade groundwater quality. For example, a reduction in aquifer recharge rates and groundwater runoff could increase contaminant concentrations in groundwater and the incidence of infectious diseases. Work carried out in the cities of Cap-Haitian and Les Cayes (Haiti) has highlighted the presence of *Cryptosporidium* oocyst in surface water [11–13] and groundwater used by the population for domestic purposes [14]. These resources are contaminated by fecal pollution and are a source of potential biological risk to the health of the exposed population. Rainfall can promote the spread of infectious agents, while temperature promotes their proliferation and survival.

2.2 State of environmental degradation in Haiti

Developing countries (DCs) face the challenges of population growth, accelerated urbanization and poverty. On one hand, socio-economic inequalities and social polarization have increased, and on the other hand, the heterogeneity of poor households has grown, including the increase in socio-economic inequalities and social polarization [15]. According to the data in the literature, some developing countries are more subject to the impacts of climatic variations, especially those with an "extreme" climate and/or those whose climate is close to that of the sea. Haiti is one of these, mainly due to its high population growth juxtaposed with conditions of economic and social poverty.

Located on the border of two tectonic plates (the North American Plate and the Caribbean Plate located under the Caribbean Sea) [16], Haiti is not only placed on the direct trajectory of extreme weather events such as storms and hurricanes, but is also the site of strong seismic activity that seriously damages its socio-economic development process [17]. In addition, in recent decades, the process of degradation of Haiti's biophysical environment and its socio-economic decline has been exacerbated by climate change. Indeed, the second national communication on climate change and recent studies on the issue have revealed the high vulnerability of the country's main strategic sectors to this occurrence. Haiti is exposed to environmental threats such as sea level rise, the intensification of extreme weather events (hurricanes, floods, droughts, etc.), erosion and coastal pollution.

The demographic explosion currently characterizing the country is leading to deforestation, resulting in impoverishment and soil degradation. This deforestation makes the country particularly vulnerable to floods and erosion. Every year it loses about 1600 t/ha of land [18]. **Figure 1** shows the impact of deforestation on the Pine Forest Biological Reserve [18].

Haiti has a geophysical environment characterized primarily by particular climatic, hydrological and biogeographic phenomena. Environmental changes such as deforestation, desertification, soil erosion and extreme poverty linked to its geographical location make the country increasingly vulnerable to climate change. According to 2014'sGerman Watch long-term climate risk index, Haiti was,

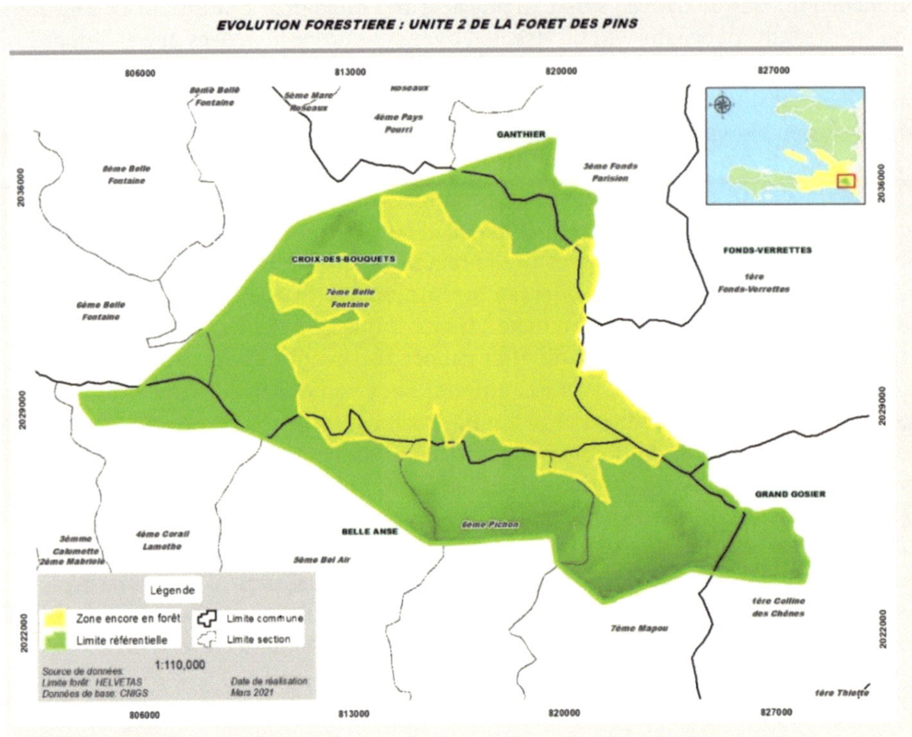

Figure 1.
Pine Forest Deforestation in Haiti [18].

between 1990 and 2008, the Caribbean country most affected by natural disasters (epidemics, floods, storms and hurricanes). These phenomena demonstrate the extent to which climate change contributes to environmental degradation, i.e. soil degradation, water scarcity, water pollution, loss of biodiversity and the occurrence of diseases. Haiti ranks third among the countries most affected by climate risks between 1993 and 2012 [19].

For developing countries, particularly Haiti, climate change represents a new threat that adds to existing risks, interacts with them and amplifies them. The negative consequences of climate change are exacerbated by the increased occurrence of extreme weather events, such as major hurricanes. These, which are increasingly intense, threaten to undermine the functioning of the various sectors associated with the country's socio-economic development, causing damage reaching alarming proportions of the national GDP. It is in this context and following the impetus provided by the Paris Agreement that the Haitian government, through the Ministry of the Environment (MDE) supported by the country's key sectors and actors, proceeded to develop the National Climate Change Policy (NCCP) following a highly participatory and inclusive process. This policy seeks to establish the major projects of the Haitian State in this area. As such, it should serve as a guide for all sectors and actors who want to contribute to the fight against climate change.

3. Impact of climate change and environmental modifications on health and vector-borne diseases

Climate change and environmental modifications are the main determinants of the changes observed in ecosystems that favor the occurrence of emerging and re-emerging animal and human diseases. More than ever, veterinary and health authorities around the world have realized the need to better understand the problem of climate loading and environmental change as it is posed in the 21st century in order to be able to prepare viable alert and response plans to these diseases, particularly vector-borne diseases whose proliferation appears to be closely linked to climatic parameters such as heat and humidity [20]. This situation is further complicated in countries such as Haiti, where significant environmental changes have been recorded in recent decades in terms of both forest cover and water resources.

Climate variability and change cause many cases of mortality and disease in humans and terrestrial and aquatic animals through the natural disasters they cause, such as heat waves, floods and droughts. The latest report of the Intergovernmental Panel on Climate Change (IPCC) has clearly shown that human activity is affecting the world's climate and has highlighted that this has multiple impacts on human and animal health.

3.1 Proliferation of vectors responsible for animal diseases and zoonosis

For about four decades, the scientific community and a large part of the civil society of developed countries have not failed to express their concern about the threat of a catastrophe looming over the planet if certain countries, major producers of greenhouse gases, persist in refusing to change their modes of industrial production which are largely responsible for the present situation. In the history of humanity, never before have there been so many massive emissions of such gases that have caused pronounced climatic disturbances that are reflected, among other things, in changes in rainfall patterns according to regions and the occurrence of extreme weather events. It is agreed that such climatic upheavals are at the root of many emerging or re-emerging infectious diseases. Indeed, it has long been known that there is a positive correlation between climate change and the occurrence of these diseases. Indeed, the temperature of arthropods/vectors generally varies according to that of the environment in which they live, hence their high sensitivity to ambient temperature variations. These temperature variations, by acting on the biology of these vectors, interact with the infectious agents that they often harbor [21].

In addition to temperature variations, other factors such as rainfall and humidity also contribute to the creation of favorable environments for vector development [3]. Changes in land use and socio-economic factors (human behavior, movement of people and goods, etc.) have also contributed to increasing ecological imbalances conducive to vector proliferation, resulting in the introduction and local transmission of new emerging pathogens in many countries [22]. However, the role of climate in the occurrence of infectious diseases, particularly vector-borne diseases, is not easily established.

This has led the IPCC to issue constant alerts about changes in the transmission of infectious diseases by vectors such as mosquitoes and ticks [23]. The sudden appearance and spread in 2007 and 2014 in many countries, tropical and temperate, of a vector-borne disease such as Chikungunya, which was facilitated by the extension of the distribution area of Aedes mosquitoes and the greater mobility of human populations. A similar scenario probably occurred in other temperate countries with other vector-borne diseases such as dengue and Zika as new areas of mosquito vector proliferation were established. Mosquito-borne diseases are climate-sensitive because the risk of epidemic disease increases or decreases in part with temperature, rainfall and humidity, which affect the life and reproductive cycle of insects [5].

3.2 Increasing prevalence and incidence rates of emerging or re-emerging diseases

Epidemic peaks are generally linked to climatic disturbances, as was the case in 2015 with the El Niño phenomenon, which led to the resurgence of malaria, chikungunya, Zika, plague and dengue fever. Since 1950, 2015 was the most important year in South America for Zika virus infection. Researchers have identified four school cases worldwide: plague and hantavirus in the United States, cholera in Tanzania, and dengue fever in Brazil, Thailand and Indonesia [3, 24]. **Figure 2** shows the emergence of several epidemic diseases around the world during the El Niño phenomenon of 2015-2016 [24].

Researchers have been interested in the high prevalence and especially the high incidence rate of Buruli ulcer observed in French Guyana since 1969. They compared the changes in rainfall in the region with the evolution of the number of Buruli ulcer cases over the past 40 years and showed that the reduction in rainfall and its runoff has led to the multiplication of areas of stagnant residual water serving as a breeding ground for the bacterium Mycobacterium ulcerans responsible for Buruli ulcer. This observation is not consistent with the generally accepted idea that reduced rainfall leads to a decrease in the prevalence of infectious diseases. On the contrary, it has been observed that swampy habitats, with the reduction of rainfall, have become more accessible and usable, thus increasing the level of human exposure to the bacteria still present in the aquatic environment.

3.3 Highlighting the interrelationships between health, biodiversity and ecosystems

Ecosystem change includes climate change, environmental change and related relationships and is believed to be closely associated with many emerging diseases [25]. The interrelationships between health, agriculture and ecosystems open a fairly broad door to the "One health" approach. They highlight how:

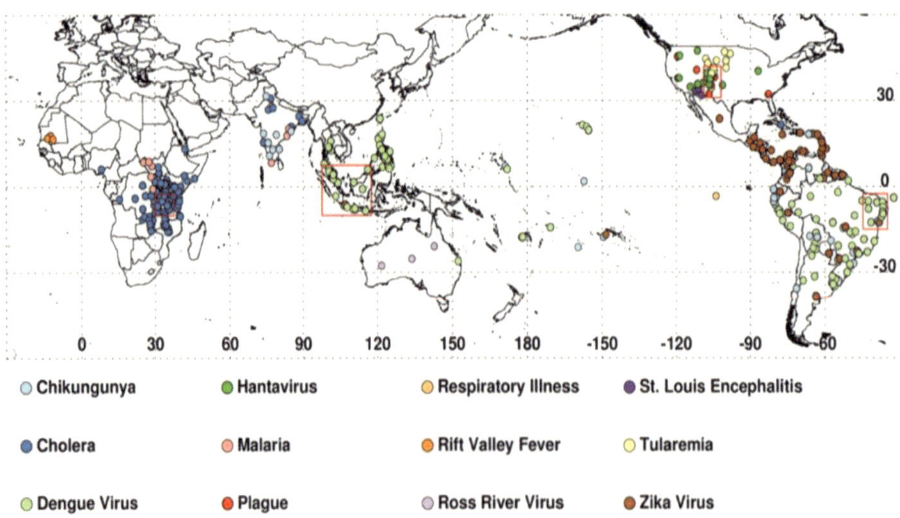

Figure 2.
Emergence of several epidemical diseases across the globe during the El Niño phenomenon of 2015–2016. The four cases studied in detail (United States, East Africa, Brazil and Southeast Asia) are boxed in red [24].

- the precarious nature of agriculture in poor regions, the strong dependence of the economy on agriculture and its vulnerability to pests/predators and pathogens can contribute to the loss of food resources, thus creating food insecurity with risks of deforestation as is the case in Haiti, and a great fragility of the population and the various livestock in terms of health due to the increased risk of infection;

- the increase in the use of the cheapest, and therefore most toxic, pesticides can have negative repercussions on the health of the population;

- Transboundary animal diseases can have a highly negative impact on international markets for animals and animal products. Indeed, diseases such as foot-and-mouth disease, bovine spongiform encephalopathy, swine fever, and avian influenza have caused economic losses in the tens of billions of dollars;

- Every hour, the oceans absorb one million tons of CO_2, creating an increase in the acidification of the environment unsuitable for marine life.

It is currently recognized that infectious and parasitic diseases have medical, social and environmental dimensions and that public health actors must strive for a holistic, comprehensive approach to better understand the dynamics of their development, particularly those that are zoonotic. To this end, a strategy should be adopted that integrates data or advances from public health, animal health, agriculture and environmental sciences in order to identify the determinants and risk factors associated with the various health states at the Human/Animal/Environment interface. Such an approach is related to the "One Health, One Health" approach and requires, to ensure its success, a new form of collaboration that requires the formation of multidisciplinary teams of scientists and the establishment of a platform for intersectoral cooperation at the institutional level.

In order to better manage the emergence or spread of zoonosis effectively, the ecological requirements of zoonotic pathogens and also the importance of anthropogenic factors must be taken into account. The unprecedented anthropogenic pressure on ecosystems in the context of global environmental change, which is constantly increasing, will continue to promote the occurrence of zoonotic diseases [26]. Thus, deforestation is a frequent source of emergence of zoonosis from wild animals. This is the case for diseases caused by West Nile virus and Nipah virus [27]. It is therefore important to consider the conditions of their emergence in relation to the environment and/or the organization of animal production chains, with particular emphasis on social factors (organization and functioning of animal husbandry and marketing structures). The governance of territories or geographical areas is another aspect that needs to be taken into consideration when organizing health management [28].

The CDC has presented a very good illustration of the impact of climate change on Human Health in the following **Figure 3** [4].

CIRAD has developed an integrated approach to health that is a little broader than the conventional concept of "One Health", which seems to us to be quite interesting, and which is based around the following major axes:

- incorporating knowledge from the human and social sciences, agronomy and environmental sciences into the approach;

- broaden the panel of conventional actors (doctors, veterinarians, public health practitioners) to include new institutional and social actors such as, on the one hand, government agents in the environmental (forestry, wildlife, water

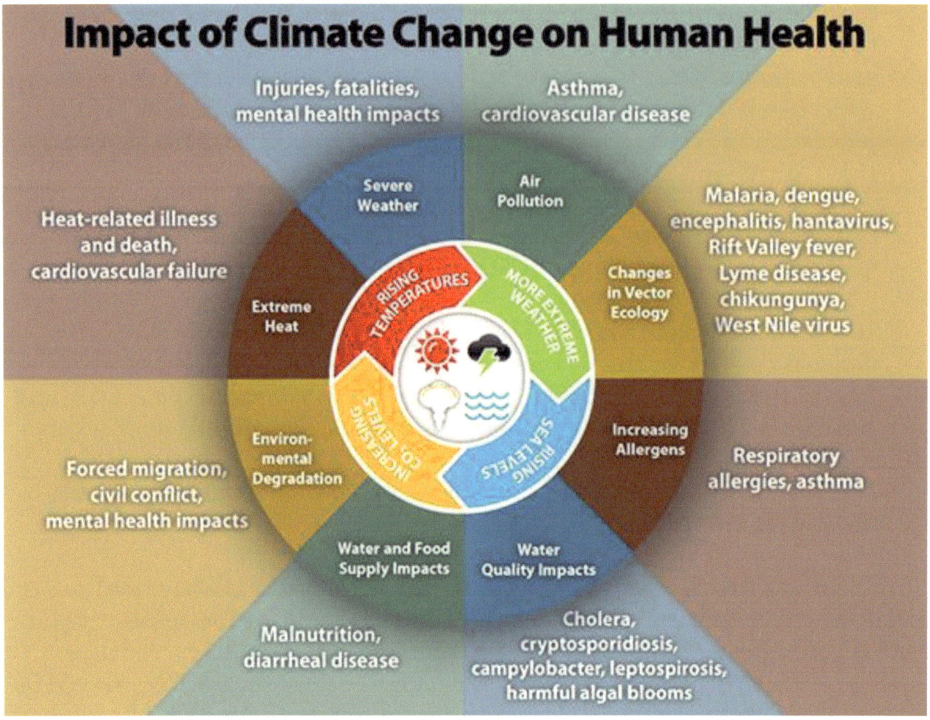

Figure 3.
Impact of Climate change on public Health [4].

management), agricultural or rural development sectors, and on the other hand, categories of social actors such as stockbreeders and farmers, peasant leaders, buyers and sellers of animal products as well as religious authorities.

The environment is continually changing. Therefore, this permanent change must be accompanied by adaptive and participatory methods to facilitate decision-making, which is quite complex for public health actors. The more complex the health problem is, the more the actors must learn to manage this uncertainty related to decision making. This is why some experts propose a participatory modeling and simulation approach to guide consultation and decision-making. This approach is largely inspired by companion modelling [28].

The tools used lead the actors concerned by health in a given territory to cooperate, even though they do not necessarily know each other or work together. These tools enable them to work together to build a shared representation of a complex situation and to simulate actions and their effects in order to build consensual solutions. This approach also offers the possibility of integrating health control and surveillance actions into the territorial context. It can therefore accompany health management interventions, such as vaccination, drug distribution or surveillance and the emergence of new clinical cases in human or animal populations.

4. Elements of Epidemiology of Vector-Borne Diseases in Haiti

In recent decades, climate change has been the central theme of several international environmental congresses. Climatologist Katharine Hayhoe has even stated that "all human beings aspire to the same thing: to live safely on our planet. So, while our work must remain objective and impartial, we are increasingly raising our voices and supporting the clear message that climate change is real, that humans are responsible for it, that its consequences are serious and that we must act immediately". It is that climate change is a multidimensional and interdisciplinary field that should be of interest to all human beings living on this planet. Its manifestations are indeed multiple, such as heat waves, warming and ocean acidification, which have important consequences on the life cycle of the main vectors responsible for animal diseases and zoonosis. It also favors the emergence of certain vector-borne diseases and the geographical extension of vector-borne diseases in temperate zones [5].

According to the World Health Organization, vector-borne diseases are responsible for more than 17% of infectious diseases and cause more than one million deaths each year [29, 30].

4.1 Scope of action of vector-borne disease epidemiology

To fight vector-borne infectious diseases in humans and animals, it is important to know their epidemiology, i.e. to have relevant information on the pathogens, vectors and manifestations of these diseases. In other words, it is important to know, for example:

- whether or not the pathogenic agent is cultivable or not;
- the sources of the pathogenic agent, i.e. animal, environment, human;
- possible reservoirs and intermediate hosts;
- how the disease is transmitted;
- the length of the incubation period;
- the duration of the transmissibility period;
- the action of physical and infectious agents;
- the susceptibility of the pathogen to available anti-infective drugs.

The epidemiology of vector-borne diseases is directly related to: the distribution, competence and capacity of vectors (the competence of a vector is its ability to infect a vertebrate host, to ensure the development of an infectious agent and to transmit this agent to another host, while capacity is associated with environmental conditions and also depends on: (i) the competence of the vector and the rate of vector-host contact; (ii) vector density and longevity; (iii) the level of infectivity of the infectious agents, their host specificity and their resistance to anti-infective; (iv) human activities, environmental and climatic conditions that may influence vector distribution and activity, and vector-human interactions and animal reservoirs [21].

In the case of Haiti, epidemiology should enable the collection of more data on the impact of climate change on the clinical and epidemiological manifestations of vector-borne diseases, and determine the consequences of climate change on ecosystems in Haiti in terms of biodiversity, vector habitats and the transmission period of certain vector-borne diseases, as well as social parameters. It would also be interesting to identify the main changes observed in Haiti in the evolution of vector-borne diseases following repeated natural disasters (cyclones) and large variations in rainfall recorded in recent years.

4.2 Vectors and infectious diseases in Haiti

As everywhere in the tropical world, mosquitoes are the most widespread vector in Haiti. But there are others such as ticks, flies, sandflies, fleas, triatomines and some freshwater gastropods such as limnea.

4.2.1 Infectious and parasitic diseases transmitted by insects in Haiti

The main insect vectors of infectious diseases in Haiti are:

- Aedes mosquitoes, vectors of Chikungunya, Dengue, Yellow Fever, Zika.
- Anopheles (Malaria)
- Culex (West Nile Virus Fever, Lymphatic Filariasis)
- Phlebotomas (Leishmaniasis)

In this chapter, we will be restricted to considering only the most important vector-borne infectious diseases such as: a. malaria, b. dengue fever, c. Chikungunya, d. Zika.

a. Malaria

Malaria is caused by Anopheles, which are responsible for approximately 219 million cases worldwide and more than 400,000 deaths each year. In Haiti, malaria is considered a major public health problem with a fairly large spatial and temporal distribution in the West departments and that of Grand-Anse.

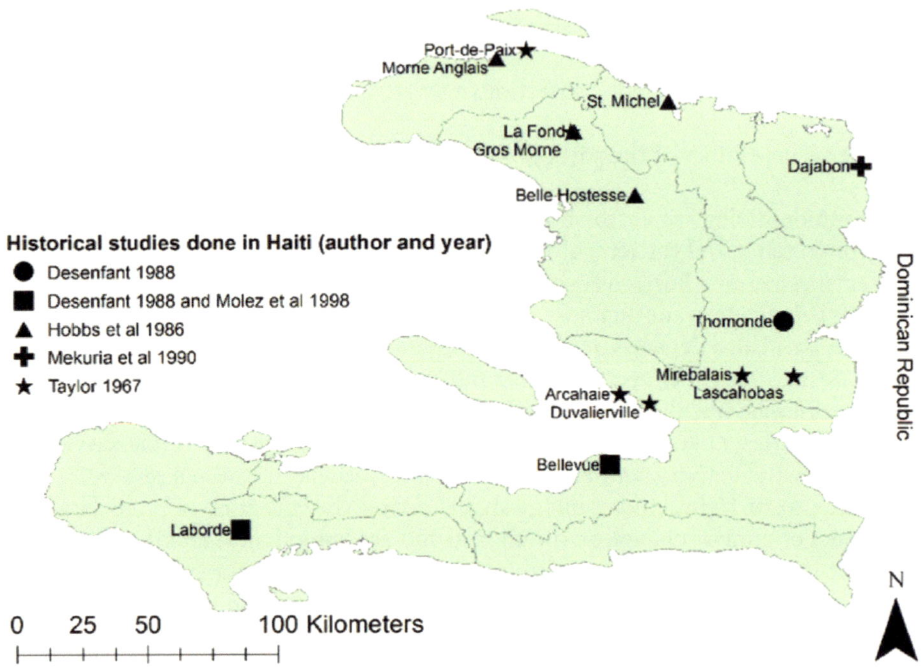

Figure 4.
Map of the sites of the mosquito behavior studies in Haiti [31].

The following **Figure 4** is an illustration of the main sites of mosquito behaviour studies.

The country has not been able to reach its goal of eliminating malaria by the year 2020 as planned. Additional information should be generated by epidemiological studies on vector ecology in order to develop strategies to facilitate the eradication of this disease [31, 32]. In order to understand the direct and indirect impacts of climate change on malaria, the variability of malaria transmission as well as climatic and anthropogenic factors need to be analyzed. The sporogonic cycle of Plasmodium is related to the increase in air temperature and the life cycle of Anopheles is related to changes in their natural breeding habitat resulting from changes in humidity following acclimatization reactions of vegetation under climate change.

The indirect impacts of temperature change on soil moisture dynamics are important and should be balanced against the direct effects of temperature change on mosquito and parasite life cycles for the prediction and future control of malaria [29, 30].

b. Dengue fever

Dengue fever is the most common infectious disease transmitted by mosquitoes of the genus Aedes, which carry the virus responsible for the disease. Although it is a tropical viral disease, it should be noted that a dengue epidemic occurred in Madeira, Portugal in 2012. This highlighted the potential for re-emergence of dengue in Europe due to global warming and the extension of vector distribution areas due to climate change. The dengue virus is circulating in Haiti, but it is not yet recognized as a major disease in the population. In 2011, to assess the prevalence of antibodies against dengue virus (DENV), serum samples were collected from infants and young children aged 7 to 36 months (n = 166) and tested by seroneutralization tests. Serotype 1 of the dengue virus infected 40% of this study population, followed by serotype 2 (12%), serotype 3 (11%) and serotype 4 (2%).It was found that 53% of infants and young children under 12 months of age had already been infected with DENV. The seroprevalence rate against DENV increased to 65% at 36 months of age. Heterotypic antibody responses were an important component of the total dengue immunity profile [33].

In October 2012, 25 cases of dengue fever, confirmed by rapid diagnostic tests (RDTs), were detected among workers of non-governmental organizations (NGOs) in Haiti based in Leogane and Port-au-Prince to determine the extent and risk factors for dengue virus infection. Of the 776 staff members of the targeted NGOs, 173 (22 percent; 52 expatriates and 121 Haitians) participated. Dengue IgM antibodies to dengue virus (DENV) were detected in 8 expatriates (15%) and 9 Haitians (7%), and the non-structural protein DENV 1 in one expatriate. Anti-DENV IgG antibodies were detected in 162 (94%) participants (79% expatriates; 100% Haitians), and confirmed by micro-neutralization tests as specific for DENV in 17/34 (50%) expatriates and 42/42 (100%) Haitians. Of 254 nymphs collected in 68 containers, 65% were AedesAegypti; 27% were Aedesalbopictus. Few NGO workers reported taking action to avoid mosquitoes (**Table 1**) [34].

A cross-sectional study of dengue virus (DENV) and West Nile virus (WNV) transmission was conducted using standard seroepidemiological methods. Blood samples (N = 673) were collected from 278 males and 395 females from three localities in the western and southeastern departments of Haiti. Serum was tested for the presence of anti-DENV and anti-WNV immunoglobulin G (IgG) antibodies using an indirect enzyme-linked immunosorbent assay (ELISA). Anti-DENV IgG antibodies were detected in 72.1% (95% confidence interval [CI] = 68.7, 75.5) of the

Variable	NGO workers with recent infection†		NGO workers without recent infection		Crude OR* (95% CI)‡	p-value
	n = 17		n = 156		n = 181	
	n	%	n	%		
Sex (male)	11	65%	120	77%	0.6 (0.19–1.59)	0.37
Expatriates	8	47%	44	28%	2.3 (0.82–6.24)	0.16
Occupation						
Indoor setting (ex. Office/admin)	1	6%	32	21%	0.2 (0.03–1.9)	0.20
Outdoor setting (ex. Construction)	8	47%	68	44%	1.2 (0.43–3.38)	0.80
Mixed setting (both indoor and outdoor)	7	41%	50	32%	1.6 (0.55–4.42)	0.42
Vaccination History (YF or JPE)	7	41%	43	28%	1.8 (0.66–5.14)	0.27
Previously lived in or traveled to Other Dengue Endemic Regions	9	53%	70	45%	1.4 (0.51–3.8)	0.61
Lived in or Travel to Dengue Endemic Regions (incl. Haiti)	15	88%	155	99%	0.48 (0.004–0.57)	0.03
Environmental factors at work place						
Screens on doors/ windows	8	47%	59	38%	1.5 (0.53–4.00)	0.60
Air-conditioning	6	35%	47	30%	1.3 (0.44–3.62)	0.78
Open water source nearby	9	53%	37	24%	3.6 (1.30–10.05)	0.02
Standing water source nearby	7	41%	45	29%	1.7 (0.62–4.82)	0.30
Reported knowledge of						
Infectious disease in Haiti (very good)	6	35%	23	15%	3.6 (1.16–10.98)	0.03
Mosquito bite prevention	9	53%	31	20%	6.2 (1.92–19.72)	0.002
Mosquito avoidance strategies employed						
Long sleeves	5	29%	50	32%	0.9 (0.30–2.64)	1.00
Long pants	5	29%	61	39%	0.7 (0.22–1.93)	0.60
Bed net	11	65%	101	65%	1.0 (0.35–2.85)	1.00
Mosquito repellent use						
multiple times a day	7	41%	26	17%	3.5 (1.22–10.04)	0.02

**OR, odds ratio.*
†Recent infection is any participant with a positive anti-DENV IgM or non-structural protein 1 (NS1) result.
‡Significance level, $p < 0.05$. Univariate analysis using Fisher's exact test was used to assess risk factors for recent infection, and 95% confidence intervals (CI) were based on the modeling accounted for the sampling design. Only significant variables with a cell size of 5 or greater were retained.

Table 1.
Risk factors for current and/or recent dengue virus (DENV) infection in non-governmental [34].

Dengue virus serotype	Derivation and height of antibody	Age groups in months (no. in sample)					
		7–12 (49)	13–18 (48)	19–24 (31)	25–30 (22)	31–36 (16)	All age groups (166)
1	Dominant	32% (15)	54% (26)	39% (12)	36% (8)	31% (5)	40% (66)
	GMT	357	448	591	615	452	465
	(95% CI)	(209–608)	(290–691)	(364–960)	(289–1,310)	(113–1,803)	(366–591)
	Cross-reactive	12% (6)	8% (4)	19% (6)	32% (7)	19% (3)	16% (26)
2	Dominant	15% (7)	6% (3)	10% (3)	18% (4)	19% (3)	12% (20)
	GMT	257	607	1286	308	389	411
	(95% CI)	(46–1,428)	(41–9,009)	(250–6,616)	(12–8,043)	(141–1,077)	(203–831)
	Cross-reactive	20% (10)	38% (18)	35% (11)	46% (10)	43% (7)	34% (56)
3	Dominant	6% (3)	10% (5)	13% (4)	18% (4)	19% (3)	11% (19)
	GMT	467	467	815	909	1807	678
	(95% CI)	(218–1,002)	(218–1,002)	(105–6,316)	(200–4,129)	(751–4,351)	(391–1,176)
	Cross-reactive	31% (15)	40% (19)	42% (13)	46% (10)	25% (4)	37% (61)
4	Dominant	2% (1)	0	3% (1)	0	5% (1)	2% (3)
	GMT	33		125		280	133
	(95% CI)	NA		NA		NA	(4–4785)
	Cross-reactive	12% (6)	15% (7)	23% (7)	22% (5)	12% (2)	16% (27)

**GMT = geometric mean titer; CI = confidence interval; NA = not available.*

Table 2.
Serotype-specific antibody to dengue virus as a function of age, Haiti [35].*

sample population; without significant differences in seroprevalence by study site, gender or age group (see **Table 2**) [35].

There was a high prevalence of anti-DENV IgG antibodies in all age groups, including the youngest age group (2–5 years), suggesting hyperendemic transmission of DENV in the western and southeastern departments of Haiti. These results undoubtedly demonstrate the endemic nature of dengue fever in the country (**Table 2**).

c. Chikungunya

Chikungunya is an infectious disease caused by an Arbovirus belonging to the Togaviridae family, which is transmitted to humans through the bite of a mosquito of the genus Aedes, mainly AedesAegypti better known as the tiger mosquito. The chikungunya virus has been known since the 1950s when it caused major epidemics in Southeast Asia and India. The wide geographical distribution of vectors has made it possible for the virus to emerge in many regions, as has been seen with other arboviruses, such as West Nile virus, which has been introduced and established on the North American continent since 1999. The first cases of chikungunya were detected in Haiti during April 2014, but the disease was detected in the Caribbean in St Martin as early as December 2013. Indeed, in a longitudinal cohort epidemiological study of 153 serum samples collected between 2011 and 2013 and another 61 collected in 2014, of those collected in 2014, none of the 153 samples were positive for IgG responses to chikungunya virus antigen, while 78.7% or 48 out of 61 were positive. In the cross-sectional sample, such responses were detected in 96 (75.6%) of the children and occurred at similar prevalence in all age groups [36].

Serological tests indicate that there has been a rapid and intense spread of the chikungunya virus in Haiti. The Ministry of Public Health and Population had reported a cumulative total of 39,343 cases between May 31 and June 16, 2014 in the 10 departments with an infection rate of 67% for the West Department. By mid-August 2014, more than 68,000 cases had been reported. However, after the peak at the beginning of June, the number of new cases per week had continued to decrease from over 12.000 to 315.

The disease left bad memories in the population because of the intense pain it caused through its clinical manifestations (signs and symptoms) including arthralgia, intense myalgia with sequelae that persisted for several months or even years. Although the clinical presentations of the diseases caused by these mosquitoes are similar, the arthralgia strongly suggests a Chikungunya virus infection [37].

d. Zika

Zika is an infectious disease caused by a flavivirus with a wide geographical distribution that is most often transmitted by the bite of an infected mosquito. The disease was first identified in the Americas in 2015 and was characterized by the occurrence of an abnormally high number of cases of congenital microcephaly in Brazil. It rapidly spread to the rest of the region and to the Caribbean including Haiti. Zika virus infection is associated with adverse fetal outcomes and rare neurological complications in adults [38]. The magnitude of the public health problems associated with Zika virus led the World Health Organization to declare the Zika virus epidemic a public health emergency of international concern on February 1, 2016 [38].

Because Zika was often an asymptomatic infection that did not necessarily require care, it was difficult to estimate the true incidence of Zika infection. However, during the period from October 12, 2015 to September 10, 2016, the Haitian Ministry of Public Health and Population (MSPP) had detected 3,036 suspected cases of infection in the general population, 22 suspected cases of Zika virus disease in pregnant women, 13 suspected cases of Guillain-Barré syndrome (GBS), and 29 suspected cases of Zika virus-associated congenital microcephaly. Nineteen patients with suspected Zika virus disease were detected, including 10 in the Western geographical department, 6 in Artibonite and 3 in the Central geographical department. These cases were confirmed by laboratory tests and included 2 pregnant women and 17 in the general population [39]. The surveillance program needs to be strengthened and supported by a functional laboratory in order to better monitor the evolution of the disease in Haiti.

5. Climate Change and The Global Health Approach

For the past fifty years or so, the world has been confronted with an unbridled population growth, a large part of which is forced to migrate to other shores to ensure its survival. At the same time, never before in history have the adverse effects of climate change and the risk of ecological disasters been so evident. These changes are accompanied by other profound alterations to the environment, such as the loss of biodiversity, deforestation, soil erosion, acid rain and ocean acidification. At the same time, the increase in life expectancy of the population and the unbridled process of urbanization have contributed to increased vulnerability to various environmental and health risks, particularly with regard to the occurrence of emerging and re-emerging vector-borne diseases for humans and animals. This has led to a holistic approach to human, animal and environmental health known as "One Health".

5.1 Nature of the "One Health, One Health" concept or approach

This concept emphasizes that public health problems that generally involve human/animal/environment interaction are so complex that they cannot be solved by a single discipline but by a multiple, transdisciplinary and multisector approach. Indeed, it is generally accepted that the environment in which human and animal populations live together has changed considerably over the years, greatly influencing the occurrence of many infectious and even non-infectious diseases.

According to the American Veterinary Medical Association, the "One Health" approach can be defined as "the joint effort of several disciplines working locally, nationally and globally to optimize the health of people, animals and the environment. In other words, it is an integrated approach that recognizes that there is a close interdependence between the well-being of humans, animals and their ecosystem health [40]. Thus, this approach promotes the principles of harmonization of human, animal and ecosystem health to better prevent and/or mitigate emerging diseases while noting that it can be applied to areas other than zoonosis, such as food safety, food security, antimicrobial resistance and response to the consequences of climate change.

Health problems are, in general, strongly linked to global environmental and socio-economic changes and to changes in production systems at the territorial level. This is what makes health management so complex as it mobilizes knowledge from both veterinary public health and agriculture and environment. Because of the emergence of new health uncertainties, unconventional actors are entering alongside the decision-makers traditionally in charge of public health [28]. In the context of climate change and outbreaks of vector-borne diseases throughout the world, including in the Caribbean including Haiti, the public health, animal health and environment sectors have three major challenges to address:

- The establishment of a platform for inter-organizational collaboration and communication to strengthen cooperation between the fields of human health, animal health and ecosystem health;
- Minimizing the impact of new emerging or re-emerging diseases by combining disease surveillance and emergency preparedness at the local, national and international levels;
- creating new methods and tools so that all of these actors can address health issues at the territorial level, the territory being understood here as a socially and politically constructed space and the seat of interactions between actors.

The real innovation of the "One Health" approach is the incorporation of the environmental component in the field of human and animal health. By using such an approach, climate change adaptation methods are more likely to contribute to solving food security problems, particularly in developing countries through the promotion of extensive livestock production systems in areas with large land areas, the increase in animal feeds, environmental sanitation and the establishment of regional integrated surveillance systems for certain vector-borne infectious diseases. It is undeniable that integrated community-based surveillance of zoonosis can be a very promising avenue for reducing the health effects of climate change [41].

5.2 Positioning of the One Health concept in relation to human and animal health

Climate change and environmental change are part of the set of changes that affect ecosystems and promote the emergence and re-emergence of animal diseases. In recent years, more than 70% of these emerging infectious zoonosis have their source in wildlife [Black and Nunn, 2009] and about 60% of emerging infectious diseases are classified as zoonotic, i.e. transmitted from animals to humans [20].

Global warming contributes to the emergence of infectious diseases in the animal and plant world by exerting a marked effect on arthropod insects (mosquitoes, aphids, sandflies, fleas), on ticks that can harbor and transport viruses, bacteria and protozoa. In addition, it causes a thermal increase that increases the risk of extending the current geographical range of these species with the risk of transmission to animals and humans of diseases against which there is no natural immunity [28]. There are a number of meteorological and climatic parameters that can affect human and animal health. In addition to heat, cold, water, ozone, air, allergens and ultraviolet rays, these include heat, cold, water, ozone, air, allergens and ultraviolet rays.

5.2.1 In men

Some authors argue that climate change is the most significant threat to human health in the 21st century, associated with an increase in chronic diseases, health problems caused by extreme heat and floods, food shortages caused by drought or floods, and various diseases including respiratory problems. The effects of climate change on human health can be both direct and indirect. They are considered direct when they are related to the physiological effects of heat and cold and indirect when they result, for example, from changes in human behavior following forced migration, major natural disasters such as floods and earthquakes, or major outbreaks of food-borne or vector-borne diseases. Not all climate-induced changes are necessarily negative for human health, especially those leading to a decrease in extreme temperatures [42].

a. Impact of heat and cold

In temperate countries, periods of high heat are sometimes accompanied by relatively high morbidity and mortality. It is estimated, for example, that in Europe, for a one-degree increase in temperature, heat-related mortality would increase by 1–4%. Heat is an immediate health risk to be considered because it has been shown that nearly three-quarters of the hot days observed since 1850 are attributable to climate change [43]. On the other hand, cold can also cause illness and death among the most vulnerable, especially the elderly and homeless. Variations in temperature, especially those that are upwardly oriented, can be the cause of some foodborne and vector-borne zoonotic diseases.

Food-borne bacterial infectious diseases such as salmonellosis and colibacillosis are generally sensitive to temperature and are becoming increasingly important every day even in developed countries such as Europe and the United States.

b. Impact of vectors

Vector-borne diseases result from the indirect impacts of climate change on biodiversity – arthropod vectors, pathogen reservoirs [44]. They are mainly transmitted by arthropods, in particular insects and ticks. They are generally responsible for animal diseases.

c. Water-related problems of climate change

Climate change induces profound changes in the volume of water available in a given area, which can materialize either through heavy rainfall and flooding or through drought leading to a scarcity of water in this area for the domestic use of the population and for animals. Floods generally carry certain infectious and parasitic diseases, including vector-borne diseases that are closely linked to the proliferation of mosquitoes and other vectors. Many outbreaks of waterborne diseases are due to the mobilization of pathogens or extensive contamination of water by fecal bacteria such as salmonella and coliforms. Thus, it is not uncommon to observe in Haiti outbreaks of anthrax or anthrax following cyclones and also an abnormally high number of gastrointestinal-dominated pathologies dominated by gastrointestinal disorders. Such contamination has generally had unfortunate consequences on the health of the population by rendering catchment waters that were intended for human consumption completely undrinkable.

Water-borne diseases are not necessarily related to floods since the lack of water can prevent daily hygiene practices, especially at the time of the new coronavirus pandemic or in countries where cholera is still prevalent. This lack of water, in some areas, can be extremely serious for the health of the population because it is important to wash your hands with soap and water several times a day to protect yourself against these two diseases.

d. Air Quality

In many industrialized countries, there is a serious air quality problem resulting from environmental degradation caused by uncontrolled industrial activities. In these countries, various pathologies of the respiratory type appear, mainly linked to the presence of ozone and particles in the air.

e. Impact of ozone on climate change

Ozone is a major pollutant in the majority of industrialized countries and its increasing concentration is dependent on climate variability and change. The Republic of Haiti, like many other poor, undeveloped countries, is experiencing the consequences of the impact of ozone on climate change, which are more attributable to the actions of neighboring industrialized countries than to its own agricultural and industrial production activities. Rising temperatures could result in local increases in peak ozone and fine particulate matter levels [45].

f. Allergens in the air

Allergens such as pollen or molds can be dangerous at certain times of the year for children and the elderly, as well as for anyone already suffering from chronic respiratory diseases such as asthma, severe allergies or chronic obstructive pulmonary disease. In a country like Haiti, the diagnosis of these disorders may not be established due to the lack of specialists in allergology.

g. The global effects of climate change on human health

It has been found that in some countries, major natural disasters have often caused severe psychological consequences for children who face such trauma. Global changes are increasing and diversifying the sources of soil and water contamination and are creating new interfaces of contact between humans, animals and their pathogens [28]. Their effects on health are generally unevenly distributed across people because the health and well-being of the population is also correlated with socio-economic factors such as income, housing, employment, education, gender and lifestyle. In addition to children, vulnerable groups include people with outdoor workplaces, the elderly, women, and those already suffering from disease or severe social inequalities [46]. Climate change also has direct impacts on the migration of people, which can be internal or national, intra-regional or international. It can have a negative impact on national economies, as the availability of food and water leads to an increasing need for humanitarian assistance and health protection for vulnerable groups [46].

5.2.2 In animals

Like humans, animals are very sensitive to the effects of climate change, which can be very negative for the health and well-being of livestock. Climate change plays a role in the establishment and geographic expansion of zoonosis [42]. However, according to several studies, the effect may, in some cases, be positive because the increase in air temperature could reduce the risk of death and improve the health and well-being of humans and livestock living in regions with very cold winters. However, extreme variations in climatic parameters such as heat, cold, humidity, and precipitation have an overall negative impact on the health and welfare of animals, resulting in a marked increase in morbidity and mortality. The negative effects of climate change are, as in humans, the consequence of combined changes in air temperature, precipitation, frequency and magnitude of extreme weather events and can also be both direct and indirect.

Heat stress can, depending on its intensity and duration, directly affect the health of animals by causing metabolic disturbances, oxidative stress and a drastic decrease in immune capacity leading to infections and death. Indirect effects are associated with the quantity and quality of feed and drinking water available to animals and the survival and distribution of pathogens and/or their vectors [47]. Indeed, animals are also highly susceptible to certain vector-borne diseases such as those transmitted by ticks like bovine anaplasmosis, piroplasmosis in dogs and cattle, cowdriosis or heartwater, equine encephalitis, African swine fever as well as by insects like Nile Valley fever or by mollusks like liver fluke. Populations of these different vectors tend to increase with climate change.

The issue of climate change, and its impacts on living beings, has become so important and relevant for life on the planet that the World Organization for Animal Health (OIE) has introduced it in recent decades into its strategies. [48, 49]. According to Vallat [48], the impact of climate change on health has often been mentioned, mainly for human health. As regards animal diseases, their relationship with climate change is more rarely mentioned, no doubt because the recent epizootics were mainly linked to highly contagious viral diseases (foot-and-mouth disease, classical and African swine fever, Newcastle disease, influenza avian, etc.) and for which the movements of animals and foodstuffs of animal origin, in particular through trade, have played a preponderant role [48].

Oyhantçaba et *al.* [49] note thet the links between animal production and climate change are complex and multi-directional. On the one hand, animal production has an influence on climate change, with mainly ruminants generating emissions of greenhouse gases. In particular, animal production is a very important source of methane and nitrous oxide released into the atmosphere. On the other hand, climate change influences livestock production by affecting the conditions governing animal production, fodder crop production and animal health. The impacts on animal health are increasingly being recognised, and this theme occupies a special section of this document, as we shall see below [49].

With the introduction and very rapid expansion of West Nile fever virus in North America, the role of wildlife has become clear. This episode highlighted the gaps in our knowledge about the ecology of this type of infection, particularly when they emerge in new settings [48].

It is a fact that the environment in which animals live plays an increasingly important role in the manifestation of diseases, particularly vector-borne diseases. Global warming has led to changes in the ecology of vectors, resulting in the disappearance of certain habitats, the appearance of new ones and, more generally, the displacement of the geographical area that hosts the habitats required by a given vector as a result of environmental changes. Such upheavals in ecosystems have had fairly serious consequences for livestock farming. Thus, we have witnessed the migration of vectors of tropical origin, often carriers of pathogenic germs, to milder and even temperate climates. But still, the causes of vector-borne diseases are multifactorial as they are generally associated not only with climate change but also with trade globalization, urbanization and deforestation [47].

In addition to vector-borne diseases, a dynamic of non-vector-borne diseases is developing, which are also subject to the influence of climate change. One example is avian influenza infections that can be influenced by the migration routes of wild waterfowl. It has been observed that some species of wild birds have reduced their migration distance as a result of global warming, which has sometimes contributed to the spread of some infectious fish diseases to areas that were previously free of them. The persistence of viruses in the environment, including in water, is also influenced by changes in temperature [44].

In general, wildlife plays a significant role in the transmission of some major animal diseases such as avian influenza, rabies, swine fever and tuberculosis. As a consequence of climate change, countries with forests or savannahs with important wildlife often face the problem of water scarcity for watering these animals. As a consequence, they are obliged to gather at the same water point, thus favoring the continuous circulation of pathogens, first among themselves and then in domestic herds due to encounters which are becoming less and less fortuitous in some countries as a result of wild deforestation and anarchic urbanization programs.

6. Methods for Combating Climate Change and Vector-Borne Diseases

Maintaining the earth's ecological system and other biophysical systems in good working order is an imperative that is part of the sustainable development option of countries to ensure the persistence or maintenance of life. It is now widely recognized that these systems are in a state of disrepair and that the resulting climate change represents one of the greatest threats to humanity in the 21st century by disrupting the well-being and health of animal and human populations. We must therefore face reality and strive to live within the norms that govern the normal functioning of our planet. Faced with climate change, which induces a whole range of diseases including vector-borne diseases and zoonosis, it is necessary to make a number of recommendations to mitigate its effects on extreme weather events and on the health of animals and humans. Special attention will be given to the major vector-borne infectious diseases that occur in the Caribbean and particularly in Haiti.

6.1 Main measures to combat climate change

It is important to restore as quickly as possible the health of ecosystems damaged by human action, through a good understanding of the relationship between climate and health, capacity building, information exchange and the promotion of research. Mitigation and adaptation measures should therefore be taken.

6.1.1 Commitment of each country to respect the recommendations of the Paris Agreement on Climate and Global Warming signed in 2016

Predictions suggest that the average global surface temperature of the earth will experience, during this century, a sharp increase of up to more than 5°C and significant changes in rainfall patterns and climate variability [50]. Each country should strive to follow the guidelines of the Paris Agreement and promote research, either at the national or regional level. Research will benefit from finding innovative methods to analyze weather and climate in relation to animal and human health. To this end, it is important to establish data series over long periods of time to better understand the mechanisms of climate change and its interaction with animal and human health or disease occurrence, and to be able to develop early warning systems to predict outbreaks and extreme weather events such as intense heat waves and rainfall, the increased risk of drought, the increase in the strength and speed of winds and tropical cyclones in certain areas such as the Caribbean, including Haiti, and the accentuation of the El Niño phenomenon.

Such work requires a firm commitment not only from the main international organizations concerned such as WMO, IPCC, WHO, OIE, UNEP but also from each country to work towards the reduction of greenhouse gases and other pollutants and to follow the principles of sustainable development required for the survival of the planet and the recommendations of the various international meetings resulting from the Paris Agreement on Climate and Global Warming.

6.1.2 An analytical approach to the impact of climate change on diseases

Evidence suggests that diseases that occur following major weather events are also conditioned by factors other than climate. This requires the collection of a baseline data set and the use of appropriate analytical methods to quantify the climate's contribution to the expression of these diseases. This requires the establishment of functional and reliable climate and disease monitoring and surveillance systems.

6.1.3 Climate change adaptation measures

The effects of climate change are objective data on which we must act quickly to complement climate change mitigation measures in order to significantly reduce their level of impact on animal and human health. These measures could address the various factors that condition the vulnerability of human populations such as population density, economic development, local ecological conditions, health status and access to health care.

6.1.4 Fight against infectious diseases

Infectious diseases, especially those of vector or waterborne origin, are very sensitive to climatic conditions. Therefore, there is a constant need to collect data on the prevalence and especially the incidence of infectious diseases to better address epidemiological studies. Only in this way will it be possible to establish any relationship between observed morbidity or mortality with a given climatic event. Multidisciplinary research teams should be formed and operate within a regional or international framework, as climate problems generally extend beyond the geographical boundaries of a single country [29].

6.2 Main vector control methods

6.2.1 Vector control guidelines

The World Health Assembly approved in 2017 "Global Action for Vector Control 2017-2030" [51]. This document provides strategic guidance to assist countries and development partners to strengthen vector control in their disease prevention and outbreak response strategies. It calls for a reorientation of vector control programs with technical capacity building, improved infrastructure, strengthened monitoring and surveillance systems and strong community mobilization. Changing the behavior of the population is considered one of the essential elements in the fight against vector-borne diseases. WHO has recognized the importance of working with partners to educate and sensitize the public and to build understanding of the need and ways to protect themselves and their communities from the various vectors. In addition, access to water and sanitation services is a very important factor in disease control and elimination.

6.2.2 Main vector control methods

Vector control methods are multiple because they change with the nature of the vectors, which present a great biological diversity. The most commonly used are: a) Biological methods which consist of using, for example, larvivorous fish at the level of water bodies and large aquaculture basins; b) Physical methods that refer to the protection of the environment, either by physical barriers (e.g., mosquito nets, window screens, etc.) or by changes in the environment (e.g., decrease in the density of copses) to cause a reduction in the vector population; c) Chemical methods which are diverse. They may use larvicides, parietal intra-household spraying, insecticide-treated nets, and space spraying; d) Sanitation which is a set of methods and techniques aimed at improving the overall health of the environment by removing the causes of unhealthy conditions.

7. Conclusion

The situation of planet earth is becoming more and more critical every day, especially in countries that care little about the problems caused by global warming and the various forms of pollution of ecosystems. The future of mankind looks very threatened and bleak due to the multifaceted impact of climate change on biodiversity, agriculture, environment and human and animal health. Indeed, the consequences of climate change on public health are today almost indisputable; they are particularly noticeable in vector-borne diseases. Slight variations in the average temperature, in the rainfall regime, in humidity, can have serious health implications, mainly in tropical developing countries because they are likely to affect the physiology of vectors.

The Republic of Haiti has suffered for years the adverse effects of climate change with a marked disturbance in the rainfall regime, the occurrence of prolonged periods of drought and an increase in air temperature. Descriptive epidemiological studies reveal significant prevalence rates of many vector-borne diseases in the country: malaria, dengue fever, chikungunya, Zika, yellow fever, Nile Valley fever, lymphatic filariasis, diseases linked to tick bites, etc. While the causal relationship between health and climate and environmental changes has not yet been clearly defined in Haiti for lack of in-depth epidemiological studies, there is no doubt that there is a positive correlation between these variables.

It is therefore high time to conduct studies on climate change at national and regional levels in order to better understand their impact on terrestrial and aquatic ecosystems and to better understand, in particular, their impact on human and animal health through analytical epidemiological research. It is therefore urgent to take the necessary steps to define a coherent framework of action and intervention strategies likely to facilitate the reversal of the accelerated trend of degradation of the environment and the health of the population, at least in areas of the country identified as high risk. This framework will include in its approach the "One health" approach, taking into account the environmental component in the field of action of human and animal health with a view to reducing the effects of climate change on human health in Haiti.

The variations observed in the epidemiology of vector-borne diseases, in particular arboviruses (dengue fever, yellow fever, Zika for example), result from social, economic and environmental changes that are largely dependent on climate change. It is important to understand the dynamics of this evolution in the country which is faced with a great lack of local meteorological and climatic data, due to the lack of stations or centers assigned to the collection of this data on a regular and systematic basis. In addition, there is also no reliable information on the biotopes of arthropod vectors, any changes that have occurred in their way of life in recent decades, the distribution of vectors at the country level, the contributing factors and/or limiting their proliferation in the Haitian context, estimates of their population according to periods of rain and drought, etc.

The country benefits from considering the opportunity to revitalize the inter-sectoral cooperation platform with a strong involvement of national and foreign universities to make it functional and capable of properly addressing the various problems related to climate change and its impact on public health by general and vector-borne diseases in particular It is in this perspective that the next actions of Quisqueya University will be oriented.

Acknowledgements

The authors are thankful to FOKAL (Fondation Connaissance et Liberté), the AOG (Association communautaire paysanne des Originaires de Grande Plaine) and the SCAC (Service de Coopération et d'Action Culturelle) of the France Embassy in Haiti for their financial support.

Author details

Ketty Balthazard-Accou[1,2,3*], Max François Millien[3], Daphnée Michel[2,3,4], Gaston Jean[3], David Telcy[5] and Evens Emmanuel[1]

1 Université Quisqueya – École Doctorale "Société et Environnement" (EDSE), Port-au-Prince, Haïti

2 Association Haïtienne Femmes, Science et Technologie, Port-au-Prince, Haïti

3 Université Quisqueya – Laboratoire de Recherche sur les Zoonoses et Intoxications Alimentaires (LAREZIA), Port-au-Prince, Haïti

4 Programme de Maîtrise en Santé Publique, Université Quisqueya – Faculté des Sciences de la Santé, Port-au-Prince, Haïti

5 Université Quisqueya, Faculté des Sciences, de Génie et d'Architecture (FSGA), Programme de Maîtrise en Aménagement et Développement Urbains des Quartiers Précaires, Port-au-Prince, Haïti

*Address all correspondence to: kettybal@gmail.com

References

[1] Parry, M., Parry, M. L., Canziani, O., Palutikof, J., Van der Linden, P., & Hanson, C. (Eds.). (2007). Climate change 2007-impacts, adaptation and vulnerability: Working group II contribution to the fourth assessment report of the IPCC (Vol. 4). Cambridge University Press.

[2] Amuakwa-Mensah, F., Marbuah, G., & Mubanga, M. (2017). Climate variability and infectious diseases nexus: Evidence from Sweden. Infectious Disease Modelling, 2(2), 203-217.

[3] Caminade, C., McIntyre, K. M., & Jones, A. E. (2019). Impact of recent and future climate change on vector-borne diseases. Annals of the New York Academy of Sciences, 1436(1), 157.

[4] Luber, G., & Lemery, J. (Eds.). (2015). Global climate change and human health: From science to practice. John Wiley & Sons. 672 p. ISBN 1118505573, 9781118505571

[5] CNEV. (2016). Influence du réchauffement climatique sur la propagation des maladies vectorielles et de leurs vecteurs. Montpellier: Centre national d'expertise sur les vecteurs, UMR MIVEGEC (IRD-CNRS-UM1-UM2. 13p. https://www.anses.fr/fr/system/files/CNEV-Ft-Fev2016-Rapport_Changement_climatique_et_maladies_vectorielles.pdf

[6] IPCC (2018). Global warming of 1.5°C. an IPCC special report on the impacts of global warming of 1.5°C above pre-industrial levels and related global greenhouse gas emission pathways, in the context of strengthening the global response to the threat of climate change, sustainable development, and efforts to eradicate poverty. Masson-Delmotte, V. et al. (Eds). World Meteorological Organization, Geneva, Switzerland

[7] Paiva, R. (2015). Brasil tem epidemia de dengue confirmada segundo índice da OMS. JORNAL HOJE. Edição do dia 04/05/2015 04/05/2015 14h17 - Atualizado em 04/05/2015 15h26. http://g1.globo.com/jornal-hoje/noticia/2015/05/brasil-tem-epidemia-de-dengue-confirmada-segundo-indice-da-oms.html

[8] (IPCC) 2001. Climate change 2001: The scientific basis, (Eds) J.T. Houghton,Y. Ding, D.J. Griggs, M. Noguer, P.J. van der Linden & D. Xiaosu. Contribution of working group I to the third assessment report of the IPCC. Cambridge University Press, Cambridge.

[9] Burkett VR, Suarez AG, Bindi M, Conde C, Mukerji R, Prather MJ, St. Clair AL, Yohe GW (2014) Point of departure. In: Field CB, Barros VR, Dokken DJ, Mach KJ, Mastrandrea MD, Bilir TE, Chatterjee M, Ebi KL, Estrada YO, Genova RC, Girma B, Kissel ES, Levy AN, MacCracken S, Mastrandrea PR, White LL (eds) Climate change 2014: impacts, adaptation, and vulnerability. Part A: global and sectoral aspects. Contribution of working group II to the fifth assessment report of the intergovernmental panel on climate change. Cambridge University Press, Cambridge, pp 169-194

[10] IPCC. (2007). Climate change 2007: Impacts, adaptation and vulnerability. Contribution of working group II to the fourth assessment report of the intergovernmental panel on climate change. Cambridge, UK: Cambridge University Press.

[11] Brasseur P, Eyma E, Li X,Verdier Ri, Agnamey P, Liautaud B,et al. Circulation des oocystes de Cryptosporidium dans les eaux de surface et de distribution par adduction publique à Port-au-Prince, Haiti. In: Colloque International Gestion

Intégrée de l'Eau en Haïti, Actes du Colloque;2002. pp. 172-175

[12] Raccurt, C. P., Brasseur, P., Verdier, R. I., Li, X., Eyma, E., Stockman, C. P., ... & Nevez, G. (2006). Cryptos poridiose humaine et espèces en cause en Haïti. Tropical Medicine & International Health, 11(6), 929-934.

[13] Damiani, C., Balthazard-Accou, K., Clervil, E., Diallo, A., Da Costa, C., Emmanuel, E., Totet, A., & Agnamey, P. (2013). Cryptosporidiosis in Haiti: surprisingly low level of species diversity revealed by molecular characterization of Cryptosporidium oocysts from surface water and groundwater. *Parasite (Paris, France)*, *20*, 45. https://doi.org/10.1051/parasite/2013045

[14] Balthazard-Accou, K., Fifi, U., Agnamey, P., Casimir, J. A., Brasseur, P., & Emmanuel, E. (2014). Influence of ionic strength and soil characteristics on the behavior of Cryptosporidium oocysts in saturated porous media. Chemosphere, 103, 114-120.

[15] Jaglin, S., 2001, L'eau potable dans les villes en développement: les modèles marchands face à la pauvreté, Revue Tiers Monde, T. XLII, 166: 275-303.

[16] Emmanuel, E., Prévil, C. (2018). Mot des coéditeurs. Cahier thématique – Gestion de l'environnement et développement durable, Haïti Perspectives, 6 (3): 15-16.

[17] Boisson, D., Emmanuel, E., Calais, E. (2020). Aléas Telluriques: Eau et Environnement en Zones Urbanisées d'Haïti. Communication orale. In Session: Eau et environnement en zones urbanisées littorales & insulaires 24 juin 2020. Conférence électronique: Favoriser les interactions et réalisations transformantes entre le RESCIF et l'IRD.

[18] HELVETAS. (2012). Préservation et Valorisation de la Biodiversité en haute altitude en Haïti. Helvetas, Direction du développement et de la coopération DDC. Port-au-Prince:HELVETAS.

[19] Fleurant, M.M. Les changements climatiques à Haïti: pour la résilience socio-écologique des populations par l'adaptation dans le domaine de l'agriculture. Possibilités et limites du droit interne et international [Thèse de Doctorat]. Québec, Canada: Université Laval; 2020. p. 412

[20] Black, P., & Nunn, M. (2009). Conséquences du changement climatique et des modifications environnementales sur les maladies animales émergentes ou ré-émergentes et sur la production animale. In Conf. OIE, pp. 1-13.

[21] Jourdain, F., & Paty, M. C. (2019). Impact des changements climatiques sur les vecteurs et les maladies à transmission vectorielle en France. Les Tribunes de la sante, 3:41-51.

[22] OMS (2017). Action mondiale pour lutter contre les vecteurs: rapport du Secrétariat. Organisation mondiale de la Santé, No. A70/26 Rev. 1.

[23] IPCC 2007. Climate Change 2007: The Physical Science – Summary for Policymakers. Contribution of Working Group I to the Fourth Assessment Report of the Intergovernmental Panel on Climate Change, 17 pp. www.ipcc.ch

[24] Anyamba, A., Chretien, J. P., Britch, S. C., Soebiyanto, R. P., Small, J. L., Jepsen, R., ... & Tucker, C. J. (2019). Global disease outbreaks associated with the 2015-2016 El Niño event. Scientific reports, 9(1), 1-14.

[25] Hanson, C., Finisdore, J., Ranganathan, J., & Iceland, C. (2008). The Corporate Ecosystem Services Review: Guidelines for Identifying Business Risks & Opportunities Arising from Ecosystem Change. World Resources Institute, Washington, USA.

http://pdf.wri.org/corporate_ecosystem_services_review.pdf

[26] Jones, K. E., Patel, N. G., Levy, M. A., Storeygard, A., Balk, D., Gittleman, J. L., & Daszak, P. (2008). Global trends in emerging infectious diseases. Nature, 451 (7181):990-993.

[27] Kilpatrick AM. (2011). Globalization, Land Use, and the Invasion of West Nile Virus. Science. 334(6054): 323-327. doi:10.1126/science.1201010

[28] Duboz, R., Binot, A., (2017). Santé des animaux et des hommes: s'entraîner à gérer l'incertitude par la modélisation et la simulation participatives. Perspective, CIRAD, 2017, N° 41, 4 p. ff10.18167/agritrop/00043ff. ffhal-01537680f

[29] OMS (2004). Changement climatique et santé humaine: risques et mesures à prendre: résumé. Genève: OMS, 40p. ISBN 92 4 259081 9

[30] Pham, T. B., Phong, C. H., Bennett, J. B., Hwang, K., Jasinskiene, N., Parker, K., ... & James, A. A. (2019). Experimental population modification of the malaria vector mosquito, Anopheles stephensi. PLoS genetics, 15(12), e1008440.

[31] Frederick, J., Saint Jean, Y., Lemoine, J. F., Dotson, E. M., Mace, K. E., Chang, M., Slutsker, L, Le Menach, A, Beier J. C., Eisele T. P., Okech, B. A., Beau de Rochars, V. M., Carter, K. H, Keating, J, Impoinvil, D. E. (2016). Malaria vector research and control in Haiti: a systematic review. Malaria journal, 15(1), 376.

[32] Raccurt, C. P., Brasseur, P., Lemoine, F., Cicéron, M., Existe, A., & Boncy, J. (2014). Caractéristiques épidémiologiques du paludisme dans la commune de Corail, Grande Anse, Haïti. Bulletin de la Société de pathologie exotique, 107(5), 337-341.

[33] Rioth, M., Beauharnais, C. A., Noel, F., Ikizler, M. R., Mehta, S., Zhu, Y., Long, C. A., Pape, J. W., & Wright, P. F. (2011). Serologic imprint of dengue virus in urban Haiti: characterization of humoral immunity to dengue in infants and young children. The American journal of tropical medicine and hygiene, 84(4), 630-636. https://doi.org/10.4269/ajtmh.2011.10-0323

[34] Salyer, S. J., Ellis, E. M., Salomon, C., Bron, C., Juin, S., Hemme, R. R., ... &Desormeaux, A. M. (2014). Dengue virus infections amongHaitian and expatriate non-governmental organizationworkers—Leogane and Port-au-Prince, Haiti, 2012. PLoSNegl Trop Dis, 8(10), e3269.

[35] Weppelmann, T. A., Burne, A., von Fricken, M. E., Elbadry, M. A., De Rochars, M. B., Boncy, J., & Okech, B. A. (2017). A Tale of Two Flaviviruses: A Seroepidemiological Study of Dengue Virus and West Nile Virus Transmission in the Ouest and Sud-Est Departments of Haiti. Am J Trop Med Hy., *96*(1), 135-140. https://doi.org/10.4269/ajtmh.16-0422.

[36] Poirier, M. J., Moss, D. M., Feeser, K. R., Streit, T. G., Chang, G. J., Whitney, M., Russell, B. J., Johnson, B. W., Basile, A. J., Goodman, C. H., Barry, A. K., & Lammie, P. J. (2016). Measuring Haitian children's exposure to chikungunya, dengue and malaria. Bulletin of the World Health Organization, 94(11), 817-825A. https://doi.org/10.2471/BLT.16.173252

[37] WHO (2016). Chikungunya fact sheet. World Health Organization, Geneva, Switzerland. https://www.who.int/news-room/fact-sheets/detail/chikungunya

[38] Chazal, M., Beauclair, G., Gracias, S., Najburg, V., Simon-Lorière, E., Tangy, F., ... & Jouvenet, N. (2018). RIG-I recognizes the 5′ region of dengue